OPERATIVE ORTHOPAEDICS

Barcode replaced July 2012

This book is due for return on or before the last date shown below.

18 MAR 2010

29-SEP-2010

- 4 MAR 2011

12 JUL 2011

31-JAN-2013

- 8 APR 2013

29 APR 2016

13-JUL-2016

29 OCT 2019

OPERATIVE ORTHOPAEDICS
The Stanmore Guide

Edited by

Timothy Briggs MD MBBS (Hons) MCH (Orth) FRCS (Eng) FRCS (Ed) MD (Res)
Royal National Orthopaedic Hospital Trust, Stanmore, UK

Jonathan Miles MBCHB FRCS (Tr & Orth)
Royal National Orthopaedic Hospital Trust, Stanmore, UK

William Aston BSc MBBS FRCS (Tr & Orth) (Edinb)
Royal National Orthopaedic Hospital Trust, Stanmore, UK

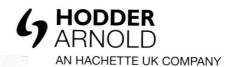
HODDER
ARNOLD
AN HACHETTE UK COMPANY

First published in Great Britain in 2010 by
Hodder Arnold, an imprint of Hodder Education,
part of Hachette UK, 338 Euston Road, London NW1 3BH
www.arnoldpublishers.com/
www.hodderarnold.com

Hachette Livre UK's Hodder Headline's policy is to use papers that are
natural, renewable and recyclable products and made from wood grown
in sustainable forests. The logging and manufacturing processes are
expected to conform to the environmental regulations of the country
of origin.

Whilst the advice and information in this book are believed to be true
and accurate at the date of going to press, neither the author[s] nor the
publisher can accept any legal responsibility or liability for any errors or
omissions that may be made. In particular (but without limiting the
generality of the preceding disclaimer) every effort has been made to
check drug dosages; however it is still possible that errors have been
missed. Furthermore, dosage schedules are constantly being revised and
new side-effects recognized. For these reasons the reader is strongly
urged to consult the drug companies' printed instructions before
administering any of the drugs recommended in this book.

British Library Cataloguing in Publication Data
A catalogue record for this book is available from the British Library

Library of Congress Cataloging-in-Publication Data
A catalog record for this book is available from the Library of Congress

ISBN   978 0 340 985 007

1 2 3 4 5 6 7 8 9 10

Commissioning Editor:	Gavin Jamieson
Project Editor:	Joanna Silman
Production Controller:	Joanna Walker
Cover Designer:	Helen Townson
Index:	Jan Ross

Typeset in 9.5pt Berling Roman by Phoenix Photosetting, Chatham, Kent
Printed and bound in India by Replika Press Pvt. Ltd.

This book is dedicated to all hard-working orthopaedic trainees whose enthusiasm for learning and patient care was our motivation for creating this book.

Tim Briggs, Jonathan Miles, Will Aston

Contents

Contributors

William Aston BSc MBBS FRCS (Ed) (Tr & Orth)
Consultant Orthopaedic Surgeon, Royal National
Orthopaedic Hospital Trust, Stanmore, UK

Timothy W R Briggs MCH (Orth) FRCS (Ed)
Medical Director and Consultant Orthopaedic
Surgeon, Royal National Orthopaedic Hospital Trust,
Stanmore, UK

Peter Calder MBBS FRCS (Eng) FRCS (Tr & Orth)
Consultant Orthopaedic Surgeon, Royal National
Orthopaedic Hospital Trust, Stanmore, UK

Richard Carrington MBBS FRCS (Orth)
Consultant Orthopaedic Surgeon, Royal National
Orthopaedic Hospital Trust, Stanmore, UK

Simon Clint BSc MBBS FRCS (Tr & Orth)
Specialist Registrar, Royal National Orthopaedic
Hospital Trust, Stanmore, UK

Michael Cooper BSc MBCHB FRCA
Department of Anaesthetics, Royal National
Orthopaedic Hospital Trust, Stanmore, UK

Nicholas Cullen BSc MBBS FRCS (Tr & Orth)
Consultant Foot and Ankle Surgeon, The Royal
National Orthopaedic Hospital Trust, Stanmore, UK

Lee A David MBBS MRCS (Eng) FRCS (Tr & Orth)
Consultant in Trauma and Orthopaedic Surgery,
Maidstone and Tunbridge Wells NHS Trust,
Maidstone, UK

Gorav Datta MD FRCS (Tr & Orth)
Specialist Registrar, Royal National Orthopaedic
Hospital Trust, Stanmore, UK

James Donaldson MBBS BSc MRCS
Specialist Registrar, Royal National Orthopaedic
Hospital Trust Rotation, Stanmore, UK

Mark Falworth FRCS (Eng) FRCS (Orth)
Consultant Shoulder Surgeon, Royal National
Orthopaedic Hospital Trust, Stanmore, UK

Mike Fox MBBS
Consultant Orthopaedic Surgeon, Royal National
Orthopaedic Hospital Trust, Stanmore, UK

Nicholas Goddard FRCS
Consultant Orthopaedic Surgeon, Royal Free Hospital,
London, UK

Omar Haddo BMedSci MBBS FRCS (Tr & Orth)
Consultant Orthopaedic Surgeon, Whittington
Hospital, London, UK

David J Harrison MB BS BSc (Hons) AKC FRCS
Consultant Orthopaedic Surgeon, Spinal Deformity
Unit, Royal National Orthopaedic Hospital Trust,
Stanmore, UK

Aresh Hashemi-Nejad FRCS FRCS (Orth)
Consultant Orthopaedic Surgeon and Clinical
Director, Royal National Orthopaedic Hospital Trust,
Stanmore, UK, and Honorary Senior Lecturer,
University College London, London, UK

Russell Hawkins BSc MBBS MRCS (Eng) FRCS (Tr & Orth)
Specialist Registrar, Royal National Orthopaedic
Hospital Trust, Stanmore, UK

Deborah Higgs FRCS (Tr & Orth)
Royal National Orthopaedic Hospital Trust, Stanmore,
UK

Max Horowitz MBBS
Specialist Registrar, Royal National Orthopaedic
Hospital Trust, Stanmore, UK

Hui Yun Vivian Ip MBCHB MRCP FRCA
Royal National Orthopaedic Hospital Trust,
Stanmore, UK

Laurence James BSc MBBS MRCS (Eng) FRCS (Tr & Orth)
Foot and Ankle Fellow, Royal National Orthopaedic
Trust, Stanmore, UK

Robert Jennings MBBS BSc MSC MFSEM (UK) FRCS ED
(Tr & Orth)
Royal National Orthopaedic Hospital Trust, Stanmore,
UK

Raman Kalyan MRCS MD FRCS (Tr & Orth) DNB ORTH
D ORTH (Eng)
Clinical Lecturer/Specialist Registrar, Royal National
Orthopaedic Hospital Trust, Stanmore, UK

Norbert Kang MBBS MD FRCS (Plast)
Consultant Plastic and Hand Surgeon, Royal Free
Hospital, London, UK

Simon Lambert BSc FRCS FRCSEdOrth
Consultant Orthopaedic Surgeon, The Shoulder and
Elbow Service, Royal National Orthopaedic Hospital,
Stanmore, UK

Jonathan Miles MBCHB FRCS (Tr & Orth)
Royal National Orthopaedic Hospital Trust, Stanmore,
UK

Sean Molloy MRCS MSc (Orth Eng) FRCS (Orth)
Consultant Orthopaedic Spinal Surgeon, Royal
National Orthopaedic Hospital Trust, Stanmore, UK

Lauren Ovens MbChb MRCS
Specialist Registrar Plastic Surgeon, Royal Free
Hospital, London, UK

Robert Pearl BSc FRCS (Tr & Orth)
Specialist Registrar Plastic Surgeon, Royal Free
Hospital, London, UK

Rob Pollock BSc FRCS (Tr & Orth)
Consultant Orthopaedic Surgeon, Royal National
Orthopaedic Hospital Trust, Stanmore, UK

Matthew Shaw MBBS FRCS
Specialist Registrar, Royal National Orthopaedic
Hospital Trust, Stanmore, UK

Dishan Singh FRCS (Tr & Orth)
Consultant Foot and Ankle Surgeon, Royal National
Orthopaedic Hospital Trust, Stanmore, UK

John Skinner MB BS FRCS (Orth)
Consultant Orthopaedic Surgeon and Honorary
Senior Lecturer, Royal National Orthopaedic Hospital
Trust, Stanmore, UK

Preface

Operative Orthopaedics: The Stanmore Guide aims to provide practical instruction in elective orthopaedic surgical procedures. Each chapter has been written by a consultant orthopaedic surgeon and a trainee. It covers the list of procedures identified by the Specialist Advisory Committee as key in the field of orthopaedic surgery and presented as they are laid out in the training syllabus.

It provides an explanation of orthopaedic surgery from preoperative planning and consent, through approaches and operative technique to postoperative care. Each procedure is described in a simple and consistent format to enable the reader to describe and carry out safe, evidence-based approaches and common operations. It contains key references and sample viva questions.

This guide will serve junior trainees as they enter their surgical training and will acts as a revision tool for trainees sitting the FRCS (Tr & Orth) examination, which has evolved into a format emphasizing the importance of surgical procedures and the relevant anatomy.

The variety of equipment and instruments available to today's orthopaedic surgeons is mind-boggling. The one essential tool for a surgeon in training is an understanding of the basic techniques, upon which all procedures depend. The consistent and organized style of this book will teach these techniques and enable its readers to think logically and 'keep a steady nerve' in the potentially stressful situations of independent operating and the FRCS (Tr & Orth) examination.

Acknowledgements

Thank you first and foremost to all of the trainees and consultants who have given generously of their time, knowledge and experiences to produce such informative writing in each chapter.

Hodder Arnold have supported us admirably from the first idea right through to final preparation of the book and their contribution has been vital to provide clear and well-illustrated guidelines for the reader.

A huge thank you to our respective wives and families for putting up with us during this project.

Final thanks go to Professor Briggs for having the idea of writing this book in the first place – another professorial idea conceived in the bath!

Anaesthesia in orthopaedic surgery

Hui Yin Vivian Ip and Michael Cooper

INTRODUCTION

The orthopaedic patient cohort is medically diverse. Patients come from the extremes of age, they may have complex causal pathology and, as they age, the patients develop multisystem co-morbidity. The breadth of surgical intervention is great, ranging from procedures such as arthroscopy causing minimal physiological disturbance, to procedures that test, and often surpass, the physiological reserve of an individual patient. As such, the conduct of an individual anaesthetic is customized to the medical demands of the patient, the requirements for the surgical technique and the limitations of the institution in which the surgery occurs.

PREOPERATIVE ASSESSMENT AND GUIDELINES

This is the process of assessing the relevance, severity and treatment of the patient's medical pathologies. This allows referral for better treatment ('optimization') and quantification of the risk of adverse perioperative events, including death, to be discussed and documented. Factors specific to anaesthesia, such as a possible difficult airway, may also be considered. Central guidelines exist to inform the ordering of preoperative laboratory tests.

FASTING

In elective surgery, standard local fasting times must be adhered to. A typical regimen is given in Table 1.1. Food includes milk and fresh fruit juices.

Table 1.1 Fasting times

	Typical foods			
	Solid food	Water	Breast milk	Formula milk
Fasting time	6 hours	2 hours	4 hours	6 hours

In trauma it is assumed that gastric emptying stops at the time of injury. Fasting time is calculated as time of intake to time of trauma. The situation is further complicated by opiate analgesics that prolong gastric emptying and render fasting times difficult to interpret. In these circumstances the need to proceed with surgical intervention may override fasting policy and surgery proceeds.

AIRWAY

A range of bedside tests exist that aim to predict difficulties in maintaining an airway or intubating an anaesthetized patient. Individual tests perform poorly and are not relevant here. Of particular relevance in orthopaedic surgery are the challenges that a rigid cervical column or an unstable cervical column may cause. The challenge of rigidity may be a difficult airway and a difficult laryngoscopy. The challenge of an unstable column is to prevent cord injury. Both are initially assessed with plain radiography. Specialized investigations to delineate pathology include computed tomography (CT) and magnetic resonance imaging (MRI).

CARDIOVASCULAR ASSESSMENT

This is aimed at quantifying the ability of the cardiovascular pump to increase work to match perioperative metabolic demands. It is an assessment of reserve and of the risk of adverse events such as an acute coronary syndrome. Key clinical markers are described below.

Exercise tolerance

For patients having major, non-cardiac surgery, inability to climb two flights of stairs confers increased risk of major postoperative complications but is not predictive of mortality.

Previous myocardial infarction

There is a risk of recurrent perioperative myocardial infarction (MI), which has a 60 per cent mortality rate. The longer surgery can be postponed after an MI, the lower the rate of recurrent MI (Table 1.2).

Table 1.2 Percentage risk of recurrent myocardial infarction (MI) at different times post MI

Time since MI	Risk of recurrent MI
<3 months	5.7 per cent
4–6 months	2.3 per cent
>6 months	1.5 per cent

Typical investigations used to quantify cardiac reserve are listed below.
- **Exercise electrocardiogram (ECG)** – helps to determine any coronary flow limitation when cardiac work increases.
- **Thallium scintigraphy and dobutamine stress echocardiography** – these dynamic 'stress tests'

are especially useful for patients who are unable to perform exercise ECG due to musculoskeletal disease or severe cardiopulmonary disease. Perfusion defects of the myocardium under physiological stress indicate coronary insufficiency.
- **Cardiopulmonary exercise testing** – this is a dynamic test that predicts the patient's anaerobic threshold. As such it tests respiratory and cardiac reserve. It reflects other factors such as motivation, mobility and nutrition. It can be used to predict the risk of surgery and obviate the need for other tests such as angiography or echocardiography.
- **Coronary angiography** – this is used to visualize coronary arterial flow and disease. This is often the end point of coronary investigation and may allow treatment by stenting and angioplasty at the same time.

Hypertension

Stage 3 hypertension (systolic blood pressure [BP] =180 mmHg or a diastolic BP =110 mmHg) should be controlled prior to surgery. A recent meta-analysis found that patients with mild or moderate hypertension and no evidence of end-organ damage were at no increased perioperative risk. End-organ damage includes left ventricular hypertrophy (ECG criteria), a history of cerebrovascular accident (including transient ischaemic attacks), renal insufficiency and retinal changes.

Heart murmurs

The valve pathology underlying murmurs may have significant implications for anaesthetic technique. Lesions that limit the cardiac output (most famously aortic stenosis) can cause profound hypotension as the heart cannot increase cardiac output to maintain blood pressure as vascular resistance drops. This is most marked with neuroaxial anaesthesia and can cause morbidity due to organ hypoxia. For example, coronary perfusion may become critically low resulting in an acute coronary syndrome. Echocardiography is useful to determine the nature and the severity of the valve lesion.

RESPIRATORY ASSESSMENT

Preoperative assessment determines the severity and potential reversibility of respiratory pathology. Disease states limit gas flow, gas exchange or both. The end point of respiratory disease is hypoxaemia and tissue hypoxia. This can precipitate organ failure with serious adverse outcomes. Common pathologies are described below.

Asthma

Stable asthma is usually benign. However, some anaesthetic agents can trigger bronchospasm and are avoided. Conversely, some result in bronchodilation and are favoured. Assessment should include spirometry and peak flow measurements. Preparation may include bronchodilator premedication, e.g. salbutamol. Some anaesthetists choose a regional technique to avoid airway instrumentation and opiate use.

Chronic obstructive airways disease

Gas flow and exchange are limited. These patients are at risk of postoperative respiratory failure due to atelectasis and segmental lung collapse. This causes hypoxaemia. Assessment should include spirometry (a forced expiratory volume in 1 second greater than 1 indicates an ability to clear secretions), oximetry (and perhaps arterial blood gases) and an assessment of exercise ability. A baseline chest radiograph may be useful but is by no means mandatory. An ECG may show signs of right heart strain and is also indicated as this group is likely to have coexistent cardiovascular disease. Preoperative and postoperative chest physiotherapy is essential. Anaesthetists will tend towards regional anaesthesia in respiratory cripples to minimize the chances of postoperative respiratory failure. Opiates are a potent source of respiratory depression and, coupled to sedation and pain, can be a powerful trigger for respiratory decompensation.

Respiratory tract infection

This is often viral. Upper respiratory tract infection is most common. Patients with productive cough or objective symptoms (pyrexia, fatigue, myalgia, anorexia) should only proceed if it is an emergency surgery. The risk of laryngospasm and bronchospasm is increased. Viral myocarditis may also occur, leading to cardiac failure or even death in the perioperative period. Guidelines commonly suggest a 4- to 6-week delay from the start of respiratory tract infection to elective surgery.

Groups at special risk

Cerebral palsy patients may have poor bulbar function and weak cough, which puts them at risk of aspiration, and they have a higher incidence of postoperative respiratory tract infection. This is exacerbated by any cognitive impairment that reduces their ability to cooperate with physiotherapy and interventions such as non-invasive ventilation. Low tone neuromuscular syndrome patients are at risk of postoperative respiratory failure and plans will include intensive care, possible postoperative ventilation and tracheostomy formation. Of note, volatile anaesthesia is usually avoided in this group due to the risk of rhabdomyolysis, renal failure and hyperkalaemic cardiac arrest.

RECOMMENDED REFERENCES

Biccard BM. Relationship between the inability to climb two flights of stairs and outcome after major non-cardiac surgery: implications for the pre-operative assessment of functional capacity. *Anaesthesia* 2005;6:588–93.
Howell S, Sear J, Foex P. Hypertension, hypertensive heart disease and perioperative cardiac risk. *Br J Anaesth* 2004;**92**:570–83.
National Institute for Health and Clinical Excellence. *Preoperative Tests: the Use of Routine Preoperative Tests for Elective Surgery*. Available at: www.nice.org.uk/Guidance/CG3 (accessed 8 April 2009).

INTRAOPERATIVE TECHNIQUES

Discussion of the selection and conduct of individual techniques is beyond the scope of this chapter. The technique chosen is dependent on the patient, hospital, procedure, surgeon and anaesthetist. There is little conformity of opinion.

GENERAL ANAESTHESIA

This is the most common option and is entirely appropriate for most procedures, environments and patients. It is a balanced technique of analgesia, muscle relaxation and sedation. This is confirmed by data review as exemplified by recent publications concerning primary joint replacement.

PERIPHERAL REGIONAL ANAESTHESIA

This is the placement of local anaesthetic adjacent to individual nerves or plexus of nerves to produce a zone of sensory and motor block. This may be the only mode of anaesthesia. More commonly, it is a pain-relieving adjunct to general anaesthesia or sedation. As such, opiate use is minimized and patients may actually mobilize earlier. Clearly, there may be conflict with masking neurological injury. Heavy-handed anaesthesia may produce prolonged motor block to the detriment of the patient. Increasingly this modality is preferred for primary arthroplasty, with clinical spill into other techniques.

NEUROAXIAL LOCAL ANAESTHESIA

For lower limb procedures, spinal, epidural or combined spinal–epidural blocks can provide complete analgesia and motor block. As above, they may be used alone or in conjunction with sedation or general anaesthesia. They are often the technique of choice in those with respiratory disease in an effort to minimize opiate-induced respiratory embarrassment. Outcome evidence is poor. However, there is some literature base to support this practice. They are a valuable tool to reduce opiate use and have been associated with a lower incidence of deep vein thrombosis and lower perioperative blood loss. This may no longer be valid in light of new advances in thrombo-embolic prophylaxis and other anaesthetic techniques available to modulate perioperative blood loss. However, these techniques are an important part of a multimodal approach to fast track surgery.

Contraindications

- Refusal
- Local or systemic infection
- Allergy to agents used
- Coagulopathy
- Anticoagulants (relative contraindication) increase the risk of haematoma at the site of infiltration, around nerves or in the epidural space. Aspirin is not a contraindication

LOCAL ANAESTHESIA

Some body surface procedures are amenable to surgery using local infiltration alone.

POSTOPERATIVE CARE

ANALGESIA

Simple analgesics

These can be very effective for mild and moderate pain. Common drugs are paracetamol and non-steroidal anti-inflammatory drugs. Best effect is gained when they are given regularly, ideally after a loading dose in theatre. In more severe pain, they are still useful adjuncts with well-documented opiate-sparing properties.

Oral opiates

These include codeine derivatives, complex agonists such as tramadol and morphine derivatives. These are well recognized for more severe pain and can be used regularly, with stronger alternatives available for breakthrough pain. Newer derivatives such as oxycodone provide excellent pharmacokinetics with twice daily dosing of modified-release compounds providing 24-hour analgesia supplemented by short-acting versions effective for breakthrough pain.

Systemic opiates

For severe pain, intravenous opiates may be given as patient-controlled analgesia (PCA). This allows the patient to titrate their own dosing. It is effective, safe and popular. Better pain scores and fewer side effects (nausea, vomiting, and sedation) are regularly received using this modality of opiate delivery compared with intermittent intramuscular dosing. Other routes such as transdermal delivery are available. These take a long time to reach a steady plasma concentration and are similarly slow to decline when discontinued. This inflexibility makes them difficult to use in the perioperative period. They are more suited to long-term use in chronic pain syndromes.

Local anaesthesia

Local anaesthetic techniques may be continued into the postoperative period. These provide excellent analgesia with minimum side effects. However, immobility may be a problem. Well-conducted blocks in units used to managing these patients are very successful and do not need to delay mobilization.

OXYGEN

Oxygen therapy should be given to patients with an epidural infusion, or PCA, which contains opiates. This supplemental oxygen maintains alveolar oxygen tension longer if respiratory depression and hypoventilation occurs. Supplemental oxygen used for the first 3 days postoperatively can also minimize the risk of perioperative ischaemic events. Clearly, patients with respiratory pathology (respiratory tract infection, atelectasis, thromboembolism) will be relatively hypoxic and oxygen therapy is an essential.

FLUID MANAGEMENT

The goal of intravenous fluid therapy is to maintain normovolaemia. This allows adequate cardiac output and, assuming a reasonable haemoglobin concentration, tissue oxygen delivery. Maintenance water and electrolytes need to be supplied and ongoing blood loss compensated for in the form of blood substitute, or blood itself. Triggers for transfusion vary. Blood is expensive, immunosuppressant, associated with worse outcome and a vehicle for disease

transmission. However, red cells are vital to oxygen delivery and haemostasis. The trigger will depend on the predicted continuing blood loss, the patient's co-morbidities and symptoms. Typically a haemoglobin concentration of 8 g/dL is taken as acceptable.

DISPOSAL

High-dependency care may benefit many orthopaedic patients. Delivery of this will depend on local protocol and infrastructure. Clearly, those at increased risk of organ failure or requiring a higher level of nursing supervision should be placed in an appropriate environment.

RECOMMENDED REFERENCES

Fischer HBJ, Simanski CJP. A procedure specific and systematic review and consensus recommendations for analgesia after total hip replacement. *Anaesthesia* 2005;**60**:1189–202.
Fischer HBJ, Simanski CJP, Sharp C, *et al.* A procedure specific systematic review and consensus recommendations for postoperative analgesia following total knee arthroplasty. *Anaesthesia* 2008;**63**:1105–23.
Fowler SJ, Symons J, Sabato S, *et al.* Epidural analgesia compared with peripheral nerve blockade after major knee surgery: a systematic review and meta analysis of randomized trials. *Br J Anaesth* 2008;**100**:154–64.

Viva questions

1. In patients with hypertension, how would you determine whether elective surgery can proceed?
2. What are the contraindications to neuraxial blockade?
3. Why is a respiratory tract infection a problem?
4. Who should receive oxygen therapy in the postoperative period?
5. When could an echocardiograph be the preoperative investigation of choice?

Tumours

William Aston and Timothy Briggs

NEEDLE BIOPSY OF BONE

PREOPERATIVE PLANNING

Indications

To **obtain a histological diagnosis** so that further treatment can be planned.

Contraindications

Lesions that are closely related to neurovascular structures, where a needle biopsy would put these structures at risk.

Consent and risks

- Neurovascular injury and infection are the main risks
- Possible tumour seeding

Patients should also be warned that a second needle biopsy or open biopsy may be necessary if inadequate tissue for histological diagnosis is obtained.

Templating

The needle entry point and tract needs careful thought and should be planned by the surgeon performing the tumour resection, as the biopsy tract will need to be excised if malignancy is found.

The type of biopsy needle should also be considered. A fine-bore needle, through which an aspiration can be taken, is usually unsuitable to make a diagnosis in bony lesions, unless pus is aspirated from a sequestrum. A thicker-bore needle (11G or 13G), capable of boring through the outside of the lesion and taking core biopsies such as a Jamshidi needle (Fig. 2.1), is preferable.

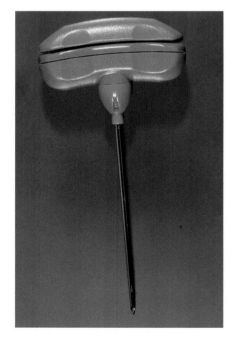

Figure 2.1 *Jamshidi needle*

For tumours that have a large soft tissue component or that have destroyed the cortex, a Trucut or Temmo (preloaded) needle can be used. These take a slice of tissue and come in 11 and 14 gauges.

Anaesthesia and positioning

Needle biopsy can be done under local, local with sedation or general anaesthesia. For children, hard lesions and lesions which may be difficult to access, a general anaesthetic should be used.

Positioning is dependent on the area to be reached and if necessary the imaging modality being used.

SURGICAL TECHNIQUE

Landmarks and incision

The line of the biopsy should be sited **in the line of a possible future surgical incision**, so that it can be excised at the time of surgery (Fig. 2.2). It must

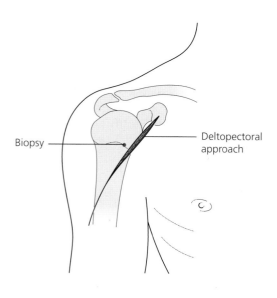

Figure 2.2 *Position of biopsy for proximal humeral tumour – in the line of the deltopectoral approach, but slightly lateral so that the needle passes through the deltoid muscle and avoids the cephalic vein*

pass directly to the site of the tumour and through only the myofascial compartment in which the tumour is located, preferably through muscle and away from the neurovascular structures at risk. It should aim to take a representative sample of the tumour, which can be identified on pre-biopsy imaging. The needle is passed after a simple stab incision in the skin, with a no. 15 blade.

Deep dissection

The needle is passed through the stab incision and directly to the area being biopsied, under radiological control if necessary.

Technical aspects of procedure

Multiple core biopsies are needed, aiming to minimize diversion from the tract. If unsure whether representative tissue has been taken, a frozen section should be undertaken. In cases where preoperative imaging is atypical or where infection is suspected, samples should also be sent for microbiology.

The needle should not be passed through the lesion into normal tissue. For lesions close to joints, the needle **must not pass through the capsule** and therefore potentially contaminate the joint. It may be necessary to drill the bone prior to needle insertion in sclerotic lesions. Careful handling of the specimens is important so as not to destroy the microarchitecture. Discussion with the histopathologist will elucidate whether they wish to receive the specimen fresh or fixed in formalin.

Closure

Use Steri-Strips.

POSTOPERATIVE INSTRUCTIONS

- Neurovascular and routine observations.
- Local pressure in the case of vascular lesions.

RECOMMENDED REFERENCES

Saifuddin A, Mitchell R, Burnett S, *et al*. Ultrasound guided needle biopsy of primary bone tumours. *J Bone Joint Surg Br* 2000;**82**:50–4.

Stoker DJ, Cobb JP, Pringle JAS. Needle biopsy of musculoskeletal lesions. A review of 208 procedures. *J Bone Joint Surg Br* 1991;**37**: 498–500.

OPEN BIOPSY OF BONE

PREOPERATIVE PLANNING

Indications

- Patients who are not suitable for a needle biopsy
- Patients in whom tissue from a needle biopsy was insufficient to make the diagnosis

Open biopsy can be incisional where a sample of the lesion is taken or it can be excisional where the whole lesion is removed. Excisional biopsy is generally reserved for lesions which, on radiology, have diagnostic features of a benign lesion.

Contraindications

Lesions where a satisfactory needle biopsy can be performed.

Consent and risks

- Neurovascular injury
- Infection
- Seeding of the tumour

Templating

The incision should be planned with the surgeon and be made in the line of the surgical approach that will be used to remove the tumour.

Thought should be given as to how to localize the tumour, e.g. with image intensifier intraoperatively if necessary.

Anaesthesia and positioning

Regional/general anaesthesia and patient positioned to enable good access.

SURGICAL TECHNIQUE

Landmarks and incision

The incision should be in the line of a possible future operative approach so that the biopsy tract can be resected with the specimen.

Dissection

Dependent on the location.

Technical aspects of procedure

It is important to minimize potential complications of biopsy such as infection and haematoma as a poorly performed biopsy **carries significant morbidity**. The tourniquet should be deflated before closure and, if a drain is used, the exit point should be in the line of any further incision.

Only one compartment of the limb should be violated during the approach. Muscles should be split and meticulous haemostasis applied to minimize haematoma formation and spread of fluid through tissue planes. The area to be biopsied should be carefully exposed, taking care not to disrupt the capsule or expose more of the tumour than is necessary. If a capsule is opened then it should be closed carefully.

A **representative sample** of tissue should be taken to include the transition from normal to abnormal tissue if possible. If there is any doubt then frozen section should be undertaken to ensure a diagnostic specimen.

Closure

Routine.

POSTOPERATIVE INSTRUCTIONS

Neurovascular observations.

RECOMMENDED REFERENCES

Ashford RU, McCarthy SW, Scolyer RA, *et al*. Surgical biopsy with intra-operative frozen section. An accurate and cost-effective method for diagnosis of musculoskeletal sarcomas. *J Bone Joint Surg Br* 2006;**88**:1207–11.

Mankin HJ, Lange TA, Sapnnier SS. The hazards of biopsy in patients with malignant primary bone and soft tissue tumours, *J Bone Joint Surg Am* 1982;**64**:1121.

Pollock RC, Stalley PD. Biopsy of musculoskeletal tumours – beware. *A NZ J Surg* 2004;**74**:516–19.

EXCISION OF BURSA

PREOPERATIVE PLANNING

Indications

Chronically infected or thickened bursae.

Consent and risks

Risks are dependent on the location of the bursa. General risks, such as infection, apply as well as stiffness of the surrounding soft tissues due to removal and postoperative scarring.

Templating

Plan and approach depends on site.

Anaesthesia and positioning

- Regional or general as appropriate
- Positioning as appropriate.

SURGICAL TECHNIQUE

Landmarks and incision

Depend on location.

Superficial dissection

Through skin and tissue planes taking care not to disrupt the bursa if chronically infected.

Deep dissection

Removal of entire bursa carefully protecting surrounding soft tissues.

Technical aspects of procedure

Depend on the location.

Closure

Routine.

POSTOPERATIVE INSTRUCTIONS

Routine and neurovascular observations.

EXCISION OF BENIGN BONE TUMOUR

PREOPERATIVE PLANNING

Common indications

- Impending fracture, e.g. aneurysmal bone cyst
- To prevent further bony destruction and/or functional loss in aggressive lesions – e.g. giant cell tumour
- Mechanical symptoms – osteochondroma
- Pain – osteoid osteoma
- Risk of malignant transformation.

Contraindications

No definitive characterization of the lesion on either imaging or pathology.

Consent and risks

Depend on anatomical location and pathology of the lesion.

Templating

The approach depends on access required to perform resection and reconstruction if necessary.

Anaesthesia and positioning

Usually general anaesthesia and routine positioning.

SURGICAL TECHNIQUE

Landmarks and incision

As per preoperative plan.

Dissection

The exposure is dependent on the anatomical location and whether the plan is to perform curettage of the lesion (intralesional excision) or to excise it (marginal excision) and reconstruct it. It is usually **unwise to** attempt tumour excision and reconstruction through 'minimally invasive' approaches.

Technical aspects of procedure

Again, these depend on procedure and location. If *en bloc* resection is planned then reconstruction options need to be available, including any autograft or allograft necessary, in conjunction with any hardware for fixation. If curettage is planned, graft or adjuvant treatments, such as cement, liquid nitrogen or phenol, may be required to fill/treat the resulting cavity.

Necessary imaging modalities need to be available, such as computed tomography for localization of an osteoid osteoma or image intensifier to localize a larger lesion.

Closure

Routine – procedure dependent.

POSTOPERATIVE CARE AND INSTRUCTIONS

- Routine
- Weightbearing and physiotherapy regimen – depend on procedure.

RECOMMENDED REFERENCE

Malawer MM, Dunham W. Cryosurgery and acrylic cementation as surgical adjuncts in the treatment of aggressive (benign) bone tumours. *Clin Orthop Relat Res* 1991;**262**:42.

BONE CYST CURETTAGE ± BONE GRAFT

PREOPERATIVE PLANNING

Indications

- Risk of fracture or repeated fracture
- Failure of other methods of treatment, such as a steroid injection into the cyst.

Contraindications

If radiology is not classical of a bone cyst, then histopathological diagnosis should be sought.

Consent and risks

- General risks and that of recurrence
- Depend on the location

Operative planning

Planning of the approach to allow good access to the whole cyst while not threatening the physis or nearby neurovascular structures.

Anaesthesia and positioning

General anaesthesia; positioning depends on the access required.

SURGICAL TECHNIQUE

Landmarks and incision

Utilization of a recognized surgical approach in most cases.

Dissection

Dissection to bone, following described approaches and avoiding neurovascular structures, exposing the periosteum over the length of the cyst. The image intensifier is often necessary to locate the lesion or to confirm the position and extent of the cavity.

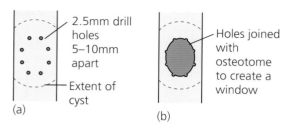

(a)   (b)

2.5mm drill holes 5–10mm apart

Extent of cyst

Holes joined with osteotome to create a window

Figure 2.3a,b *Technique for making a cortical window for curettage of a bony lesion*

Technical aspects of procedure

Once the cyst has been located, a 2.5 mm drill bit is used to drill (at 5–10mm intervals) the outline of a cortical window through which curettage is going to take place. By drilling it confirms the presence of the cyst and avoids stress risers in the bone or the propagation of a fracture. The holes are joined up with a small osteotome or saw blade (Fig. 2.3).

Once the cyst is entered, thorough curettage can take place, attempting to remove tissue from all bone surfaces. A communication is made from the cyst to the medulla of the bone to allow the cyst to fill with blood (which reduces recurrence rate). Screening with an image intensifier (Fig. 2.4) confirms that the whole cavity has been treated.

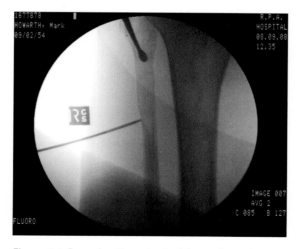

Figure 2.4 *Screening the extent of the cavity to be curetted*

If the cyst is close to the growth plate, the cortical window is made distant to the physis; curettage of the growth plate is avoided as this may lead to a growth disturbance. The cyst can be grafted with a cancellous or corticocancellous autograft from the ileum, tibia or fibula. An allograft may also be used to fill the defect.

The cortical window, if large enough, may be replaced and held with a screw or periosteal sutures.

Closure

Routine.

POSTOPERATIVE INSTRUCTIONS

Restoration of the range of motion of neighbouring joints is undertaken as soon as possible. Weightbearing status is dependent on the anatomical location and the size of the defect.

RECOMMENDED REFERENCE

Aboulafia AJ, Temple HT, Scully SP. Surgical treatment of benign bone tumors. *Instr Course Lect* 2002;**51**:441–50.

MALIGNANT TUMOUR PRINCIPLES

PREOPERATIVE PLANNING

Common indications

- Excision of an isolated primary tumour
- Excision of a primary tumour with metastatic disease depending on life expectancy
- Excision of isolated metastases
- Excision of a fungating tumour for local control
- Excision of tumour recurrence.

Contraindications

- Poor life expectancy
- Co-morbidities
- Malignancies treatable by chemotherapy alone such as lymphoma.

Consent and risks

Depend on the anatomical location and magnitude of the procedure.

Operative planning

The tumour, the surrounding compartments and the whole bone must be satisfactorily imaged to allow adequate planning of the procedure and reconstructive method. This will usually involve plain films, computed tomography and magnetic resonance imaging.

Planning of the surgical approach needs to enable sufficient access to remove the tumour and any structures to be sacrificed to **ensure tumour clearance with wide margins**, which means removal of a layer of the normal tissue surrounding the whole tumour (Fig. 2.5).

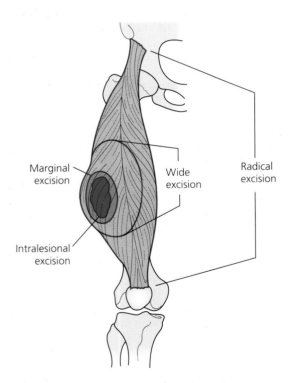

Figure 2.5 *Intralesional, marginal, wide and radical margins for the excision of bone and soft tissue tumours. (Note the diagram shows a soft tissue lesion)*

Structures at risk and the method of reconstruction have to be considered. Surgical approaches that are not routinely used may have to be employed and plastic surgical techniques may be necessary to provide soft tissue coverage after resection. In cases of highly vascular tumours or particularly renal and thyroid metastases, preoperative embolization should be considered to reduce the intraoperative blood loss.

Anaesthesia and positioning

General or regional anaesthesia as appropriate and positioning to allow sufficient access.

SURGICAL TECHNIQUE

Landmarks and incision

Depend on anatomical location of the tumour.

Dissection

Dissection must enable **removal of the tumour en bloc with a layer of normal tissues surrounding it** to provide a wide margin. In some cases neurovascular structures may be preserved and therefore a marginal excision around these structures is performed. Postoperatively, an opinion regarding adjuvant therapy is obtained. However, if cure is sought, and the neurovascular structures are involved then they must be sacrificed. This may mean an amputation or reconstruction of the vessels.

Technical aspects of procedure

Margins and structures to be sacrificed can usually be anticipated from good-quality imaging. However, during the procedure the surgeon needs to decide, based on experience and the feel of the tissues, what has to be sacrificed, in conjunction with the imaging.

The parts of the procedure that have the easiest anatomical access are undertaken first. Samples from remaining surrounding tissues are sent for histology if the resection margin is questionable. Intraoperative frozen section can be used to ensure an adequate resection margin if there is any doubt.

The wound should be thoroughly washed with water (as water is highly hypotonic, it may aid in lysis of any spilled tumour cells) after removal of the tumour. If any spillage of the tumour or invasion of the capsule of the tumour has taken place intraoperatively then after washing, new instruments, gloves and gowns should be used for reconstruction and/or closure.

If it is found postoperatively on histological examination that an inadequate margin has been taken then a repeat wide local excision should be considered.

Closure

- Routine closure
- Drains to be placed in line of incision to facilitate tract excision if re-excision is necessary.

POSTOPERATIVE CARE AND INSTRUCTIONS

- Routine

- Weightbearing and physiotherapy – depend on procedure.

RECOMMENDED REFERENCE

Enneking WF, Maale GE. The effect of inadvertent tumour contamination of wounds during the surgical resection of musculoskeletal neoplasms. *Cancer* 1988;**62**:1251.

RECOMMENDED REFERENCES (FOR WHOLE CHAPTER)

General information relating to all of the above topics can be found in:

Enneking WF. *Musculoskeletal Tumour Surgery*. New York: Churchill Livingstone, 1983.

Malawer MM, Sugarbaker PH. *Musculoskeletal Cancer Surgery Treatment of Sarcomas and Allied Diseases*. Dordrecht: Kluwer Academic Publishers, 2001.

Sim FH, Frassica FJ, Frassica DA. Soft tissue tumours: diagnosis, evaluation and management. *J Am Acad Orthop Surg* 1994;**2**:202–11.

Viva questions

1. What do you know about the biopsy of a tumour?

2. How would you perform a biopsy of a bony lesion?

3. How would you perform a biopsy of a soft tissue lesion?

4. How would you choose between a needle biopsy and an open biopsy?

5. What must be avoided during biopsy?

6. How would you excise a bursa?

7. How would you make a cortical window in bone?

8. How would you treat a benign bone cyst?

9. What are the indications for excision of a benign bone tumour?

10. What considerations have to be taken into account when excising a benign bone tumour?

11. What are the indications for excision of a malignant bone tumour?

12. How would you plan the excision of a malignant bone tumour?

13. What are the principles involved in the excision of a malignant bone tumour?

14. What is the difference between an open biopsy and an excision biopsy?

15. What does a marginal resection mean?

16. What is the difference between a wide and a radical resection?

17. How would you ensure that you have an adequate biopsy?

18. What do you understand by the term limb salvage?

19. Why might it not be possible to salvage a limb?

20. Where and by whom should a biopsy be carried out?

3

Surgery of the cervical spine

Raman Kalyan and David J Harrison

Halo vest fixation

Cervical spine	Clinical range of motion	Radiological upper spine (C1–C2) range of motion	Radiological lower spine (C3–C7) range of motion
Flexion	45°	15°	40°
Extension	55°	15°	25°
Lateral bending	40°	0°	50°
Axial rotation	70°	40°	45°

Position of arthrodesis

- Maintain the sagittal contour (lordosis) and avoid local kyphosis
- During anterior inter-body fusion surgery, the graft or artificial cage selected is wedge shaped with greater anterior vertebral height
- The rods are contoured into lordotic shape during posterior fusion/stabilization procedures

ANTERIOR APPROACH TO THE CERVICAL SPINE (C3–T1)

PREOPERATIVE PLANNING

Indications

- Anterior decompression for spinal canal or foraminal stenosis:
  - Presenting symptoms – myelopathy, radiculopathy, neurological deficit
  - Herniated disc from degenerative or traumatic causes
  - Osteophytes
  - Bony element (traumatic causes)
  - Subluxation of the vertebra due to degenerative process
  - Tumour
  - Infection
  - Congenitally narrow canal
  - Ossification of posterior longitudinal ligament
- Anterior intervertebral fusion:
  - Degenerative pathology
  - After anterior decompression for above indications
- Anterior stabilization
  - Trauma
  - Degenerative subluxation
  - After decompression/fusion
- Cervical disc replacement
  - Degenerative disc disorders
- Biopsy/excision/drainage of collection
  - Tumour
  - Infection.

Consent and risks

- Dysphagia: 50 per cent in short term; 10 per cent long term (more common in multilevel surgery, longer retraction time, older patients). This complication can be reduce by keeping retraction time to a minimum, using smooth contour retractors, lower profile plate, good tissue handling and haemostasis.
- Recurrent laryngeal nerve injury: 0.2 per cent; it produces paralysis of one side of the vocal cord, and leads to hoarseness of the voice, airway problems and aspiration. **More common in the right-sided approach.** The reason for its vulnerability on the right side is because of its course, as it crosses from lateral towards the trachea in the midline, in the lower part of the neck. Some consider it to occur due to the dual compression of the nerve from the self-retaining deep retractor on the lateral aspect and medially by the cuff of the endotracheal tube within the trachea. This can be avoided by relaxing the retractor often and deflating and reinflating the cuff after application of the retractor
- Other neurological injuries: superior laryngeal nerve, hypoglossal nerve, sympathetic nerve and stellate ganglion
- Spinal cord injury
- Vascular injury: inferior thyroid artery, common carotid artery, vertebral artery, internal jugular vein
- Haematoma
- Visceral injury: oesophagus, trachea
- Infection: 0.5 per cent
- Cerebrospinal fluid (CSF) leak and fistula: 0.1 per cent
- Death: 0.1 per cent

Risks for fusion/stabilization

- Bone graft donor site morbidity
- Non-union/pseudarthrosis: 4–20 per cent in single level fusion, 25–50 per cent in multilevel fusion
- Implant pull out/failure
- Anterior graft migration

Operative planning

An image intensifier should be available from the start of the procedure. If an operative microscope is to be used it should be pre-booked. Some prefer to use magnification loupes, along with headlights for improved illumination of the operative field.

All radiological investigations should be available. Check/pre-order the specific implants and instrumentation.

If iliac bone crest graft is required, then the side and draping need to be pre-planned; a tri-cortical graft is best. In high-risk cases, the spinal cord integrity is monitored intraoperatively using evoked potentials (somatosensory or motor) and this needs to be organized.

ANAESTHESIA AND POSITIONING

The operation is performed under general anaesthesia. The head end of the patient is positioned opposite to the anaesthetist; therefore, long tubing is needed which requires to be safely placed and well secured. The outer end of the endotracheal tube is positioned and fixed away from the side of the incision. Prophylactic antibiotics are given as per protocol.

Place the patient in a supine position on the operating table with or without Mayfield skull clamp attachment. Head ring and adhesive tape are used to position the head securely if the Mayfield clamp is not used. The Mayfield skull clamp attachment provides a three-point rigid cranial fixation and allows greater flexibility in positioning of the cervical spine and better visualization during imaging. It is particularly useful in surgery for cervical spine fracture. It enables better control of cervical spine position and allows change in position and manipulation during surgical procedure.

A rolled up pad or saline bag or sandbag is placed between the scapulae to enable slight extension of the cervical spine as desired. The head is minimally rotated to the opposite side of the planned approach to enable better access. The head end of the table is tilted up to minimize venous bleeding. The foot end of the bed may need levelling to prevent migration of the patient down the bed. To enable adequate visualization of the lower cervical spine an image intensifier is used and for improved access, broad strips (10 or 15 cm [4 or 6 inches]) of adhesive are used to pull the shoulders down and anchor them to the operation table.

The accessibility of the image intensifier and the ability to visualize the required field must be checked. The positioning of the image intensifier and the microscope during the procedure needs to be planned.

SURGICAL TECHNIQUE

Choosing the side for the approach

For the upper and middle cervical spine, the right- or left-sided approach can be used. Right-sided approach is usually preferred by the right hand dominant surgeon and vice versa. The site of the pathology (for example in tumour) can sometimes influence the choice.

For the lower cervical spine (C6 and below), some prefer the left-sided approach, because of the increased risk of injury to the recurrent laryngeal nerve injury with the right-sided approach.

If previous surgery has been carried out on one side of the neck, then the opposite side will be the preferred choice of approach.

Choosing the incision

Depending on the number of vertebral levels to be exposed, the incision can be transverse, oblique or longitudinal. For fewer vertebral levels transverse or oblique incisions are used and for broader exposure longitudinal incision is preferred.

The cosmetic appearance is better with transverse and mild oblique incision along the neck's skin creases/cleavage lines.

Landmarks

Few palpable structures in the anterior aspect of the neck, give an approximate estimation of the vertebral level and incision (Fig. 3.1). It is common practice to use an image intensifier to identify the level of the incision and the incision site is marked.

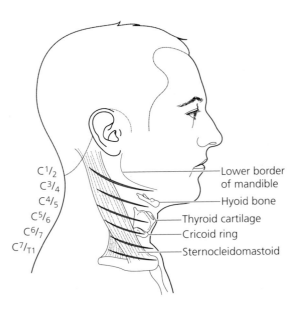

Figure 3.1 *Anatomical landmarks and levels in the anterior approach to the cervical spine*

The following guidelines can be applied for the transverse incision for the approaches to the following vertebral levels:
- C3 and C4 level – level of the hyoid bone or two finger breaths below the mandible
- C4 and C5 level – level of the thyroid cartilage
- C5 and C6 level – level of the cricoid cartilage
- C6 and below – two finger breaths above the clavicle.

The anterior border of the sternocleidomastoid muscle and the midline are identified and marked.

Incision

The skin incision extends from the posterior border of the sternocleidomastoid muscle to the midline, extending further if necessary.

Superficial dissection

Structures at risk

- Longitudinal and traversing veins in deep cervical fascia

- Inferior thyroid artery
- Carotid sheath (enveloping the common carotid artery, internal jugular vein and vagus nerve)
- Trachea and the oesophagus
- Recurrent laryngeal nerve and superior laryngeal nerve

The platysma muscle is cut in the same direction as the skin incision or split longitudinally along its fibres. The platysma is supplied by the cervical branch of the facial nerve and it receives its branches in the mandibular region, superior to the incision site. However, dividing the platysma does not cause any significant morbidity.

The anterior border of the sternocleidomastoid is identified and the deep cervical fascia is incised medially. The longitudinal and traversing vein may need retraction or ligation. The sternocleidomastoid muscle is gently retracted laterally and the strap muscles and thyroid gland are retracted medially. The superior belly of the omohyoid

muscle can be divided if it traverses the operating field or if an extensive approach is required.

This dissection exposes the carotid sheath and the pretracheal fascia (Fig. 3.2). The carotid pulse is palpated and the pretracheal fascia incised medial to the carotid sheath using blunt dissection (peanut surgical swab). **The carotid sheath enveloping the common carotid artery, internal jugular vein and vagus nerve are retracted laterally and the trachea and the oesophagus are retracted medially.** The prevertebral fascia and the longus colli muscle are visualized.

Deep dissection

Structures at risk

- Vertebral artery
- Sympathetic nerve and stellate ganglion
- Spinal cord injury

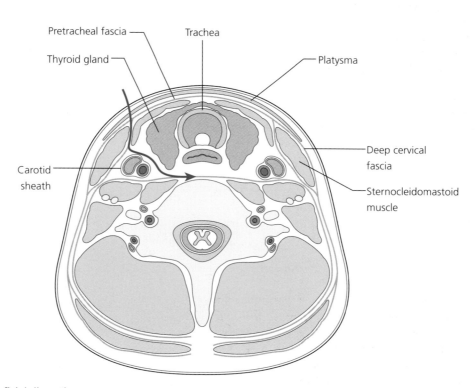

Pretracheal fascia

Thyroid gland

Trachea

Platysma

Carotid sheath

Deep cervical fascia

Sternocleidomastoid muscle

Figure 3.2 *Superficial dissection*

The prevertebral fascia is incised with blunt dissection to expose the anterior surface of the cervical spine with the two longus colli muscles. The right and left longus colli muscles are stripped subperiosteally from the anterior vertebral bodies, using cautery and maintaining good haemostasis (Fig. 3.3). The smooth-ended retractor blades are placed underneath the two longus colli muscles to improve the exposure; this helps to protect the oesophagus, recurrent laryngeal nerve, trachea and carotid sheath from injury by the retractors.

The appropriate level is identified using a bent needle as a marker (bent at about 1 cm to act as a stop) seen on a lateral radiograph using an image intensifier. After the level is identified, the further procedure of decompression, fusion or stabilization is carried out.

Closure

After removal of the retractors, special attention is paid to haemostasis of all the layers, as a retractor could have acted as a temporary tamponade. Also, check for any injury to the visceral structures.

A deep drain is placed with care and kept for 24 hours. The platysma is approximated well by interrupted suture. The subcutaneous layer is closed by 2–0 Vicryl. Skin is closed by subcuticular stitches or skin clips. Check for bleeding at the Mayfield clamp pin site and apply Opsite spray or dressing as required.

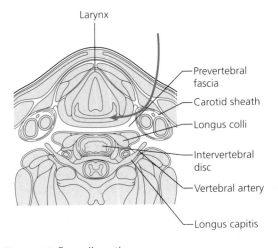

Figure 3.3 *Deep dissection*

POSTOPERATIVE CARE AND INSTRUCTIONS

Prescription of neck collars varies according to the pathology, type of surgery/stabilization and surgeon's choice.

POSTERIOR APPROACH TO THE CERVICAL SPINE (C2–C7)

PREOPERATIVE PLANNING

Indications

- Posterior stabilization/fusion:
  - Trauma, degenerative subluxation, after decompression/fusion
- Posterior decompression of the spinal canal or foraminae stenosis:
  - (Presenting symptoms – myelopathy, radiculopathy, neurological deficits)
  - Degenerative pathology – facet joint arthritis, osteophytes, ligamentum hypertrophy, instability
  - Trauma (instability, bony and disc encroachment)
  - Others – congenital stenosis, ossification of posterior longitudinal ligament, tumour, etc.
  - (Posterior decompression is preferred to anterior decompression in multilevel (>2 levels) degenerative stenosis if suitable)
- Biopsy/excision/drainage of collection:
  - Tumour
  - Infection.

Consent and risks

- Haemorrhage: usually caused by straying away from subperiosteal plane and entering intermuscular plane. Extension of the exposure lateral to facet risks bleeding from the segmental vessels and venous plexus. Cervical canal also has a rich epidural venous plexus which can bleed profusely
- Dural tear
- Cord or nerve root damage: (rare). It is important to use bipolar cauterization while controlling bleeding near the cord and nerve roots. Cord

handling needs to be kept minimal and care taken not to plunge instruments into the interlaminar space. The laminae can be surprisingly thin and fragile

- Vertebral artery injury: (rare). Vertebral artery is at risk when the exposure extends over the transverse process and in surgery involving C1 and C2. Injury bilaterally endangers the blood supply to the hindbrain
- General morbidity and mortality are shown to be increased in patients of older age and those with myelopathy

Operative planning

An image intensifier should be available at the start of the procedure, for example to check for spine alignment during positioning in patients who have instability of the cervical spine. The image intensifier is also used perioperatively to identify level, check spinal alignment, and check implant, screw and graft position. For other considerations at this stage, see 'Anterior approach to the cervical spine' (p. 14).

Anaesthesia and positioning

The operation is performed under general anaesthesia. The patient is placed in the prone position on the operating table. The head end of the patient is positioned at the opposite side to the anaesthetist. The long anaesthetic tubing is secured safely.

The head is positioned in a special head ring or brace, or held by a Mayfield skull clamp attachment, which provides three-point rigid cranial fixation, allows greater flexibility in positioning and better visualization during imaging. The eyes should be protected appropriately during prone positioning. During exposure the neck is positioned in slight flexion, to allow easier dissection and avoid skin creasing.

The spinal stability needs to be taken into account and the spinal alignment to be checked with imaging if necessary. As with the anterior approach, broad strips (10 or 15 cm [4 or 6 inches]) of adhesive tape are used to pull the

shoulders down, and the position of the image intensifier and microscope is checked. The head end of the table is tilted upwards to minimize venous bleeding.

SURGICAL TECHNIQUE

Landmarks

Identification of the level is important to avoid unnecessary dissection of the wrong levels. The external occipital protuberance and the longer spinous processes of C2, C7 and T1 vertebrae are easily palpable landmarks to guide the location of the incision. An image intensifier can also be used to verify the level as needed.

Incision

A midline straight incision centring over the exposure required. The skin in this area is vascular and thick and adrenaline can be injected to reduce bleeding.

Superficial dissection

Structures at risk

Segmental vessels and venous plexi (bleeding is much worse if dissection strays from the midline or into muscle. Lateral extension of the dissection beyond the facet joint risks bleeding from the segmental vessels).

The fascia is incised at the midline. Retractors and palpation are used to keep dissection in the midline. The nuchal ligament is split in the midline and the spinous process is reached. The spinous processes of C3, C4, C5 and C6 are normally bifid.

Using Cobb elevators and diathermy, further dissection is carried out in the subperiosteal plane reflecting the paracervical muscles off the spinous process and the lamina, either bilaterally or unilaterally as required. The extent of lateral extension depends on the procedure planned, e.g. need to expose the facet joint or transverse process.

Deep dissection (Fig. 3.4)

Structures at risk

- Dura
- Cord and nerve root
- Vertebral artery
- Epidural venous plexus

Care should be taken to avoid plunging instruments into the interlaminar space. If required, the ligamentum flavum is detached from the inferior lamina using a spatula, Kerrison punch or triple zero curette. Further laminotomy, laminectomy or laminoplasty are carried out as needed.

Closure

- Approximation of fascia with musculature and the nuchal ligament
- Approximation of the subcutaneous tissue and the skin. The posterior neck skin is thick and, owing to skin creases, it is better to keep the neck in slight flexion if possible to attain better approximation, typically with subcutaneous sutures.

POSTOPERATIVE CARE AND INSTRUCTIONS

Prescription of neck collars varies according to the pathology, type of surgery/stabilization and surgeon's choice.

POSTERIOR APPROACH TO THE UPPER CERVICAL SPINE (C1–C2)

The approach is very similar to that of the lower cervical spine and it is recommended that this section is read in conjunction with the previous one.

PREOPERATIVE PLANNING

Indications

- Posterior stabilization and fusion (C1–C2, occipitocervical):
  - Trauma

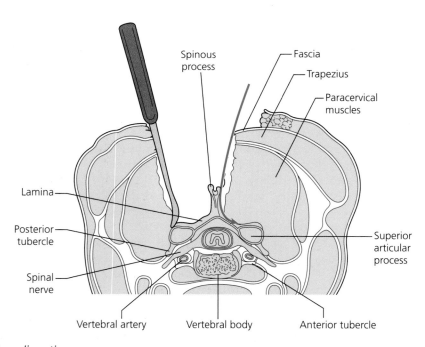

Figure 3.4 *Deep dissection*

- Degenerative subluxation
- Following decomposition from other causes
- Posterior decompression:
  - Spinal canal stenosis from various aetiologies, e.g. rheumatoid arthritis, trauma, degeneration, tumour.

Consent and risks

- Similar to posterior approach of C2 to C7
- Haemorrhage: the venous plexi are rich around the C2 nerve root and posterior to C1–C2 facet and they tend to bleed profusely
- Vertebral artery injury: vulnerable at C1 level, passing through the foramen transversarium of the C1 it turns medially and runs in the groove of C1 to pierce the posterior atlanto-occipital membrane and enter the foramen magnum
- Nerve injury: the greater occipital nerve (branch of posterior rami of C2), third occipital nerve (branch of posterior rami of C3) and suboccipital nerve are prone to injury if you stray away from the subperiosteal plane, while dissecting laterally

Operative planning

This is similar to the posterior approach of C2–C7. Three-dimensional computed tomography (CT) reconstruction is needed to plan the appropriate angle for C1–C2 transarticular screw fixation.

Anaesthesia and positioning

See 'Posterior approach to the cervical spine' (p. 18).

SURGICAL TECHNIQUE

Landmarks

- External occipital protuberance in the posterior aspect of the skull in the midline (midpoint of the superior nuchal line)
- The spinous process of C2 vertebra (the longest in the upper cervical spine).

An image intensifier can also be used to verify the level as needed.

Superficial dissection

Structures at risk

- Suboccipital venous plexus
- Vertebral artery

See 'Posterior approach to the cervical spine' (p. 18). The Cobb elevator and diathermy are used to separate the musculature from the occiput (superior nuchal line to superior margin of foramen magnum). Subperiosteal dissection is carried out separating the muscles from the C1 and C2 spinous processes and lamina, taking care of the interlaminar spaces, venous plexus and vertebral artery.

Deep dissection

If required, the ligamentum flavum is detached between C1 and C2 and the posterior atlanto-occipital membrane between occiput and C1, using a triple zero curette, spatula or Kerrison punch.

POSTOPERATIVE CARE AND INSTRUCTIONS

Prescription of neck collars varies according to the pathology, type of surgery/stabilization and surgeon's choice.

HALO VEST FIXATION OF THE CERVICAL SPINE

PREOPERATIVE PLANNING

Indications

- Cervical spine trauma (temporary or definite stabilization), e.g. odontoid and upper cervical spine fracture, fracture of the occipital condyles
- External stabilization following surgery as a primary stabilizer or as an adjuvant, e.g. after osteotomy for ankylosing spondylitis
- Instability due to infection or tumour

- Paediatric patients – trauma, post fusion, scoliosis and other pathologies
- Halo traction (halo-gravity traction, halo-wheelchair traction, halo-pelvic traction) – trauma, scoliosis, post surgery, etc.

Contraindications

- Active infection at the pin site area or in the area of the skin covered by the vest.
- Patients with conditions where pin purchase in the skull bone is unlikely to provide adequate support for the required duration, e.g. rheumatoid arthritis
- Doubt about patient compliance, understanding and ability to cope, e.g. dementia
- Patients experiencing recurrent, significant falls.

Consent and risks

- Pin loosening: 36–60 per cent (The pin should be retightened regularly using 8 inch-pounds torque (2–5 inch-pounds torque for children). It is retightened 48 hours after initial application and thereafter every week. If the resistance is not met after a few full turns, then a fresh pin is applied in a new adjacent location as appropriate. This complication can be minimized by selecting appropriate pin insertion site on the skull, adopting perpendicular pin insertion angle and using the correct pin insertion torque
- Pin site infection: 20 per cent
- Pin migration and dural puncture
- Loss of reduction: More common in anterior column insufficiency/poor reduction/poorly fitted vest mainly in obese or very thin individuals
- Pressure sores and skin problems underlying the vest area
- Restricted ventilation and pneumonia
- Restricted arm elevation
- Scar
- Dysphagia: 2 per cent. Can be prevented by avoiding immobilization at extreme range of neck extension

Operative planning

Templating

The patient's head circumference and chest circumference are measured to determine the crown and vest size, respectively. The manufacturer of the halo vest provides a rough guidance with regard to selection of the sizes (paediatric, small, medium and large). The halo ring can be trialled to check that it provides a **clearance all round the head circumference of 1–2 cm**. Availability of the correct size of the crown and vest, and other equipment and materials, is confirmed.

Three or more people are usually needed for the application of the vest and for log rolling the patient, if required. The nature and type of the neck instability should be taken into account by the surgeon. An image intensifier can be used, if needed, to assess cervical position. A crash trolley should be available for emergency resuscitation.

Anaesthesia and positioning

The operation is performed under local anaesthesia, enabling recognition of any changes in the neurological status during the procedure and manipulation. General anaesthesia is occasionally required if concomitant surgical procedures are carried out.

A hard cervical spine collar is applied for provisional additional support, to improve stability and prevent neurological deterioration. The patient is positioned supine, with the head close to the edge or beyond the edge of the bed, so that the posterior portion of the ring can be positioned appropriately. Most modern systems have either the posterior position of the ring open or curved superiorly to enable easy positioning. If slight extension of the cervical spine is desired to improve alignment, then a saline bag is placed between the scapulae.

The positioning of the image intensifier during the procedure needs to be planned. The accessibility of the image intensifier and the ability to visualize the required field must be checked.

SURGICAL TECHNIQUE

Selection of pin insertion sites

Anterior pin sites

Anterolateral aspect of the skull, about 1 cm superior to the supraorbital rim, above the lateral two-thirds of the eyebrows (Fig. 3.5). This site is optimal (relatively safe zone) for the following reasons:

- It is lateral to the frontal sinus, supratrochlear nerve and supraorbital nerve (structures at risk)
- It is medial to the temporalis muscle (pin penetration can lead to pain during mastication and speaking), temporalis fossa (thin bone) and zygomaticotemporal nerve
- There is adequate skull thickness
- It is below the equator (largest circumference) of the skull (prevent cephalad migration).

Posterior pin sites

Postero-lateral aspect of the skull at the 4 o'clock and 8 o'clock positions, roughly diagonal to the contralateral anterior pins (Fig 3.5). These sites are:

- Below the equator of the skull, but still 1 cm above the upper tip of the ear
- Where the skull is more uniformly thick
- Away from at risk neurological and muscular structures.

Halo application

Appropriate sterile precautions are undertaken during halo ring application using sterile pins and ring. Care is taken to avoid injury to the eye during the procedure.

The halo ring is positioned about 1 cm above the superior ear tip and eyebrows, but below the equator of the skull. They are temporarily stabilized using three positioning baseplates (Fig. 3.6) at the 12 o'clock, 5 o'clock and 7 o'clock positions. The appropriate locations for the pin sites and the corresponding holes in the ring are identified. Hair is shaved or trimmed over the posterior pin sites, if required. The skin over the chosen pin site area is prepared with antiseptic

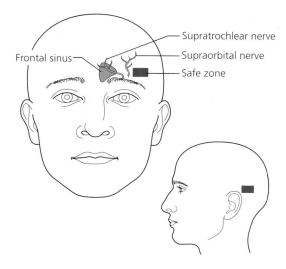

Figure 3.5 *Safe zones for anterior and posterior pin placement*

solution and is infiltrated with local anaesthetic solution.

The pins are positioned in the corresponding holes and advanced through the skin as perpendicular as possible to the skull surface. (A perpendicular bone–pin interface enables increased contact area of the pin tip and so better purchase). The patient should gently close the eyes and relax the forehead when the anterior pins are fixed. This avoids skin tethering and problems with eyelid closure. Direct insertion of pins into the skin without a prior skin incision is preferred. A single-use torque-limiting device, which breaks off when a torque of eight inch-pounds is reached, is available in some halo systems. These are used to advance the pins if available; if not a torque-limiting screwdriver is used.

The pins are tightened in diagonal fashion, by working on the contralateral pins concurrently (see Fig. 3.6). Each pin is secured using a locknut to prevent loosening. The locknuts are tightened gently, as over tightening can result in backing out of the pin. After the locknut comes in contact with the ring, it is tightened further by one-eighth turn with the spanner supplied. If skin tenting is noted around the pin, a skin release can be performed with a scalpel. Now the secured halo ring can be used to control and position the cervical spine for further procedures.

Vest application

The posterior and anterior halves of the vest are separated, but left connected to their respective two upright posts. The bolts, nuts and the connectors are loosened but dismantling of various parts of the vest is best kept to a minimum, to avoid confusion and save time. After the neck is stabilized to the trunk manually, the trunk is lifted or log rolled for the placement of the posterior vest and the two upright posts.

The anterior vest is applied next. Both halves of the vest are connected and tightened to a level that will allow two fingers to slide between the vest and chest. The patient should be able to breathe comfortably. Both the shoulder straps are also fixed and tightened. The two right posts are connected loosely to the right connector and similarly the left two posts are connected to the left connector. Both the connectors are then slackly fixed to the halo ring. The head and neck are positioned and all the bolts and nuts are tightened after placing the posts and connectors in the appropriate position. Attach the spanner to the front of the anterior vest for quicker access, to deal with any emergency that requires vest removal.

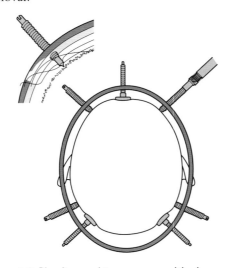

Figure 3.6 *Pin sites and temporary positioning baseplates*

An image intensifier may be used to check the cervical spine position and to enable correction under image guidance. All of the fixations are retightened when a satisfactory position is achieved.

Halo application in children

Multiple pins and low torque techniques are used. For older children, the torque used for pin application is 2–5 inch-pounds. Six pins or more can be used. For children under 3 years, 10–12 pins can be used. A CT scan of the skull helps to plan pin placements, by avoiding thin bone and suture lines. The pins are hand tightened only. Custom-made halo vest components may be required or a plaster jacket can be applied instead.

POSTOPERATIVE CARE AND INSTRUCTIONS

If an image intensifier was not used, a radiograph is used to check the alignment.

Forty-eight hours after application the locking nuts are unlocked and all of the pins retightened to 8 inch-pounds. The locking nuts are retightened. The pins and other fixations must be rechecked regularly – at least every 2 weeks thereafter. Regular care is required for the pin sites and the skin under the vest. Regularly check imaging as appropriate, as loss of reduction is common. One spanner should always be attached to the anterior vest and the rest of the application tools and spares to be kept by the patient.

RECOMMENDED REFERENCES

Bauer R, Kerschbaumer F, Poisel S. *Atlas of Spinal Operations*. New York: Thieme Medical Publishers, 1993.
Clark CR. *The Cervical Spine*, 3rd edn. Philadelphia: Lippincott Raven Publishers, 1998.
Nordin M, Frankel VH. *Basic Biomechanics of the Musculoskeletal System*, 3rd edn. Philadelphia: Lippincott Williams & Wilkins, 2001.

Viva questions

1. How do you position a patient for anterior cervical spine surgery?

2. Describe the steps of the anterior cervical approach and the reasons behind them.

3. What are the structures at risk in anterior cervical surgery and how are they avoided?

4. Describe the radiological signs indicating cervical spine instability.

5. Describe how you will position a patient for the posterior approach to the cervical spine.

6. What are the structures at risk during a posterior approach to the lower cervical spine and how can they be avoided?

7. What are the structures at risk during a posterior approach to the upper cervical spine and how are they avoided?

8. How do you apply a halo to stabilize the cervical spine?

9. What complications occur in halo stabilization of the cervical spine?

10. How is a halo vest looked after following application?

4

Surgery of the thoracolumbar spine

Matthew Shaw and Sean Molloy

THORACIC ANTERIOR DECOMPRESSION/FIXATION/FUSION

PREOPERATIVE PLANNING

Indications

Anterior instrumentation of the spine is indicated in degenerative, traumatic or pathological processes that cannot be addressed adequately with a posterior approach or by a posterior approach alone. These include:
- Fractures of the middle and anterior columns, whereby the vertebral body is unable to take load thus leading to further collapse/kyphosis (Fig. 4.1)
- Compressive pathologies, including fracture, tumours and disc prolapses compressing the cord anteriorly.

Contraindications

- Poor respiratory function (likely to lead to increasing morbidity)
- Medical resources not able to deal with complications and morbidity of procedure.

Consent and risks

- Mortality: <1 per cent
- Respiratory infection (common)
- Anterior chest wall pain
- Major vessel damage: 2–15 per cent
- Neurological compromise
- Cosmesis of scar
- Thromboembolism: <1 per cent
- Back pain
- Wrong level surgery

Operative planning

Recent radiographs must be available with appropriate scans (computed tomography [CT]/magnetic resonance imaging [MRI]). The thoracic spine is a common site for wrong level surgery, and radiological markers can be used if it is thought that level identification may be a problem. Appropriate vascular/cardiothoracic advice and assistance should be on hand.

Anaesthesia and positioning

Anaesthesia is general, with or without the use of a double lumen endotracheal tube (depending on whether the lungs need individual intubation). The lateral position is used. A sand or bean bag is commonly placed underneath the operative site to aid exposure and to open the disc spaces.

The patient is secured using an anterior superior iliac spine (ASIS) support with a posterior support on the lower back. A support is placed high on the thoracic spine posteriorly and the patient further secured using tape fixation and an arm gutter for the top upper limb. The operation table should have the ability to be able to 'break' and the patient positioned over this in order to manipulate the operative site preoperatively and intraoperatively.

SURGICAL TECHNIQUE

Landmarks

The approach should go through the bed of the rib two levels above the superior vertebra that needs to be instrumented. It is possible to extend the incision to reach an inferior level but much more difficult to get higher in the spine once the incision is made.

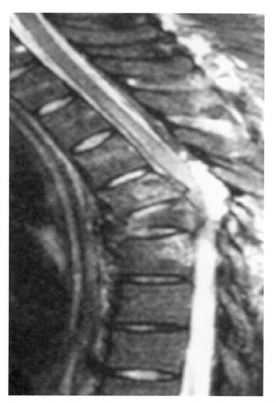

Figure 4.1 *A thoracic flexion compression fracture with kyphosis*

Approach

An incision is made in line with the selected rib. The fat and superficial muscles are cut in line with the rib. Occasionally, some muscles can be split in line with their fibres to provide a minimal access approach. The periosteum is dissected off the rib (with an elevator) and the rib is circumferentially freed from the underlying soft tissue. Rib cutters are used to remove the rib and the underlying pleura is carefully incised and the lung protected with a chest pack. A rib spreader is then positioned.

The posterior pleura is incised and a plane developed protecting the segmental blood supply. The spine, discs and segmental vessels are now exposed.

Procedure

The segmental vessels in the area of interest may need to be sacrificed. The discs are incised and removed piecemeal, removing the cartilaginous endplates aiding fusion. If performing a vertebrectomy/corpectomy, the discs above and below the vertebra in question are removed before removing it piecemeal. Implants can then be positioned.

Closure

On closure, a chest drain is inserted and the chest closed in layers. First, 1 Vicryl is applied to the pleura and transverse thoracis and then each individual layer is sutured. Second, 2-0 Vicryl is placed into the fat layer and a subcuticular layer applied to the skin to give the best cosmetic result.

Postoperative care and instructions

Adequate analgesia is achieved by means of patient-controlled analgesia (PCA), intercostal blocks or paravertebral catheter. Neurovascular observations are continued. The chest drain is left on free drainage and removed when drainage is satisfactory – this is often taken as less than 125–150 mL/24 hours.

A postoperative chest X-ray is mandatory to check that the lung is fully inflated.

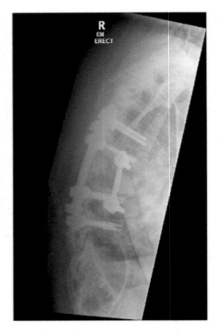
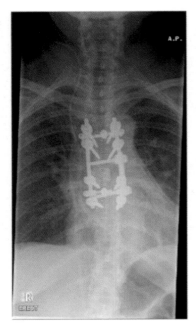

Figure 4.2 *Thoracic vertebrectomy with posterior stabilization for a solitary metastasis*

RECOMMENDED REFERENCE

Ikard RW. Methods and complications of anterior exposure of the thoracic and lumbar spine. *Arch Surg* 2006;**141**:1025–34.

THORACIC POSTERIOR DECOMPRESSION/FIXATION/FUSION

PREOPERATIVE PLANNING

Indications

- Unstable thoracic fracture (often in association with a sternal fracture) (Fig. 4.3)
- Posterior cord compression from a tumour or degenerative process
- Palliative procedure for an anterior tumour or compressive pathology, where the patient's condition does not allow for an anterior approach
- Disc pathology as part of costotransversectomy
- Coronal or sagittal deformity correction.

Contraindications

- Respiratory status does not allow for prone positioning
- Coagulopathy.

Consent and risks

- Mortality
- Infection: 2 per cent
- Neurological injury (higher rate in the thoracic spine as canal dimensions smaller)
- Wrong level surgery
- Blindness: 0.02–0.2 per cent
- Thromboembolism
- Respiratory infection
- Failure/fracture of fixation

Operative planning

Recent radiographs should be available and a CT or MRI scan available in theatre at the time of surgery. Identifying the correct level in the thoracic spine is more of a challenge as the reference points

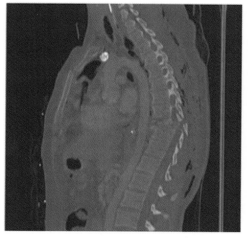 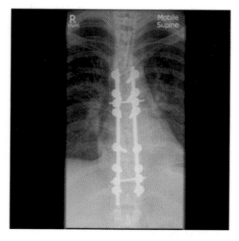

Figure 4.3 *A fracture dislocation of the thoracic spine stabilized with posterior thoracic rods and screws*

of the sacrum or C2 are not there to refer to. It is important to check the number of ribs a patient has on plain X-ray, as these can be used to mark the skin using fluoroscopy prior to incision.

Anaesthesia and positioning

The patient is positioned prone over a Montreal mattress, Jackson table, four-post frame or similar. The arms can be placed by the patient's side or out in front (depending on the level of surgery and the need to use X-ray). It is important that the shoulders are not hyperflexed or abducted (<45° abducted and <90° flexed) and there is no

pressure on the patient's axilla, which could cause a nerve palsy. Padding is used under the patient's elbows to avoid an ulnar nerve palsy. There must be no pressure on the eyes and, if possible, the table should be slightly head up to decrease central venous pressure.

SURGICAL TECHNIQUE

Landmarks

Figure 4.4 provides useful reference points in identifying the correct levels. In thin patients, the ribs can easily be felt and counted. The vertebra

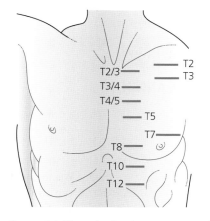

T2 Superior border of scapula.
T2/3 Suprasternal notch.
T3 Medial end of spine of scapula. Spine of T3 is posterior end of oblique fissure lung.
T3/4 Top of arch of aorta.
T4 End of arch of aorta. Azygos vein enters SVC.
T4/5 Manubriosternal junction. (angle of Louis). Start of arch of aorta.
T5 Thoracic duct crosses midline.
T7 Inferior angle of scapula.
T8 Caval opening in diaphragm. (IVC & right prenic nerve) Left phrenic pierces diaphragm. Hemi-azygos veins cross to left.
T10 Oesophageal opening in diaphragm. (oesophagus, branches of left gastric vessels, vagus nerves)
T12 Aortic opening in diaphragm. (Aorta, azygos vein, hemi-azygos vein, thoracic duct) Coeliac axis.
Splanchic nerves pierce crura. Sympathetic trunk passes behind medial arcuate ligament. Subcostal bundle passes behind lateral arcuate ligament.

Figure 4.4 *Thoracic structures corresponding to various vertebral levels*

prominens can also be used as a reference to centre the incision. In general, either the ribs or the spinous processes can be counted to obtain the correct level.

Incision

An incision is made in the midline, centred on the appropriate vertebra. Note the pedicle entry point will be above the spinous process of the vertebra counted and therefore the incision should allow for this.

Approach

Skin, fat and fascia are incised and haemostasis obtained. The paraspinal musculature is then stripped from the spine. The orientation of the transverse processes is more vertical in the thoracic spine and the facets more horizontally positioned relative to the lumbar spine with the patient prone.

The important landmarks to identify are the transverse process, the medial and lateral borders of the facet joint and the pars. All three landmarks need to be seen in order to be able to safely instrument the spine.

Procedure

The entry point for pedicle screws varies throughout the thoracic spine. From T12 to T8, the entry point becomes more cranial and more medial, and then above this it becomes lower and more lateral again. The medial and lateral borders of the facet joints give the medial and lateral starting points for the pedicle screws. In general, this is at the junction of the medial two-thirds and lateral one-third of the joint. All screws are angled medially. In the craniocaudal plane the pedicle angulation is approximately 90° to the trans-lamina line (a line drawn across the lamina above and below the screw insertion).

Decompression can be undertaken using this approach. If instrumentation is planned, the authors prefer to do this before the decompression begins as this allows some protection of the neural elements. There are many ways of decompressing the spinal cord; the

authors preferred method is one of piecemeal removal of the spinous process followed by removing the lamina using an up-cutting punch. The pars should be left intact, with at least 5 mm remaining laterally if instrumentation is not undertaken or this will cause destabilization of the spine.

Closure

Closure is in layers. A drain may or may not be inserted.

POSTOPERATIVE CARE AND INSTRUCTIONS

Adequate analgesia is provided by means of a PCA or epidural. Neurovascular observations are continued, and the patient is allowed to sit up to any angle.

Postoperative X-rays are obtained (chest radiograph may be needed if costotrans-versectomy was performed and a chest drain inserted). The patient is initially given a walking programme and a list of exercises. Lifting anything heavier than a kettle is not recommended for the first 6 weeks.

RECOMMENDED REFERENCES

Cinotti G. Pedicle instrumentation in the thoracic spine. A morphometric and cadaveric study for placement of screws. *Spine* 1999;**24**:114–19.

Kim YJ, Lenke LG, Bridwell KH. Freehand pedicle screw placement in the thoracic spine: is it safe? *Spine* 2004;**29**:333–42.

SCOLIOSIS SURGERY

PREOPERATIVE PLANNING

Indications

- Severe deformity
- Curve progression
- Radicular pain or neurological deficit (degenerative cases)
- Back pain failing conservative management (rare – degenerative cases more common)

- Neurological conditions where progression is certain and respiratory function affected
- Cosmesis.

Contraindications

- Minor curves
- When the patient's expectations do not match the surgeon's
- Poor respiratory function likely to lead to prolonged ventilation
- Spinal dysraphism, leading to a high rate of neurological complications (relative).

Choice of approach

- There is an increasing trend towards posterior-only surgery. However, much depends on the characteristics of the curve and on the surgeon's training and preference
- Thorough discectomy is only possible with an anterior approach and thus very stiff curves may benefit from anterior release prior to posterior surgery.
- Thoracolumbar/lumbar curves are often treated with anterior instrumentation, especially if there is no thoracic curve.
- Posterior instrumentation allows fixation to the pelvis – an advantage in long fusions in the elderly and in non-walking patients with neuromuscular-type curves.

Consent and risks

Complications will depend on the approach.
Anterior approach for idiopathic scoliosis:
- Mortality: 0.03 per cent
- Respiratory dysfunction/chest infection
- Neurological deficit: complete 0.03%; incomplete 1.5 per cent
- Non-union needing metalwork revision: 5 per cent
- Failure to achieve complete correction with residual curve or rotation
- Damage to sympathetic chain leading to neurovascular change in the leg
- Infection: 1–2 per cent
- Inequality of spinal balance and uneven shoulder height

- Imbalance can occur in either the sagittal or coronal planes
- Back pain (fortunately uncommon)
- Injury to the thoracic duct
- Major vessel injury
- Blindness: 0.028–0.2 per cent

For posterior procedures:
- All of the above complications apply to posterior approaches to surgery, however, neurological complications are probably slightly more common in the posterior approach and obviously there is no risk of damage to the thoracic duct
- Posterior approaches involve a significant scar, which sometimes stretches from T2 to the pelvis
- Blood loss with this approach can be considerable if not controlled adequately
- Wound infection rates are probably slightly higher with this approach

Operative planning

Scoliosis surgery is a major undertaking which should be performed in specialist centres. This chapter cannot cover every condition related to scoliosis and their management but aims to give some general guidelines and advice to the orthopaedic trainee.

Scoliosis is a diverse condition being mainly divided into degenerative, idiopathic, congenital and neurological causes. Planning for these groups will obviously be different but there are some general principles:
- All patients should be seen by a specialist experienced in the treatment of scoliosis. All patients should have a full history and examination including birth and family history and any other medical problems likely relating to their scoliosis.
- All patients should initially have anteroposterior and lateral films of the whole spine. This will help in the overall planning of surgery and assess spinal balance. If surgery may be indicated, the patient should be counselled with regard to the risks involved and a whole spine MRI performed. This test, in the authors' view, is a mandatory requirement prior to surgery to exclude abnormalities of the spinal column which could lead to an increase in

neurological complications. These include syrinx, cord tethering and Chiari malformations of the brainstem.

- Following a (normal) MRI scan, patients are again counselled with regard to the risks and benefits of surgery. A multidisciplinary team is needed, especially in the neurological scoliosis group.
- Patients need to be medically assessed if they have co-morbidities.
- Paediatric review is important and social issues need to be resolved before surgery, as do the issues of care following the procedure. Recovery is often lengthy in these patients.
- Lung function tests are useful as well as a chest X-ray and electrocardiogram (ECG). Anaesthetic involvement is required early to optimize the patient preoperatively.
- Bending scoliosis films should be performed prior to surgery. The purpose of this investigation is to assess the flexibility of the curve which will in turn help the surgeon decide which levels need to be fused. Curves are tremendously variable in their shapes as well as their flexibility. This is dependent on the patients' underlying condition as well as the age of the curve.
- Cord monitoring should be used during the procedure and an intensive care bed should be booked prior to the procedure.

Anaesthesia and positioning

Anterior procedure

The patient is positioned in the lateral position with the convexity of the curve facing upwards. The patient should be placed over a 'break' in the table in order that this can be manipulated during the procedure. A sandbag should be placed under the apex of the curve. The patient should be supported on the table by means of a side support behind the pelvis and behind the shoulder blades. The patient is padded with gel mats in order to avoid local nerve compression syndromes. A pillow is placed between the patient's legs.

Elastoplast tape is used to secure the patient on the table. The patient is then rolled back slightly to allow ease of access to the surgeon. Opening the convexity of the curve allows for ease of

access to the discs that are to be removed. An indwelling urinary catheter should be placed pre operatively.

Patients receive a general anaesthetic. Hypotension during anaesthesia is advantageous as this may decrease blood loss. A double lumen endotracheal tube is helpful but not always necessary.

Posterior procedure

For posterior procedures, the patient is laid prone, often on a Montreal mattress. This mattress has a central cut-out that allows the abdomen to hang free. This decreases the epidural venous pressure and the intraoperative bleeding. Arms should be placed with the shoulders no more than 90° abducted and the elbows should be bent to no more than 90°.

Gel pads should be used to pad the medial epicondyles of the elbows to prevent ulnar nerve injury. The patient's position should be slightly head up to decrease venous pressure around the head and there should be no pressure around the eyes. Cut-out foam or gel head supports are useful in controlling the head while avoiding pressure on the eyes.

Pillows should be placed underneath the patient's legs with the knees slightly bent. In all spinal procedures, mechanical deep vein thrombosis (DVT) prophylaxis should be considered.

SURGICAL TECHNIQUE

Anterior procedure

Landmarks

Prior to surgery, the appropriate planning X-rays should have been performed and the levels of fusion decided. It is common for anterior procedures to be combined with posterior procedures and the anterior procedure may simply involve a release and removal of the proposed discs or may involve instrumentation.

Ribs should be counted on a plain anteroposterior X-ray. Ribs should then be counted up from T12 if this is palpable. The rib bed that should be entered should be two levels above the superior vertebra being instrumented due to the downward slope of the rib cage. For example, if T9 needed to be instrumented and this was the most superior level, the incision should be made through the bed of the seventh rib (Fig. 4.5).

The authors find it useful to use a marking pen and to mark the spinous processes of the thoracolumbar spine. The incision is then marked inside the extremes of the curve.

Approach

An incision is made in line with the proposed rib. Skin, fat and muscle are incised in line with the rib. Haemostasis is obtained and self-retainers are placed. The periosteum is split on the rib and retracted off the rib. The rib is circumferentially cleared of periosteum and followed posteriorly as far back as possible. Anteriorly, the rib is exposed to the costochondral junction, and then cut and removed. The underlying pleura is exposed and carefully incised, opening the chest and exposing the lung. Wet chest packs can be used to retract the lung superiorly. The posterior pleura is then visible and this is incised taking care not to damage the underlying segmental vessels.

If the planned release or instrumentation will cross the thoracolumbar junction, the diaphragm will need to be taken down. Either before or after

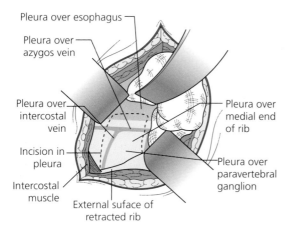

Figure 4.5 *The selection of rib level in anterior scoliosis surgery*

entering the pleural cavity, the costal cartilage is incised and the abdominal musculature divided inferomedially to allow exposure of the lumbar levels. Care must be taken to avoid damage to the peritoneum. The retroperitoneal fat is entered deep to the costal cartilage, and the peritoneum then reflected anteriorly with careful finger dissection and the use of gauze swabs as necessary. Dissection is carried down to the spine, anterior to the psoas muscle. The diaphragm is divided with electrocautery, leaving a peripheral cuff of around 2 cm of diaphragm to repair to later. Marking sutures may be inserted to help the repair later. The great vessels and viscera are carefully reflected anteriorly and protected with blunt retractors throughout the procedure.

Procedure

Once the spine is exposed, individual segmental vessels can be tied, cauterized or preserved. Disc material is then removed piecemeal until the posterior longitudinal ligament is seen. Sympathetic nerves should be preserved if possible.

It is important to appreciate the rotation in the spinal column as this considerably alters the normal anatomy and whereabouts of the spinal canal. Cartilaginous endplates are removed using a Cobb, osteotome or curette. Ideally, bony endplates should not be breached as this markedly increases blood loss.

When performing an anterior release or instrumenting the spine anteriorly, the removal of disc material provides an excellent fusion bed. The removed rib can be broken into pieces and used as autograft. When instrumenting the spine it is important to understand the rotation of the curve and the relationship of the vertebral body to the spinal canal. In the thoracic spine rib heads are a good guide to the screw insertion point and give the posterior margin at which the screw can be inserted. Following disc removal it is possible to guide screws in parallel with the endplates of the vertebra being instrumented.

In correcting scoliosis it is important to achieve a 'cadence' of screw insertion with the apical screw being most posterior. This will assist in the derotation of the spine. Bicortical fixation is beneficial and aids stability. Following screw insertion a rod is applied. The screw and rod are applied to the convexity of the curve and therefore compression in between individual screws aids reduction (Fig. 4.6). Following reduction, the screw heads are given a final tighten.

Closure

The posterior pleura may be left open or closed depending on the surgeon's preference. The chest wall is closed in layers and a chest drain inserted and sutured in.

Posterior procedure

Landmarks

It is vital to identify the appropriate levels in the thoracic spine. C7 is usually the most prominent spinous process around the neck and this can often be palpated. It is possible to count down from this level to identify the most superior vertebra that will be instrumented. Alternatively, an X-ray can be used or a shorter incision made and the ribs identified intraoperatively and counted upwards from T12.

Incision

An incision is made to the required level as previously described.

Dissection

The subcutaneous fat and fascia are incised. The spinous processes are identified and subperiosteal dissection is performed. This is extremely

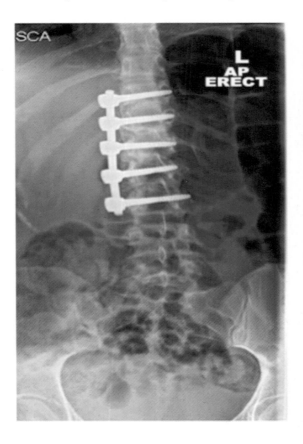

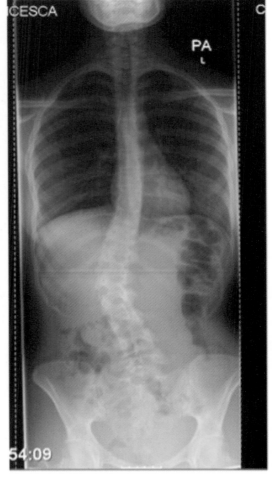

Figure 4.6 *Anterior scoliosis correction*

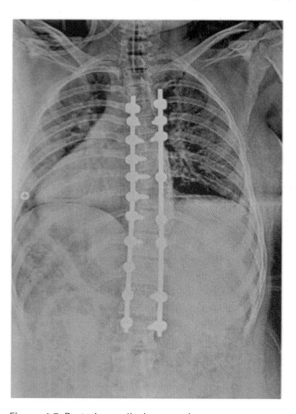

important with such large wounds, as dissection in the wrong plane will lead to excessive bleeding.

Gauze is used to pack the wounds on each side to limit blood loss. Gel foam combined with adrenaline can also help in this regard. Dissection is carried out laterally in the lumbar spine to the transverse processes in order that pedicle screw entry points can be identified. In the thoracic spine, the dissection is carried laterally to identify the transverse processes and the lateral edges of the facet joints.

Procedure

Pedicle screw fixation in scoliosis is challenging. Rotation makes for difficult pedicle screw placement. In the sagittal plane, screw angles can be judged from a 90° line to the lamina above and below the level being instrumented. In the transverse plane, screw angles may be judged from a Kocher placed on the spinous process. This technique gives a guide to the amount of rotation in a particular segment. In general, the screw

trajectory is more horizontal in the curve concavity and more vertical in the curve convexity because of the associated rotation of the spine in scoliosis. Spinal cord monitoring is mandatory throughout this procedure.

Screws need not be inserted at every level. Screw sizes are usually between 5 mm and 7 mm in diameter and vary in length from around 25 mm to 50 mm. Every surgeon will have a particular construct which he or she uses. In the upper thoracic spine, pedicle screws can be used alone or in combination with lamina, pedicle or transverse process hooks.

Before rod placement, de-cortication is extremely important. Facets are destroyed and lamina de-corticated in order for fusion to occur. Rods are then inserted. There are several ways to reduce the spine, and the authors' preferred method is by derotation of the construct sequentially from superior to inferior.

Pedicle screw fixation is a very powerful technique for reducing spinal deformity (Fig. 4.7).

Figure 4.7 *Posterior scoliosis correction*

Cross-links can be added to the construct to increase strength and load sharing. Many alternatives exist for bone grafting with some surgeons preferring local bone graft alone whereas others use a variety of bone graft substitutes/allograft and types of bone morphogenic protein (not to be used in the growing spine).

Closure

The spine is closed in layers with a watertight closure being of great importance.

Thoracoscopic anterior correction

This technique is not commonly used. It offers the ability, by means of a minimal access approach, to correct scoliosis with the use of a thoracoscope. This leaves the patient with four 2 cm cuts overlying the ribs laterally, which certainly gives a good cosmetic result. This technique has a steep and long learning curve with extended operating times in the initial phase. Some concerns remain with regard to the degree of correction obtained and the success of fusion with this approach.

POSTOPERATIVE CARE AND INSTRUCTIONS

- Neurovascular observations and analgesia are used as needed.
- Oral intake begins with clear fluids and signs of ileus are watched for.
- Postoperative haemoglobin and renal function levels are checked.
- The chest drain is removed when 24-hour drainage is satisfactory, e.g. <125 mL.
- The patient can sit to any angle and mobilize as pain allows.
- Postoperative chest and spine X-rays are taken.
- Some surgeons fit their patients with a custom-moulded thoracolumbar orthosis for up to 6 months postoperatively. This requires casting a few days after surgery, once the patient can stand for 10–15 minutes.
- Neurological injury – in patients waking up with complete motor and sensory loss the hardware should be removed immediately, with adequate blood pressure maintained, and steroids should be considered. Patients in whom root compression/injury is suspected should

have a CT scan to identify the position of the metalwork.

RECOMMENDED REFERENCES

Baig MN. Vision loss after spine surgery: review of the literature and recommendations. *Neurosurg Focus* 2007;**23**:E15.
Weiss HR, Goodall D. Rate of complications in scoliosis surgery – a systematic review of the Pub Med literature. *Scoliosis* 2008;**3**:9.

CAUDAL EPIDURAL

PREOPERATIVE PLANNING

Indications

- Acute/chronic sciatica
- Spinal stenosis (though they are more commonly treated with nerve root blocks or lumbar epidurals).

Contraindications

- Coagulopathy
- Previous failed procedures.

Consent and risks

- Failure of procedure to work
- Epidural haematoma
- Temporary loss of bladder and bowel function

Operative planning

All X-rays and scans should be in theatre at the time of surgery; a preoperative MRI scan is often performed.

Anaesthesia and positioning

There are many different ways of performing this procedure. A caudal epidural can be performed under local, sedation or general anaesthesia. The authors recommend a short general anaesthetic, with the patient positioned prone over a Montreal mattress.

SURGICAL TECHNIQUE

Landmarks

The insertion point for the caudal needle lies at the most superior margin of the gluteal cleft and is felt as a 'defect' or opening in the sacrum, the sacral hiatus.

Procedure

Fluoroscopy is used in a lateral position to check the needle position, and 5 mL of Omnipaque 300, mixed with an equal volume of saline, is inserted and an epidurogram taken (Fig. 4.8). Once the needle is seen to be in a good position, the local anaesthetic mixed with steroid is injected.

POSTOPERATIVE INSTRUCTIONS

The patient can be discharged on the day of surgery, once they can pass urine postoperatively. An outpatient review of the result of the epidural is arranged in 4–6 weeks.

LUMBAR DECOMPRESSION/FIXATION/FUSION

PREOPERATIVE PLANNING

The area of spinal fusion is controversial and a discussion of all the arguments for and against its use in spinal practice is beyond the scope of this chapter. It is fair, however, to state that there is no

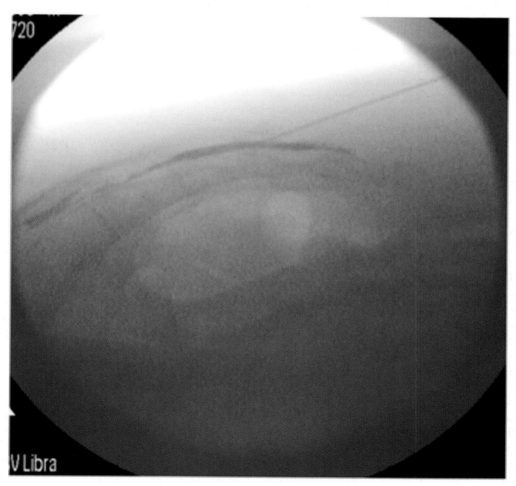

Figure 4.8 *An epidurogram from a caudal epidural*

ideal solution for back pain and most procedures with or without fusion are performed for leg symptoms. Fusion is needed in cases of instability or where decompression is likely to cause instability in the long term.

Indications

- Spondylolisthesis
- Lumbar spinal trauma
- Spinal stenosis associated with instability or degenerative disc disease
- Degenerative deformities.

Contraindications

- Smoking (may lead to non-union)
- When the patient's expectations are not in line with the surgeon's views
- Waddell's abnormal illness behaviours, e.g. widespread non-anatomical pain, pain on axial compression or rotation, straight leg raise which improves with distraction and general over-reaction to pain
- Back pain is the main symptom (proceed with caution).

Consent and risks

- Nerve injury: 1 per cent
- Cauda equina injury: 0.1 per cent
- Infection: 1–2 per cent
- DVT/pulmonary embolism: 1 per cent
- Improvement in symptoms: 85 per cent for leg pain; no change 10 per cent; worsening 5 per cent
- Non-union: 5 per cent
- Dural tear

Operative planning

- A full history and examination is taken from the patient. Specifically, symptoms of spinal stenosis, nerve root compression, involvement of bladder and bowels are enquired about
- Plain X-rays are taken to exclude deformity and fracture, and to use as a baseline for levels intraoperatively

- An MRI scan is ordered preoperatively. Blood tests may be indicated preoperatively to exclude infection where discitis is suspected. Scans should be reviewed with the patient. All forms of conservative treatment must be exhausted before spinal fusion is considered. The patient's expectations must be managed in order to achieve the best result. It is sensible for the surgeon to meet the patient several times pre operatively.
- An anaesthetic assessment may be needed preoperatively. A cell saver should be considered for extensive fusions and if deformity correction is to be performed, spinal cord monitoring should be undertaken

Anaesthesia and positioning

The patient should be preferably positioned prone and on a Montreal mattress or Jackson frame. The mattress has a central cut-out, allowing the abdomen to be free during the operation. This may well contribute to limiting blood loss. If fusion is not planned the spine can be flexed to facilitate the decompression. The arms are placed on arm boards with the shoulders at 90°. It is important to check that there is no pressure on the eyes or the ulnar nerves at the elbow and that the shoulders are safely positioned.

Anaesthetic is general, postoperative pain relief can be augmented with an intraoperative epidural and the catheter can be left in postoperatively. Hypotensive anaesthesia is useful in reducing intraoperative blood loss.

SURGICAL TECHNIQUE

Landmarks

For a guide to surface anatomy please see Figure 4.9 – note that the thoracic levels relate to the scapula and thus will change if the arms are not by the sides. In addition, the level of the top of the iliac crests varies from the L3/4 disc to the L4/5 disc, especially with transitional lumbosacral vertebrae, and correlation with plain X-rays is important. X-ray guidance can be used at the start of the operation to mark levels and, once a level is confirmed, it is possible to count up or down on the spinous processes.

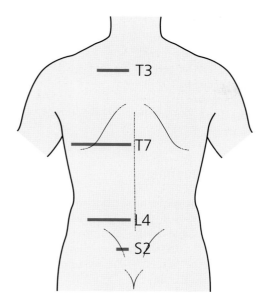

Figure 4.9 *Anatomical levels in the lumbar spine*

Incision

Following adequate positioning of the patient and level identification, a midline longitudinal incision is made.

Dissection

Subcutaneous tissues, fat and fascia are incised in line with the skin. Haemostasis is obtained. A Cobb retractor is used to put the paraspinal musculature under tension. Diathermy is then used to resect the musculature off the posterior vertebra. On an initial first pass the muscles are dissected from the spinous processes and laminae onto the medial border of the facets. It is important not to damage the facet joints and while performing a fusion, the superior facet joint in the fusion should be protected and not violated.

The wound is packed on each side and deeper retractors inserted. When performing an instrumented fusion it is important that the pedicle entry points are clearly seen. In the lumbar spine this involves the visualization of the pars, and the junction of the transverse process and the facet.

Soft tissue is stripped off the spine laterally until the transverse process is clearly seen. A Holman retractor can be placed over the lateral edge of the transverse process to aid in retraction. The pedicle in the lumbar spine corresponds to the junction of the transverse process, superior facet and the pars. The superior facet can be removed to aid visualization of the pedicle entry point as long as this is not at the top level of the fusion. Bleeding must be controlled at all times.

Procedure

Structures at risk

- Dura
- Nerve root

Once dissection is complete, it is important to use X-ray guidance to mark the correct level. This can be done by means of a marker on a spinous process or pedicle.

Once the level is identified, screws can be inserted as necessary. Screws are inserted at the confluence of the pars, transverse process and facet (see Fig. 4.11, p. 36). Following screw insertion, rods can be inserted and distraction or compression applied as needed. Following instrumentation, decompression can be undertaken if required.

There are many ways of performing this procedure, and the authors' preference is to use a burr and an osteotome to remove the lamina. Nerve roots are then explored and an undercutting facetectomy can be performed using an osteotome or up-cutting punch. It is important that nerves are decompressed both in the lateral recesses and out through the foramen. The foramen can be enlarged by applying distraction through the screw construct.

Dural breach occurs in up to 5 per cent of procedures and can be repaired using 5-0 Prolene suture by means of an interrupted or continuous technique. Other options include blood, fascia or fat patches, dural 'glues' or membranes designed to seal dural leaks, such as DuraGen.

The wound is closed in layers. If a dural leak has

occurred it is advisable to either not insert a drain or if a drain is inserted to have it on free drainage to encourage the leak to seal. Maintain the patient supine for 24–48 hours following the operation to encourage healing of the tear and to avoid the complication of low-pressure headache. Mobilization should not begin until the patient can sit without headache.

POSTOPERATIVE CARE AND INSTRUCTIONS

Neurovascular observations are undertaken, and drains, if used, are removed at 24 hours. The patient may mobilize as able and can sit to any angle (if there is no dural leak). Analgesia, postoperative bloods and X-rays are recommended.

RECOMMENDED REFERENCE

Malter AD, McNeney B, Loeser JD, *et al*. 5-year reoperation rates after different types of lumbar spine surgery. *Spine* 1998;**23**:814–20.

LUMBAR DISC SURGERY

PREOPERATIVE PLANNING

Indications

Lumbar discectomy is indicated for patients who have failed 6 weeks of conservative measures in the treatment of an acute disc prolapse. Early surgery may be indicated for patients who are incapacitated by pain or in those who have painful motor loss or symptoms of cauda equina.

Contraindications

- Coagulopathy
- Waddell's abnormal behaviour signs (relative)
- Neurological symptoms not matching MRI and clinical findings.

Consent and risks

- Nerve root injury: 1 per cent

- Epidural haematoma
- Dural tear: 5 per cent
- Infection: 1–2 per cent
- Wrong level surgery: <1 per cent
- Cauda equina: 0.01 per cent
- Ongoing pain
- Post-discectomy instability leading to back pain
- Blindness

Operative planning

An MRI scan is performed prior to surgery. Plain X-rays are useful in assessing transition levels in the lumbar sacral spine. Symptoms should be reviewed prior to surgery, as there is a good chance that the patient will have improved since last being seen in clinic.

Anaesthesia and positioning

General anaesthesia is used. Hypotension during the anaesthesia procedure is useful as this may reduce epidural bleeding. The patient can be positioned in one of several ways, and the authors' preference is to position the patient in the knees to chest position (Fig. 4.10). This position is initially difficult to master but has the advantage of opening the interspinous spaces and allowing easier access to the disc in question. The patient's knees are moved so they are under the patient's abdomen and a box is placed underneath the chest. Side supports are used to stabilize the patient. A bar is placed behind the patient's buttocks to support the trunk. Positioning of the patient on a Montreal mattress, a Wilson frame or a Jackson table is also acceptable.

In the knees to chest position it is important to adequately pad the patient's pressure points including ulna nerves, shoulders, knees and feet. The eyes must be free of obstruction.

SURGICAL TECHNIQUE

Landmarks

The authors prefer to mark the level pre- and intraoperatively. A needle is placed in the prepared skin at the point which it is estimated that the target level sits. A cross-table lateral X-ray

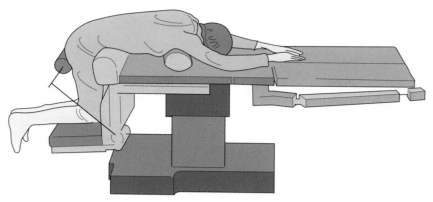

Figure 4.10 *The knees to chest position for lumbar discectomy*

is taken. The needle is adjusted and inserted onto the spinous process of the correct level. An estimate of disc level can be taken from the surface landmarks (see Fig. 4.9, p. 39).

Incision

The level involved is marked with a needle, and the skin incision is centred on the marker.

Approach

The fat and fascia are incised in line with the skin. Diathermy is then used to dissect the musculature off the posterior elements of the spine. Haemostasis is obtained. The soft tissue is swept laterally using a Cobb elevator. The outer aspects of the facet joints are identified.

It is important for the operating surgeon to be able to identify the important landmarks as well as the correct level. The lamina of the vertebra above the disc is identified and the inferior edge delineated. The ligamentum flavum should be identified and then incised. A McDonald elevator can be used to protect the underlying dura. If it is difficult to expose the dura, or there is a very narrow interlaminar window, it is sometimes helpful to start removing the inferior border of the superior lamina. The ligamentum inserts into the underside of the lamina and therefore once the attachment has been released the ligamentum opens like a 'curtain'. Once the canal has been opened it is important to again check the operative

level and therefore cross-table fluoroscopy is used with a McDonald elevator in the canal.

An interlaminar window is then developed. In some cases very little bone needs to be removed in this process. In arthritic spines the dissection can be difficult and a substantial amount of bone is resected. It is important not to remove more than one-third of the facet as this may cause instability warranting further procedures.

The dura is carefully exposed and, as the window is expanded, the nerve root is found and protected. Before the disc material is removed, it is essential that the nerve root is identified. Sometimes the disc lies below the posterior

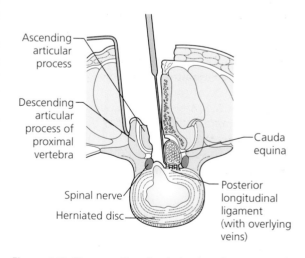

Figure 4.11 *The operative view in lumbar discectomy*

longitudinal ligament (PLL) and at other times, with large prolapses, the disc will have 'broken through' this layer. When the PLL is not breached this will need to be incised before the disc is removed.

Procedure

Nerve root retractors are used to protect both the cauda equina and the nerve root as the disc is incised. The disc is then removed piecemeal. The amount of disc that is removed from the disc space is highly variable and surgeon dependent.

For large discs it can be very difficult to retract the cauda equina enough to expose the disc. In these cases it is sensible to extend the size of the interlaminar window and possibly even perform hemi- or total laminectomy. This manoeuvre will then allow adequate retraction and visualization of the disc and nerve root.

The authors like to wash out the operative field with saline and insert an epidural catheter for a 'one shot' epidural for postoperative pain relief. The catheter is then removed.

Closure

The fascia is closed with continuous 1 Vicryl and the fat opposed with 2-0 Vicryl. Then 3-0 Monocryl is applied to the skin with Steri-Strips and an Opsite dressing.

MINIMAL ACCESS SURGERY

Over the past decade there has been a drive by industry and surgeons to perform procedures through smaller incisions in the hope that by minimizing local trauma to the tissues, recovery improves and postoperative pain reduces.

The term microdiscectomy has been coined for discectomies using a microscope. This improves visualization of anatomy through a smaller incision. The basic technique remains the same.

Newer retractors are also becoming more widely available. These retraction tubes allow for incisions of 2–3 cm and often have inbuilt lights and even cameras to improve visualization. These retractors may come more into widespread use in the next few years.

DISC REPLACEMENT SURGERY

Over the past 2 decades there has been increasing interest in the use of lumbar disc replacement. Several types exist using different bearing surfaces including metal on metal and metal on polyethylene. Centres of rotation can be fixed or mobile. The long term outcome of these prostheses is still unknown and the authors advice is to use these with care; fusion still remains the most widely accepted treatment for discogenic lower back pain. Disc replacements are inserted via an anterior extraperitonneal approach which is beyond the scope of this chapter.

POSTOPERATIVE CARE AND INSTRUCTIONS

Neurovascular observations and analgesia as required are provided. The patient is allowed to sit to any angle and should be seen in the clinic in 6–8 weeks.

RECOMMENDED REFERENCES

Tafazal SI, Sell PJ. Incidental durotomy in lumbar spine surgery: incidence and management. *Eur Spine J* 2005;**14**:287–90.

Weinstein JN, Tosteson TD, Lurie JD *et al*. The Spine Patient Outcomes Research Trial (SPORT) *JAMA*. 2006;**296**(20):2441–2450.

FACET INJECTION

PREOPERATIVE PLANNING

Indications

- Lower back pain with facet joint arthrosis
- Pain in the lower back on extension
- Failure of conservative treatments, including physiotherapy.

Contraindications

- Coagulopathy
- Inability to tolerate injections or have anaesthetic/sedation.

Consent and risks

- Failure of treatment/short-lived effect (high risk)
- Infection (uncommon)

Operative planning

All patients should have at least a plain X-ray prior to the procedure. In reality, most patients have had an MRI scan before injection.

Anaesthesia and positioning

Patients are placed prone. The procedure can be performed under local anaesthesia, sedation or general anaesthesia.

SURGICAL TECHNIQUE

Approach and procedure

The authors' preferred method is to perform facet blocks under CT control with an experienced radiologist. Without this facility, blocks can be performed with fluoroscopy in theatre. The angle of the C-arm needs to be adjusted in order to allow for the obliquity of the facets in the lumbar spine. Needles can be placed within the facet joint and checked by means of insertion of Omnipaque dye. The authors advocate performing up to three bilateral levels in one sitting; 2 mL of local anaesthetic and steroid combined are introduced into the facet joints.

POSTOPERATIVE CARE AND INSTRUCTIONS

Neurovascular observations are carried out. The patient is allowed home when comfortable (same day) and asked to keep a post-procedure pain diary. A clinic appointment is made for 6 weeks to review symptoms.

NERVE ROOT BLOCK

PREOPERATIVE PLANNING

Indications

- Known nerve compression, seen on MRI, not responding to normal analgesics or conservative treatments
- As a diagnostic test for an equivocal MRI scan
- Patient in the acute phase of a disc prolapse in severe pain and unable to mobilize.

Contraindications

- Coagulopathy
- Inability to tolerate injections or have anaesthetic/sedation.

Consent and risks

- Failure of treatment/short-lived effect (high risk)
- Infection (uncommon)

Operative planning

All patients should have at least a plain X-ray prior to the procedure. In reality most patients have an MRI scan before injection. Nerve root blocks can be instigated on a clinical basis alone if there is delay in obtaining an MRI.

Anaesthesia and positioning

Patients are placed prone. The procedure can be performed under local anaesthesia, sedation or general anaesthesia.

SURGICAL TECHNIQUE

Procedure

The authors' preferred approach is to use CT fluoroscopy and an experienced radiologist to perform this procedure, but it can be performed in theatre using X-ray guidance. A 22G spinal needle is manoeuvred, via a posterolateral approach, into the spinal foramen. Omnipaque dye can be used as a position check, before injecting local anaesthetic and steroid locally.

POSTOPERATIVE CARE AND INSTRUCTIONS

As per facet injections.

RECOMMENDED REFERENCE

Wagner AL. Selective nerve root blocks. *Tech Vasc Interv Radiol* 2002;5:194–200.

Viva questions

1. Describe the relevant surgical landmarks when planning an anterior approach to the T10 vertebral body.

2. What are the indications for performing an anterior approach to the spine?

3. Describe where the segmental blood supply of the vertebral body lies in relation to the disc.

4. At what level of the thoracic spine does the inferior border of the scapula lie when the arms are by the sides? Where, in relation to the spinous process, does the corresponding pedicle of the same vertebra lie?

5. Describe what steps you would take to minimize wrong level surgery in the thoracic spine.

6. What role do chest drains have in thoracic spinal surgery?

7. What factors are involved in selecting patients for scoliosis surgery?

8. Give a brief account of the preoperative management of a patient due to undergo scoliosis surgery.

9. Describe the positioning and the peripheral nerves at risk from prone positioning of a patient.

10. Which nerve runs in the lateral recess at the L5/S1 level?

11. Describe your intraoperative and postoperative management of a dural tear.

12. What might be the presentation and management of an acute epidural haematoma?

13. Describe the approach for a lumbar discectomy.

14. What nerve root would be compressed by an L4/5 far lateral disc?

15. An L4/5 left-sided paracentral disc protrusion will impinge on which nerve root?

16. What is the incidence of nerve root injury with a discectomy?

17. Describe the orientation of the facet joints at different levels of the spine.

18. Following temporary success of facet blocks, which other radiological procedure can be performed with potential for longer-lasting benefit?

19. Which nerve root leaves the spinal canal via the L4/5 foramen

5

Surgery of the peripheral nerve

Gorav Datta, Max Horowitz and Mike Fox

CARPAL TUNNEL DECOMPRESSION

PREOPERATIVE PLANNING

Indications

- Median nerve compression neuropathy at the wrist
- As part of a fasciotomy for compartment syndrome/decompression after distal radial fracture
- Drainage of sepsis.

Contraindications

- Active overlying skin infection
- Uncertainty over diagnosis – may warrant further investigation before proceeding.

Consent and risks

- Nerve injury: median nerve injury <1 per cent; palmar cutaneous nerve injury <1 per cent
- Radial artery injury: <1 per cent
- Failure to relieve symptoms: 1–10 per cent; the incidence is highest in heavy/repetitive manual workers
- Pillar pain: quoted at up to 10 per cent, this is tenderness around the site of ligament release
- Scar tenderness: the incidence is reduced by massage in the postoperative period
- Complex regional pain syndrome (rare)
- Infection

Operative planning

History and clinical examination remain the mainstay of diagnosis. It is essential to examine the entire limb as well as the cervical spine to exclude a 'double-crush' lesion. Nerve conduction studies are useful and should be available on the day of surgery. They are considered essential in cases of recurrent carpal tunnel syndrome and complex upper limb lesions. Prolonged sensory latency is the earliest and most reliable nerve conduction abnormality. Magnetic resonance imaging (MRI) is rarely indicated, unless there is clinical evidence of a space-occupying lesion causing the symptoms. Conventional radiography is not generally indicated. Consideration should be given to extraneous causes such as diabetes mellitus, rheumatoid and other arthritides, amyloidosis and thyroid dysfunction; where appropriate these may also require investigation prior to operation.

Anaesthesia and positioning

The procedure may be carried out under local, regional or general anaesthesia. Most primary decompressions are performed under local anaesthesia. A local anaesthetic consisting of 1 per cent lidocaine and 0.5 per cent bupivacaine in a 1:1 mixture is infiltrated into the wound prior to surgical draping. General anaesthesia is usually reserved for revision procedures.

The patient is positioned supine on an operating table and the arm is positioned on an arm table in supination, with a padded lead hand used to maintain finger extension. A tourniquet is inflated to 250 mmHg. In obese patients, a forearm tourniquet is recommended.

SURGICAL TECHNIQUE

Landmarks

The tendon of palmaris longus (absent in about 10 per cent) is easily seen and palpated by opposing the thumb and little finger and then flexing the wrist to around 30°. The distal end of the tendon bisects the anterior surface of the carpal tunnel. Other useful landmarks include the thenar skin crease (running at the base of the thenar eminence) and the transverse skin crease of the wrist joint (running parallel to the joint line). The transverse wrist crease marks the proximal border of the flexor retinaculum. If the thumb is outstretched to 90° a parallel line drawn across the palm in line with its distal border represents the surface marking of the superficial palmar arch: this is known as Kaplan's cardinal line (Fig. 5.1).

Incision

The incision runs a few millimetres to the ulnar side of the thenar skin crease, in the line of the long axis of the ring finger. This ensures that any scarring is well away from the median nerve and

ensures that proximal extension avoids the palmar cutaneous branch of the median nerve. The extent is from the distal volar wrist up to a few millimetres proximal to the superficial palmar arch. In revision surgery, the proximal extent is increased: this is curved to run along the ulnar side of the palmaris longus tendon (Fig. 5.2). This avoids crossing the wrist joint crease at a right angle and, once again, minimizes any damage to the palmar cutaneous branch of the median nerve.

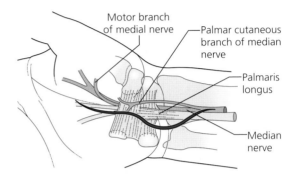

Figure 5.2 *Extended incision for revision/complex carpal tunnel decompression*

Dissection

Structures at risk

- Palmar cutaneous branch of the median nerve is at risk if the skin incision is angled to the radial side of the forearm
- Deep motor branch of the median nerve (due to variation in its course) – staying on the ulnar side of the median nerve minimizes the risk of damaging the structure
- Superficial palmar arch
- Median nerve

The exposure continues in line with the skin incision until the superficial palmar fascia is exposed deep to subcutaneous fat. Occasionally the belly of flexor pollicis brevis (FPB) is superficial to the fascia and is divided. The fibres of the superficial palmar fascia are incised in the same line.

Retraction of the skin flaps will reveal the

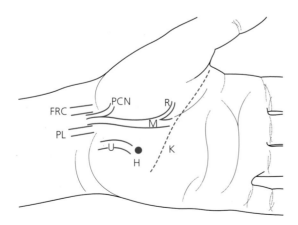

Figure 5.1 *Surface anatomy of the wrist and hand. K, Kaplan's cardinal line; M, median nerve; R, recurrent motor branch; PCN, palmar cutaneous nerve; U, ulnar nerve; H, hook of hamate; PL, palmaris longus tendon; FCR, flexor carpi radialis tendon*

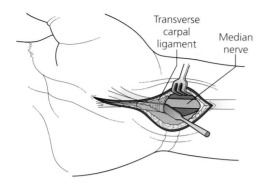

Figure 5.3 *Release of the flexor retinaculum*

insertion of palmaris longus into the flexor retinaculum. If it is in the way, it can be retracted to the radial side: this exposes the median nerve. Careful dissection through the flexor retinaculum is recommended until the nerve is visualized. A McDonald tissue dissector is passed between the plane of the flexor retinaculum and the median nerve. The dissector must be used with caution and should elevate the retinaculum and not press down on the nerve. The flexor retinaculum is incised with a scalpel, cutting down onto the McDonald tissue dissector, which lies over the nerve and protects it (Fig. 5.3).

The nerve is released from proximal to distal. In revision surgery the nerve should be dissected out proximal to the wrist crease. The perivascular fat pad is the distal border of the flexor retinaculum. This must be retracted to visualize the distal end of the ligament to ensure complete decompression. The proximal end of the wound should also be retracted to ensure complete release under direct vision with either tenotomy scissors or a blade.

The deep motor branch of the median nerve can have a variable course. Usually, it arises on the radial side of the median nerve as the nerve exits the carpal tunnel. The nerve continues radially, entering the thenar muscles between abductor pollicis brevis and FPB. However, variations may include a motor branch arising from the median nerve within the carpal tunnel, running distally to pierce the retinaculum supplying the thenar muscles. Bearing this in mind during the

dissection, it is prudent to stay on the ulnar side of the median nerve to prevent damage to the motor branch.

External neurolysis need only be performed if the nerve is adherent to adjacent structures. Internal neurolysis is not performed.

The tourniquet should be released prior to wound closure. It is important to check for reperfusion of the nerve and to ensure adequate haemostasis before skin closure.

Extensile measures

These are generally not necessary for standard carpal tunnel surgery and are reserved for specific indications.

Proximal

The approach may be extended proximally to expose the median nerve in the forearm. This may be required in cases of fracture fixation with concomitant carpal tunnel decompression. Extension is gained between the tendons of flexor carpi radialis and palmaris longus. The nerve lies on the deep surface of flexor digitorum superficialis in the forearm. The median nerve is retracted to the ulnar side and pronator quadratus incised to access the distal radius.

Distal

The incision may be extended distally with a zigzag incision (Brunner incision) to access any digit, providing a complete palmar exposure. This is useful in procedures requiring the drainage of sepsis.

Closure

Skin closure is performed with 4-0 interrupted nylon sutures. An occlusive dressing is applied, followed by a compressive hand dressing. The compression dressing should allow immediate mobilization of the fingers and wrist and should not be excessively bulky.

ENDOSCOPIC DECOMPRESSION

Endoscopic decompression may be performed through the Brown two-portal or the Agee single portal technique. The main proven benefits of the endoscopic procedure are restoration of normal grip and absence of a painful scar in the early postoperative period. The procedure, however, has a steep learning curve with complications ranging from nerve injury and an inability to see anatomical variations to incomplete release.

POSTOPERATIVE CARE AND INSTRUCTIONS

The bandage is removed 3–7 days following surgery. The sutures are removed and advice on scar massage given 10–14 days postoperatively. It is imperative that patients are encouraged to mobilize their fingers from day 3 onwards. They should also be counselled that it takes 6 weeks to regain their pinch grip and 3 months to achieve a power grip.

RECOMMENDED REFERENCES

Cobb T, Dalley B, Posteraro R, *et al.* Anatomy of the flexor retinaculum. *J Hand Surg Am* 1993;**18**:91–9.

Graham B. The value added by electrodiagnostic testing in the diagnosis of carpal tunnel syndrome. *J Bone Joint Surg Am* 2008;**90**:2587–93.

Green DP. *Green's Operative Hand Surgery*, 5th edn. Philadelphia: Elsevier, 2005.

Hankins CL, Brown MG, Lopez RA, *et al.* A 12-year experience using the brown two-portal endoscopic procedure of transverse carpal ligament release in 14,722 patients: defining a new paradigm in the treatment of carpal tunnel syndrome. *Plast Reconstr Surg* 2007;**120**:1911–21.

Rotman MB, Donovan JP. Practical anatomy of the carpal tunnel. *Hand Clin* 2002;**18**:219–30.

Smit A, Hooper G. Elective hand surgery in patients taking warfarin. *J Hand Surg Br* 2004;**29**:206–7.

Steinberg DR. Surgical release of the carpal tunnel. *Hand Clin* 2002;**18**:291–8.

Thoma A, Veltri K, Haines T, *et al.* A systematic review of reviews comparing the effectiveness of endoscopic and open carpal tunnel decompression. *Plast Reconstr Surg* 2004;**113**:1184–91.

Upton ARM, McComas AJ. The double crush in nerve entrapment syndromes. *Lancet* 1973;**ii**:359–62.

ULNAR NERVE DECOMPRESSION AT THE WRIST

PREOPERATIVE PLANNING

Decompression of the ulnar nerve at the wrist is a relatively uncommon procedure. Nerve compression may be associated with space-occupying lesions, anomalous muscles or trauma. It is imperative that the patient is examined from the cervical spine downwards, and clinical findings should be correlated with neurophysiology.

Indications

- Decompression of the canal of Guyon
- Ulnar nerve repair at the wrist (e.g. laceration).

Contraindication

Active overlying skin infection.

Consent and risks

- Nerve injury
- Vascular injury
- Infection
- Failure to relieve symptoms
- Stiffness
- Scar tenderness and hypersensitivity

Anaesthesia and positioning

The procedure may be carried out under local, regional or general anaesthesia. A local anaesthetic consisting of 1 per cent lidocaine and 0.5 per cent bupivacaine in a 1:1 mixture is infiltrated into the wound prior to surgical draping. There should be a low threshold for general anaesthesia if more than a simple exploration is being considered.

The patient is positioned supine on an operating table and the arm is positioned on an arm table in supination, with a padded lead hand used to maintain finger extension. A tourniquet is inflated to 250 mmHg.

SURGICAL TECHNIQUE

Landmarks

The hypothenar eminence and transverse wrist skin crease are important surface landmarks. The bony landmarks of Guyon's canal (Table 5.1) are palpated and marked; the hook of hamate lies 1 cm radial and distal to the pisiform, which is easily palpated at the base of the hypothenar eminence.

Table 5.1 Boundaries of Guyon's canal

Floor	*Pisohamate and pisometacarpal ligaments, flexor retinaculum and opponens digiti minimi*
Roof	*Volar carpal ligament and palmaris brevis*
Medial wall	*Pisiform, flexor carpi ulnaris and abductor digiti minimi*
Lateral wall	*Flexor digiti minimi, hook of hamate and flexor retinaculum*
Proximal extent	*Flexor retinaculum*
Distal extent	*Fibrous arch of the hypothenar muscles*

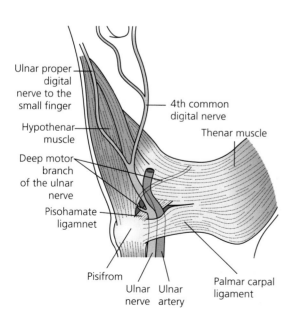

Figure 5.4 *The relations of Guyon's canal*

Incision

The incision lies in between the two landmarks (hook of hamate and pisiform) and runs distally for approximately 4 cm and proximally for 3 cm (Fig. 5.5). It is curved to the ulnar side, on crossing the wrist flexor crease, to overlie the tendon of FCU.

Superficial dissection

Structure at risk

A crossing cutaneous nerve between the ulnar nerve and the skin exists in 15 per cent of cases and must be protected.

The subcutaneous fat is incised to the deep fascia of the forearm. The tendon of flexor carpi ulnaris (FCU) is identified and the fascia is incised on its radial border. The FCU tendon is retracted to the ulnar side revealing the ulnar nerve and artery (the artery lies radial to the nerve). If necessary, the incision is followed proximally to release the distal aspect of the antebrachial fascia.

Deep dissection

Once the nerve and artery are identified proximally, they are traced distally where they enter Guyon's canal. The volar carpal ligament is incised taking care not to damage the nerve or artery (Fig. 5.6). The hook of hamate is then identified. Incising the edge of the hypothenar muscles reveals the deep motor branch as it continues around the hook of hamate.

Incising the volar carpal ligament, the palmaris brevis muscle and the hypothenar fibrous tissue will decompress the ulnar nerve within Guyon's canal. The nerve need not be completely circumferentially dissected out as this may devascularize it. Distally, the interval between the pisohamate and pisometacarpal ligaments is explored for any masses, fibrous bands or fracture fragments. The superficial branch passes superficial to the fibrous arch of the hypothenar muscles. The ulnar artery must be examined at this point to ensure that it is free of aneurysm or thrombus – it should be smooth and not tortuous.

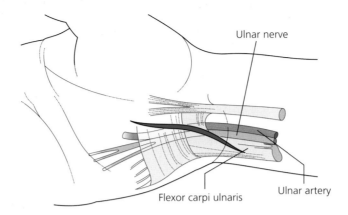

Figure 5.5 *The incision for ulnar nerve decompression at the wrist*

Despite the ability to accurately diagnose the site of compression, surgical decompression should involve exposure of the nerve from the distal forearm to the hand distal to the bifurcation. The commonest causes of compression are ganglia, other space-occupying lesions, fracture fragments and a thrombosed ulnar artery. The tourniquet should be deflated to ensure that there is no iatropathic injury of the ulnar artery and to achieve haemostasis.

Extensile measures

The incision may be extended proximally to the forearm. The deep fascia is incised on the radial border of FCU. A plane is developed between the FCU and the flexor digitorum superficialis (FDS), retracting the FCU to the ulnar side, revealing the ulnar nerve.

Closure

Skin closure is performed with 4-0 interrupted nylon sutures and a bulky, compressive hand dressing is applied.

POSTOPERATIVE CARE AND INSTRUCTIONS

The bandage is removed 3–7 days following surgery, and active finger motion is encouraged at all times. Sutures are removed at 10–14 days postoperatively.

RECOMMENDED REFERENCES

Green DP. *Green's Operative Hand Surgery*, 5th edn. Philadelphia: Elsevier, 2005.
Polatsch DB, Melone CP, Beldner S, *et al*. Ulnar nerve anatomy. *Hand Clin* 2007;**23**:283–9.
Waugh RP, Pellegrini DV. Ulnar tunnel syndrome. *Hand Clin* 2007;**23**:301–10.

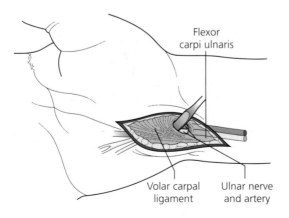

Figure 5.6 *Incision of the volar carpal ligament*

ULNAR NERVE DECOMPRESSION AT THE ELBOW

PREOPERATIVE PLANNING

Indications

- Ulnar nerve compression with or without recurrent subluxation of the nerve
- Exploration of the ulnar nerve in trauma.

Contraindication

Active overlying skin infection.

Consent and risks

- Nerve injury to the ulna, median or the medial antebrachial nerve (the commonest at 4 per cent)
- Medial elbow tenderness: 10 per cent
- Failure to relieve symptoms and recurrence: 10 per cent
- Elbow stiffness: 5–10 per cent
- Elbow instability associated with medial epicondylectomy: 1–5 per cent

Operative planning

A full neurological examination of the upper limb must take place. This should include an examination of the cervical spine as well as eliciting Tinel's sign at the elbow and wrist. Unlike in carpal tunnel disease, neurophysiological examination should be performed in almost all cases.

It is the authors' preferred choice to manage the majority of cases with simple decompression. Other options include partial medial epicondylectomy or nerve transposition procedures (which can be subcutaneous or submuscular). Partial medial epicondylectomy can be useful where there is significant extrinsic pressure on the nerve (e.g. an osteophyte). Transposition remains controversial because of an increased incidence of haematoma and infection without convincing improvements in results.

Anaesthesia and positioning

The procedure may be carried out under regional or general anaesthesia.

The authors prefer a medial approach as this avoids incision directly over the nerve. It also allows early visualization of the medial antebrachial cutaneous nerve of the forearm. The patient is positioned supine on an operating table and the arm is positioned on a padded arm table, in supination, with the shoulder externally rotated. If a posterior approach is used, the patient is positioned in the lateral decubitus position with the arm placed in front of the chest, resting on a padded arm gutter. If a tourniquet is used it is inflated to 250 mmHg. The authors do not routinely use a tourniquet as pre-infiltration with local anaesthetic mixed with adrenaline provides excellent postoperative analgesia as well as a clear field for surgical dissection.

SURGICAL TECHNIQUE

Landmarks

The olecranon can easily be palpated posteriorly as it is a subcutaneous structure. Similarly the medial epicondyle is easily palpated. The nerve runs between these two structures and is at its most superficial at this point. Figure 5.7 shows the relations of the ulnar nerve at the elbow.

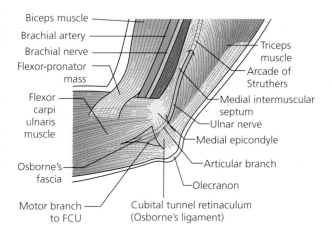

Figure 5.7 *The relations of the ulnar nerve*

Medial approach

The medial incision starts 5 cm proximal to the medial epicondyle and extends distally to lie medial to the ulna distal to the elbow joint. It is advisable to place the skin incision anterior to the medial epicondyle so that the nerve does not lie directly under the skin wound. This prevents scarring directly over the nerve and the medial cutaneous nerve of the forearm branch can be visualized. It is also less likely that a painful medial pressure area will occur. Subcutaneous tissues are reflected proximally and distally exposing the cubital tunnel retinaculum.

Posterior approach

This is recommended for the identification of the nerve in complex elbow trauma.

A longitudinal incision is made in the midline approximately 5 cm above the olecranon. The incision is curved laterally around the lateral side of the olecranon process and then curved medially so that the incision lies over the middle of the ulna distally. Curving the incision laterally moves the suture line away from the midline and avoids any potential pressure area over the olecranon process. The subcutaneous tissues are then dissected medially to expose the medial epicondyle. The advantage of the posterior approach is that frequently patients may have other elbow disorders requiring surgery (e.g. rheumatoid arthritis) and further incisions may be performed through the same scar. The disadvantage is that considerable dissection is necessary to expose the medial side adequately.

Deep dissection

The ulnar nerve is identified proximal to the cubital tunnel by blunt dissection. It is first released at the arcade of Struthers (the hiatus in the medial intermuscular septum through which the ulnar nerve enters the posterior compartment). The roof of the cubital tunnel is Osborne's ligament (the cubital tunnel retinaculum) proximally and Osborne's fascia (the deep component of the aponeurosis of the two heads of FCU) distally. The nerve is followed distally and Osborne's ligament is incised from proximal to distal. The veins lying on the dorsal surface of the medial intramuscular septum should be identified and coagulated. The nerve is traced into the two heads of the FCU to ensure release distally. At this stage it is important to identify and protect the motor branch to the FCU.

The nerve should not be dissected from its groove as this may lead to subluxation and devascularization. After release, the elbow is moved through its full range; the nerve should be lax in full extension and should remain in the groove in full flexion. Residual adherent structures should be released and if subluxation is a problem then medial epicondylectomy or subcutaneous transposition should be considered.

Medial epicondylectomy

This procedure is useful in patients with a medial epicondyle fracture non-union or space-occupying lesions within the cubital tunnel (e.g. medial osteophyte, exostosis or ganglion). Routine decompression is performed, after which the common flexor origin is elevated off the medial epicondyle in a subperiosteal manner.. A sleeve is left around the bone to ensure smooth closure and haemostasis. A partial medial epicondylectomy is performed with a narrow osteotome; bone wax can be placed on the exposed cancellous bone. The periosteal sleeve is closed over the epicondyle stump with a heavy Vicryl suture; this should be done in full extension so that an extension lag is avoided.

The anteroinferior medial collateral ligaments must be avoided and no more than 20 per cent of the depth of the epicondyle should be excised to prevent elbow instability.

Subcutaneous transposition

The theory behind transposing the nerve is to reduce tensile stress on the nerve. This occurs during traction on the nerve in flexion and leads to an increased intraneural pressure and flattening of the nerve around the medial epicondyle. This increased pressure may cause temporary ischaemia.

The medial intramuscular septum must be divided to ensure tension-free transposition. It is essential that the longitudinal vascular supply of the nerve is left intact and that the motor branches are protected and allowed to move with the main body of the nerve.

Once the nerve is decompressed and easily transposable anterior to the medial epicondyle, a subcutaneous fascial flap is elevated with a scalpel. The nerve is placed anterior to the deep surface of the flap and the distal flap edges are sutured to deep dermal tissue with an absorbable 3-0 Vicryl suture. The wound is then closed as normal.

Closure

The wound is closed with interrupted 2-0 Vicryl sutures for the subcutaneous layer and a running subcuticular monofilament suture for skin. If a tourniquet has been used it should be released and followed by meticulous haemostasis. A sterile dressing should be applied and then a compressive dressing over it.

POSTOPERATIVE CARE AND INSTRUCTIONS

Dressings are removed at 3–4 days. Range of motion exercises within the limits of comfort should be started at the same stage. Active hand and wrist motion is encouraged at all times.

The wound should be checked at 2 weeks and the patient advised on appropriate care of the scar. Heavy lifting should be avoided for 1 month. It is important to counsel the patient that not all symptoms may be relieved by the surgery and that recovery may take up to 6 months.

RECOMMENDED REFERENCES

Catalano LW, Barron OA. Anterior subcutaneous transposition of the ulnar nerve. *Hand Clin* 2007;**23**:339–44.

Mowlavi A, Andrews K, Lille S, *et al.* The management of cubital tunnel syndrome: a meta-analysis of clinical studies. *Plast Reconstr Surg* 2000;**106**:327–34.

O'Driscoll SW, Jaloszynski R, Morrey BF, *et al.* Origin of the medial ulnar collateral ligament. *J Hand Surg Am* 1992;**17**:164–8.

Osterman AL, Spiess AM. Medial epicondylectomy. *Hand Clin* 2007;**23**:329–37.

Waugh RP, Zlotolow DA. *In situ* decompression of the ulnar nerve at the cubital tunnel. *Hand Clin* 2007;**23**:319–27.

PRINCIPLES OF SURGERY ON PERIPHERAL NERVES

PREOPERATIVE PLANNING

The aims of surgery are:
- To confirm a diagnosis and establish prognosis
- To restore function
- To relieve pain.

Indications

- Closed traction injury of the brachial plexus leading to severe paralysis
- Associated nerve and vascular injury
- Nerve injury with an associated fracture requiring early internal fixation
- Increasing progression of a neurological injury or an entrapment neuropathy
- Failure of recovery of a lesion within an expected timeframe
- Failure of recovery in conduction block within 6 weeks of injury
- Persistent pain following injury
- Severe paralysis of a nerve following blunt trauma.

Contraindications

- Active infection
- Function unaffected by nerve injury.

Consent and risks

- Infection
- Nerve damage/failure of repair
- Vascular injury
- Specific to the site of operation, e.g. local structures at risk

Operative planning

Earlier surgery following nerve injury permits easier identification of tissues (due to less scar tissue) and therefore any repair is easier as it is possible to visualize and match the arrangement of the cut ends of the nerve fascicles. The results of prompt repair are also markedly better due the favourable biological environment for nerve healing. A nerve stimulator should be available. Magnification of at least three times with loupes is helpful. If nerve grafting is likely to be performed, a suitable donor graft should be identified preoperatively and the patient made aware of the need.

Anaesthesia and positioning

Surgical procedures involving the exploration/repair of peripheral nerves should be performed under general anaesthesia, with antibiotic cover to minimize the chance of any postoperative infection. Where possible, a tourniquet is used to achieve a completely bloodless field, facilitating ease of identification of structures. Remember that after approximately 15 minutes of ischaemia, nerve conduction becomes abnormal so any tourniquet should be released when stimulating a nerve.

SURGICAL TECHNIQUE

Incision

The course of cutaneous nerves should always be remembered when planning a skin incision. A painful neuroma may result from a transected cutaneous nerve and lead to considerable morbidity to the patient.

Nerve assessment

When nerves have been damaged and surgery has been delayed, a neuroma will have formed. The consistency of a neuroma is important when assessing nerve injury, as a hard neuroma may represent an abundance of connective tissue and little in the way of nerve tissue. Making an incision through the damaged epineurium permits visualization of any nerve bundles present, and stimulation of the nerve proximally. This may give some indication as to likely recovery. Stimulating the nerve proximally and recording from the nerve distally gives the best guide for recovery. An

absence of recording distally is a relative indication to resect and repair the nerve, depending on the macroscopic fascicular structure seen. Care should be taken not to undertake excessive mobilization, as this may lead to devascularization of a nerve.

Bipolar diathermy should be used at all times when coagulating blood vessels around nerves.

METHODS OF REPAIR

Primary repair

The ends of an injured nerve are cut back progressively until the cut surfaces show bulging healthy nerve bundles. An end-to-end anastomosis is performed, which is possible if the resection gap has been small, little mobilization of the nerve has been necessary, and the nerve is not under tension. Flexing a nearby joint reduces tension on a nerve, and extra length can be gained by transposition (e.g. anterior transposition of the ulnar nerve) of a nerve. The two principal types of primary repair are **epineural** repair and **fascicular** repair. Epineural repair is technically less demanding and faster to complete. Fascicular repair (Fig. 5.8) is performed if there has been a clean transection of a nerve trunk (e.g. in the brachial plexus). In each method of repair the true epineurium is exposed. In a fascicular repair the matched bundles are opposed and sutured with perineurial 11-0 nylon sutures and then 10-0 nylon sutures are passed through the perineurium and epineurium. This is done circumferentially to complete the repair. In an epineurial repair (Fig. 5.9), the fascicular groups in the nerve ends are matched as closely as possible and the ends are then sutured with 10-0 nylon sutures through the epineurium. An initial suture is placed at each of the lateral ends of the nerve, with interrupted sutures subsequently placed on the anterior and posterior aspect of the nerve to complete the repair.

Nerve grafting

Cable grafts (Fig. 5.10) are the gold standard for bridging gaps between two cut ends of a nerve where primary repair is not possible. Nerve bundles are matched to bundles; this is achieved by viewing and matching the nerve ends either

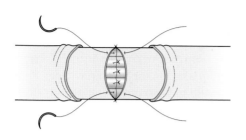

Figure 5.8 *Fascicular nerve repair*

using loupes or a microscope, using magnification to get the best possible match. Cable grafts consist of multiple cutaneous nerve strands from a donor nerve. The commonest donor nerves used are the medial cutaneous nerve of the forearm and the sural nerve in the lower limb. As many grafts as required are used to give good coverage of the cut face of the nerve. The length of the graft should be approximately 15 per cent longer than the gap to be bridged. The grafts can either be fixed with a tissue glue or sutured in place. If a gap to be bridged is greater than 10 cm, grafting is unlikely to be of great benefit.

If a nerve has been severely damaged to the extent that repair and grafting are not possible, nerve transfer (neurotization) is performed: a distal nerve is reinnervated using an intact donor proximal nerve.

POSTOPERATIVE CARE AND INSTRUCTIONS

After nerve decompression, patients are told to leave their bulky dressings in place until they have a wound inspection 2 weeks postoperatively. Instruction to begin early hand and finger mobilization is encouraged in upper limb surgery.

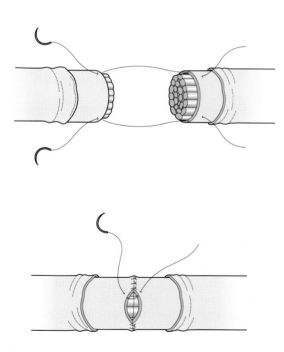

Figure 5.9 *Epineural repair*

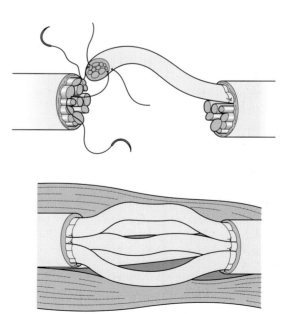

Figure 5.10 *Cable nerve grafting*

After nerve repair and grafting, the limb is generally protected in a plaster with a sling (or crutches in the lower limb) for a period of between 3 and 6 weeks. Either outpatient or inpatient therapy (as in the case of a brachial plexus repair) is required to overcome any residual stiffness and deformity. This may include appropriate splintage and is often multidisciplinary, with occupational therapy, physiotherapy and pain team input.

PRINCIPLES OF BRACHIAL PLEXUS SURGERY

PREOPERATIVE PLANNING

The principles of brachial plexus surgery are similar to those of other peripheral nerve operations (see previous section).

The five roots of the brachial plexus lie in the posterior triangle of the neck between scalenus anterior and scalenus medius muscles. Injuries between the posterior root ganglion and the spinal cord are termed preganglionic. The three trunks of the brachial plexus lie in front of one another and in the posterior triangle of the neck. The divisions of the plexus lie posterior to the clavicle. The medial, lateral and posterior cords of the plexus are related to the second part of the axillary artery deep to pectoralis minor.

Indications

- Section/rupture/avulsion of the plexus
- Associated vascular and nerve injuries
- Open wounds
- Compressive neuropathy.

Anaesthesia and positioning

The procedure is performed under general anaesthesia, with the patient supine and the head elevated to approximately 30°.

SUPRACLAVICULAR APPROACH TO THE BRACHIAL PLEXUS

- Cervical and brachial plexus (root/trunk) surgery

- Spinal accessory nerve surgery
- Suprascapular nerve surgery
- Sympathetic chain surgery.

Landmarks

The landmarks for the supraclavicular approach are those of the posterior triangle of the neck. The base is formed by the clavicle, the medial border is formed by the medial border of the sternocleidomastoid muscle, and the lateral border by the edge of the trapezius muscle.

Incision

Structure at risk

- Supraclavicular nerves

The skin incision is made approximately one finger's breadth above the clavicle in line with the bone. Care must be taken not to damage the supraclavicular nerves, as a painful neuroma may develop.

Dissection

Skin flaps are raised exposing the apex of the posterior triangle superiorly and the clavicle inferiorly. Next the plane between external jugular vein and the sternocleidomastoid is developed, with the omohyoid muscle displayed inferiorly in the wound. The muscle is divided and reflected. Deep to the fat pad, the transverse cervical artery is present and is at risk; it is ligated. The phrenic nerve is visualized running across scalenus anterior. The nerve is followed proximally, revealing C5. The deep cervical fascia is incised and C5 and C6 are seen emerging from the lateral aspect of scalenus anterior; C7 is visualized between scalenus anterior and the upper trunk. The lower trunk is seen following division of scalenus anterior. C8 and T1 are visualized by following the plane between the subclavian artery and the lower trunk.

INFRACLAVICULAR APPROACH TO THE BRACHIAL PLEXUS

Indications

- Complete exposure of brachial plexus (when combined with supraclavicular approach)
- Infraclavicular brachial plexus repair.

Dissection

Essentially this is analogous to the deltopectoral approach to the upper humerus. The difference lies in mobilizing the cephalic vein medially and detaching and reflecting the pectoralis minor muscle from the coracoid process. In a full exposure, the pectoralis major insertion on the humerus may also be detached.

FIOLLE DELMAS APPROACH

Indications

The Fiolle Delmas approach combines the supraclavicular and infraclavicular approaches and is useful in an extensive injury to the plexus.

Incision

The platysma, with skin flaps is elevated and the mid-portion of the clavicle is exposed superiorly and inferiorly. An extension is made of the collar incision to expose the supraclavicular portion (Fig. 5.11). This extension starts at around the mid-portion of the supraclavicular incision and extends distally over the mid-portion of the clavicle running over the delto-pectoral groove to the axilla. It is a true extensile approach and can be continued distally, if necessary, as the anterior approach to the humerus. When the infraclavicular is combined with the supraclavicular approach, full exposure is given from the second part of the subclavian artery to the terminal portion of the axillary artery, with exposure of the brachial plexus from the spinal nerves to terminal branches of the plexus.

Dissection

A clavicular osteotomy may be required to

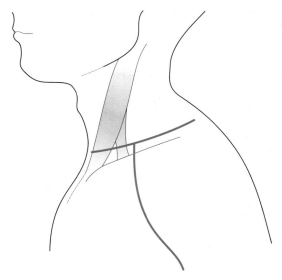

Figure 5.11 *Incision for the Fiolle Delmas approach to the brachial plexus*

facilitate access, especially if there is a vascular injury. In this case a plate should be precontoured and holes predrilled for easy fixation at the end of the procedure, remembering that the bone will be shortened by the thickness of the saw blade. Distally the pectoralis major muscle is detached from the humerus in its upper portion or, if required, its entirety. The muscle is then reflected medially exposing the clavicle, pectoralis minor muscle and the clavipectoral fascia (Fig. 5.12). The pectoralis minor muscle is divided at its tendon taking care not to damage the musculocutaneous nerve. The subclavius muscle is divided with the suprascapular vessels (once ligated). This exposes the entire plexus and vasculature from the first rib to the axilla.

POSTOPERATIVE CARE AND INSTRUCTIONS

Following nerve repair/transfer, the limb may require immobilization in a cast for 3 weeks after which the patient can start motion progressively. In the case of brachial plexus surgery, a sling is applied with a body strapping for 3 weeks, followed by readmission for a week at 6 weeks post index operation to start the rehabilitation process.

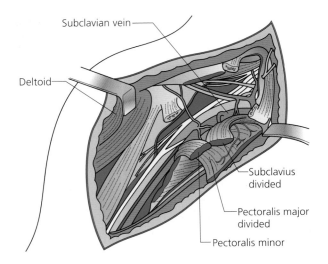

Subclavian vein

Deltoid

Subclavius divided

Pectoralis major divided

Pectoralis minor

Figure 5.12 *Dissection in the Fiolle Delmas approach to the brachial plexus*

RECOMMENDED REFERENCES

Birch R, Bonney G, Wynn Parry CB. *Surgical Disorders of the Peripheral Nerves*. London: Churchill Livingstone, 1998.

Henry HK. *Extensile Exposure*, 2nd edn. Edinburgh: Churchill Livingstone, 1957.
Tupper JW, Crick JC, Mattich LR. Fascicular nerve repairs. *Orthop Clin North Am* 1988;**19**:57–69.

Viva questions

1. Describe the landmarks and incision for a carpal tunnel decompression.

2. Describe the main structures at risk in a carpal tunnel decompression.

3. What are the sites of compression of the ulnar nerve at the elbow?

4. What are the surface landmarks for Guyon's canal?

5. Which structures commonly cause ulnar tunnel compression neuropathy at the elbow?

6. Describe the techniques used in primary nerve repair.

7. What options are available if primary repair is not possible?

8. What are the principal considerations for successful nerve transfer surgery?

9. What are the priorities in gaining function after brachial plexus injury?

6

Surgery of the shoulder

Omar Haddo and Mark Falworth

Shoulder	Range of motion
External rotation	*80°*
Internal rotation	*90°*
Flexion	*180°*
Abduction	*180°*

Position of arthrodesis

- Internal rotation 30°
- Flexion 30°
- Abduction 30°

DIAGNOSTIC SHOULDER ARTHROSCOPY

PREOPERATIVE PLANNING

Common indications

Diagnosis is often made on the basis of history, examination and investigations. However, diagnostic shoulder arthroscopy remains a useful tool in the armament of the orthopaedic surgeon as some pathologies remain difficult to diagnose with standard non-invasive investigations. Diagnostic arthroscopy therefore offers the opportunity to establish or confirm a diagnosis with the possibility to proceed to treatment with the appropriate consent.

Diagnostic arthroscopy is most frequently used for:
- Undiagnosed shoulder pain
- Complex instability, including humeral avulsion of the glenohumeral ligaments (HAGL) lesions
- Small/partial thickness rotator cuff tears.

Contraindications

- Infection of overlying skin
- Lack of proper arthroscopic instrumentation
- Gross osteoarthritis is a relative contraindication.

Consent and risks

- Nerve injury: the musculocutaneous nerve (anterior portal) and the axillary nerve (lateral portal) are most at risk. The suprascapular nerve can be damaged by the inexperienced arthroscopist
- Chondral or labral injuries: relatively uncommon
- Fluid imbalance due to fluid extravasation
- Infection: very rare
- Vascular injury: very rare

Operative planning

Recent radiographs and when relevant, ultrasound, computed tomography (CT) and magnetic resonance (MR) images (± arthrograms), should be available. Although only basic equipment is necessary for a diagnostic procedure standard equipment should be available so that therapeutic treatment can be undertaken if necessary. This includes:
- Camera with imaging and recording equipment
- Xenon light source
- Fluid management system (pump set at 30–70 mmHg)
- 5 mm 30° scope with high-flow sleeve
- Shaver
- Vaporizer
- Arthroscopic instruments
- Cannulas
- Arthroscopic implants.

Anaesthesia and positioning

General anaesthesia is preferred with the use of an interscalene block if certain procedures are planned. The choice of patient positioning is very much surgeon dependent:

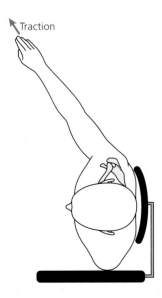

Figure 6.1
Positioning and traction for shoulder arthroscopy

- If the lateral position is used, the patient should be as far back towards the edge of the table as possible, with 15° of posterior tilt (horizontal glenoid). Front and back supports are required to secure the patient. The patient's head is placed in a gel ring. Four kilograms of longitudinal skin traction is applied with the arm in 30–50° abduction and 20–30° forward flexion (Fig. 6.1). The brachial plexus should be palpated to ensure that it remains soft and that excessive traction is not being applied
- If the beach chair position is used, the appropriate operating table (with removable lateral corner) is required. The patient's head is appropriately secured. Traction can be added based on surgeon preference. This approach is helpful if progressing to an open procedure.

The surgical field is prepared with a germicidal solution and waterproof drapes are used with adhesive edges to provide a seal to the skin.

SURGICAL TECHNIQUE

Landmarks

- Spine of the scapula
- Posterolateral corner of the acromion, lateral acromion, and anterolateral corner of acromion
- Distal clavicle and acromioclavicular joint (ACJ)
- Tip of the coracoid.

Portals

The accurate placement of arthroscopic portals is essential in shoulder arthroscopy. A variety of portals can be used. The commonest viewing portal is the posterior portal. A stab incision to the skin is placed 2 cm medial and 2 cm inferior to the posterolateral corner of the acromion. This correlates to a palpable soft spot which denotes the plane between the infraspinatus and teres minor.

To access the glenohumeral joint, the scope is aimed inferomedially towards the tip of the coracoid. The glenoid rim and the humeral head can be palpated and the scope can be pushed between them. A popping sensation is usually felt as the joint is entered. Once the posterior portal is established all other portals are made using an outside-in technique in which a spinal needle is used to determine the exact location and angle of entry into the joint.

A standard low anterior portal can also be used for passing instruments into the joint. It is placed above the lateral half of the subscapularis but medial to the medial biceps pulley. Once the needle has been placed in the appropriate position the portal is made using a size 11 scalpel, which is inserted in the same direction as the needle taking care to avoid the long head of the biceps (LHB).

To enter the subacromial space, the same posterior portal skin incision is used; however, the scope is aimed superolaterally towards the anterolateral corner of the acromion. The scope must enter the bursa and show the acromion and the bursal aspect of the cuff clearly. If cobweb-like tissue is seen, then the scope is outside the bursa and should be repositioned. This is important as the bursa helps to contain the irrigation fluid, thus limiting soft tissue swelling around the shoulder.

The lateral portal is 5 cm (three fingers breadth) distal to the acromion and 1 cm anterior to the mid-lateral line (in line with the posterior line of the ACJ). This portal is used for instrumentation of the subacromial space (Fig. 6.2).

Other portals can be made on demand. These include the anterosuperolateral, accessory anterior, accessory lateral, accessory posterior and Neviaser (superior) portals. A cannula may be used if proceeding to a therapeutic procedure. Clear cannulas are recommended as they allow visualization and aid in suture management.

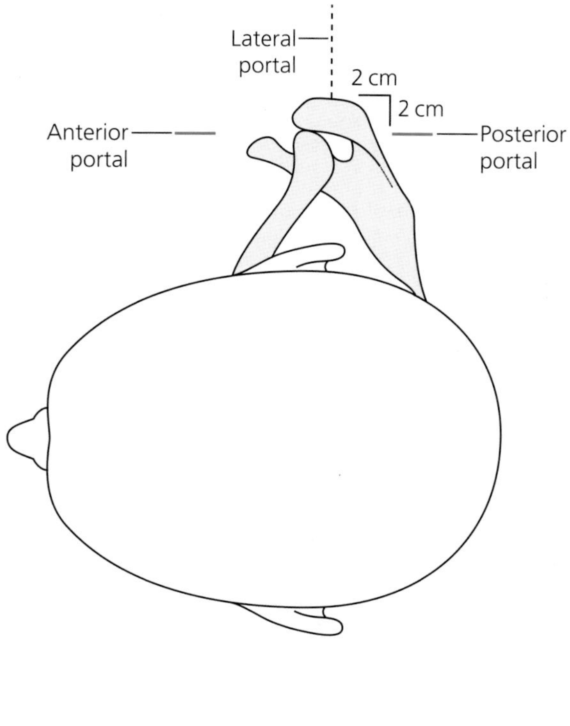

Procedure

A systematic approach is essential if pathology is not to be missed.

With the scope in the posterior portal, the glenohumeral joint is assessed first. By using the LHB tendon as a reference, the camera is adjusted so that the image is shown in the correct supero-inferior plane. The authors recommend the following systematic way of assessing the shoulder:

- The LHB should first be assessed at its insertion at the superior glenoid tubercle. By raising the arm in 90° abduction and 90° external rotation, the presence of a SLAP (superior labrum from anterior to posterior) tear can be assessed as the labrum rolls off the glenoid rim (peel-back sign). The scope can then be turned laterally and the intra-articular portion of the LHB, and that portion of the biceps tendon that lies within the inter-tubercular grove, can be assessed.
- The stability of the LHB can then be visualized by internally and externally rotating the shoulder. The medial sling/pulley can then be inspected before examining the subscapularis tendon, superior glenohumeral ligament and rotator interval in more detail. The subscapularis

Figure 6.2 *Common arthroscopic portals*

tendon insertion can be best visualized with the arm in internal rotation.

- By gently withdrawing the scope and looking laterally, the posterior pulley of the LHB can be viewed and then the supraspinatus and infraspinatus tendons can be examined. The bare area and any Hill–Sachs lesions can now be identified.
- As the arthroscope is taken further inferiorly it enters the inferior recess. The reflection of the inferior capsule and the posterior band of the inferior glenohumeral ligament (hammock effect) can be seen. By then rotating the scope, the posterior inferior labrum can be visualized and then the entire posterior and superior labrum examined before assessing the chondral surfaces of both the humeral head and glenoid.
- The anterior stabilizing structures can now be examined. Superiorly the sublabral foramen, labrum and the middle glenohumeral and anterior band of the inferior glenohumeral ligaments can all be visualized.
- An anterior portal can be made through the rotator interval for the introduction of a probe for further assessment of any soft tissue pathology or if any glenoid bone loss needs to be further assessed.
- The subacromial space should then be examined. Superiorly the acromion is seen, anteriorly the coracoacromial ligament and inferiorly the bursal side of the rotator cuff. The presence of bursal side rotator cuff tears, impingement lesions and acromial and ACJ pathology can all be assessed.

This is just one example of a systematic assessment of arthroscopic shoulder anatomy. Each surgeon can develop their own system, however, it is essential that all surgeons are familiar with arthroscopic anatomy and normal variations.

Closure

Portals can be left unsutured or closed with subcuticular 3/0 Monocryl sutures.

POSTOPERATIVE CARE AND INSTRUCTIONS

If the procedure is purely diagnostic no sling is necessary. The patient is encouraged to mobilize as soon as possible.

RECOMMENDED REFERENCE

Levy O, Sforza G, Dodenhoff R, *et al*. Evaluation of the impingement lesion: pathoanatomy and classification. Arthroscopic evaluation of the impingement lesion: pathoanatomy and classification. *J Bone Joint Surg Br* 2000;**82B**(Suppl 3):233.

ANTERIOR ACROMIOPLASTY – OPEN

PREOPERATIVE PLANNING

Common indications

- Impingement with failure of conservative management
- In association with: rotator cuff repair, shoulder arthroplasty, malunion of greater tuberosity fracture.

Contraindications

Relative: Irreparable cuff tear to avoid superior escape of the humeral head. (A limited decompression can be undertaken).

Consent and risks

- Infection
- Neurovascular injury
- Stiffness
- Fracture of the acromion: can occur if the osteotomy is performed in the wrong plane or if excess bone is resected
- Detachment of the deltoid
- Failure of procedure: wrong indications, incomplete decompression, missed cuff tear

Operative planning

Recent radiographs and, if necessary, ultrasound or MRI for rotator cuff assessment.

Anaesthesia and positioning

Anaesthesia is usually general, regional or combined. Where general anaesthesia is used alone, local anaesthetic is recommended for pain relief. The patient is in the beach chair position. A small sandbag is put under the operated shoulder. An arm board can be attached to the side of the table to rest the arm on. The surgical field is prepared and adequately draped.

SURGICAL TECHNIQUE

Landmarks

* Acromioclavicular joint
* Anterolateral corner of acromion
* Tip of the coracoid.

Incision

This procedure is rarely performed as an isolated open procedure as it is most commonly performed arthroscopically or in association with a larger open procedure. As such, the skin incision will be dictated by the other procedure, however, if it is to be performed as an isolated open procedure, a 2–3 cm anterosuperior incision is made over the anterior acromion.

Dissection

The incision is continued through subcutaneous fat and down to deltoid fascia. The anterior deltoid raphe is split in the line of its fibres. The anterior acromion is located and then an osteoperiosteal flap raised such that a strong deltoid repair can be performed at the end of the procedure.

Procedure

Deep to the anterolateral tip of the acromion is the coracoacromial ligament. A swab can be used to sweep the soft tissue medially further exposing

the ligament and separating its medial border from the clavipectoral fascia. An oscillating saw is used to excise the anteroinferior acromion. The osteotomy is aimed so that it is in continuation with the undersurface of the acromion (Fig. 6.3). The bony fragment, with its attached coracoacromial ligament, is excised. Traction is applied to the patient's arm and the under surface of the acromion is smoothed using bone nibblers. The underlying rotator cuff should then be examined for any associated pathology.

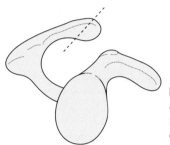

Figure 6.3 *The correct orientation for the acromion osteotomy*

Closure

A good deltoid reconstruction is essential. If the quality of the osteoperiosteal flaps is poor, a transosseous repair using no. 2 Ethibond is performed followed by subcutaneous 2/0 Vicryl and 3/0 Monocryl to skin.

POSTOPERATIVE CARE AND INSTRUCTIONS

Passive/active-assisted exercises are started from day 1 to 90° forward elevation and 30° external rotation for 3 weeks increasing to full range by 6 weeks. Strengthening exercises can be started at 6 weeks and repetitive overhead exercises at 3 months.

RECOMMENDED REFERENCES

Bigliani LU, Morrison D, April EW. The morphology of the acromion and its relationship to rotator cuff tears. *Orthop Trans* 1986;**10**:228.

Neer CS. Anterior acromioplasty for chronic impingement syndrome in the shoulder – a preliminary report. *J Bone Joint Surg Am* 1972;**54**:41–50.

ARTHROSCOPIC SUBACROMIAL DECOMPRESSION

PREOPERATIVE PLANNING

See 'Anterior acromioplasty – open' (p. 62).

SURGICAL TECHNIQUE

See 'Diagnostic shoulder arthroscopy' (p. 60) for positioning and portals.

Procedure

Structure at risk

- Acromial branch of the coracoacromial artery

The arthroscopic pump is set between 30 mmHg and 70 mmHg. The arthroscope is introduced through the posterior portal and a diagnostic arthroscopy performed. It is then introduced into the subacromial bursa. The bursal surface of the cuff is inspected to confirm the presence of an impingement lesion (inflammation, roughening and fibrillation). Next, the undersurface of the acromion is examined for a corresponding 'kissing' lesion. The acromion can be further assessed using an arthroscopic probe for any acromial hooks or spurs. The coracoacromial ligament is also inspected.

The lateral portal is used for instrumentation. A spinal needle is used for the outside-in technique of portal placement. Although this portal is at the level of the axillary nerve, the nerve is not usually threatened as the instruments are aimed proximally towards the acromion. No cannula is required.

Soft tissue resection and haemostasis can be performed with an electrocautery probe/vaporizer. The soft tissue on the undersurface of the acromion is then resected and the

coracoacromial ligament detached. The lateral edge of acromion must be exposed to ensure adequate lateral decompression.

A barrel burr/shaver is used for bone resection. If the acromion has a lateral down-slope then a lateral bevel is performed. The decompression is then performed by excising the anterior acromion, from lateral to medial. The acromial branch of the coracoacromial vessel is at risk at this stage. Anterior resection is usually approximately 4 mm (the width of the burr) or until the anterior deltoid attachment is reached. Medially, the resection is limited by the ACJ. The undersurface of the acromion is then chamfered, to smooth out any ridges (Fig. 6.4).

Further refinement of the acromioplasty can be performed by placing the arthroscope in the lateral portal and the shaver posteriorly. Any residual bone can be resected using the posterior acromion as a 'cutting-block', thus creating a flat undersurface to the acromion.

Closure

See 'Diagnostic shoulder arthroscopy' (p. 60).

POSTOPERATIVE CARE AND INSTRUCTIONS

See 'Anterior acromioplasty – open' (p. 62).

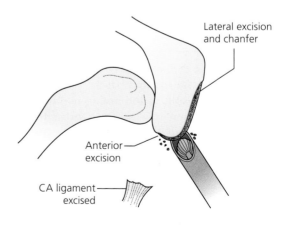

Figure 6.4 *Arthroscopic subacromial decompression; CA, coracoacromial*

RECOMMENDED REFERENCES

Levy O, Sforza G, Dodenhoff R, *et al.* Evaluation of the impingement lesion: pathoanatomy and classification. Arthroscopic evaluation of the impingement lesion: pathoanatomy and classification. *J Bone Joint Surg Br* 2000;**82B**(Suppl 3):233.

Gartsman GM. Arthroscopic acromioplasty for lesions of the rotator cuff. *J Bone Joint Surg Am* 1990;**72**:169–80.

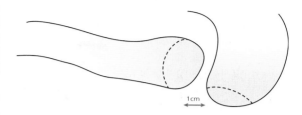

Figure 6.5 *Excision of the acromioclavicular joint*

ACROMIOCLAVICULAR JOINT EXCISION

PREOPERATIVE PLANNING

Indications

- Symptomatic ACJ arthritis not responsive to conservative treatment
- Large inferior osteophytes with secondary impingement
- Symptomatic ACJ intra-articular disc tear.

For contraindications/consent and risks/operative planning/anaesthesia and positioning, see 'Anterior acromioplasty' (p. 62).

SURGICAL TECHNIQUE

Open

Approach

If performed in combination with an open acromioplasty the same approach as previously described is made, although the incision and subsequent dissection, will need to be extended medially. If performed in isolation, a 2–3 cm strap incision is made over the distal clavicle and then a transverse incision is made in the delto-trapezoidal fascia to expose the ACJ.

Procedure

Retractors are placed to expose the distal clavicle and then an oscillating saw is used to resect enough distal clavicle such that there is a 10 mm gap between the medial acromion and the resected distal clavicle (Fig. 6.5). Care must be taken not to resect too much distal clavicle otherwise distal clavicular instability can occur. Any osteophytes on the undersurface of the acromion are trimmed with bone nibblers and any residual meniscus removed.

Closure

The superior acromioclavicular ligament and delto-trapezoidal fascia is then repaired. If performed in association with an acromioplasty, the deltoid is repaired in the manner already discussed.

Arthroscopic

Approach

See 'Arthroscopic subacromial decompression' (p. 64). An anterior portal is required. This is first localized with the insertion of a needle. This portal is 2–3 cm inferior to the level of the ACJ.

Procedure

The ACJ is identified through the arthroscope by palpating the distal clavicle. A shaver or vaporizer can be used through the lateral portal to expose the ACJ. Scar tissue and the remnants of the meniscus are resected and any inferior osteophytes excised. To ensure adequate visualization of the ACJ the fibrofatty tissue in the region of the scapular spine and distal clavicle should be resected. An anterior portal is made using an outside-in technique ensuring accurate placement of the portal such that ACJ excision is possible.

A barrel burr is used to excise the distal clavicle from inferior to superior and from lateral to medial. To ensure that adequate bone is resected, especially posteriorly, the entire circumference of the resected distal clavicle must be visualized. This is often only achieved if both the anterior and posterior acromioclavicular ligaments are excised. However, care must be taken not to excise the superior acromioclavicular ligament or to resect too much bone as this can destabilize the joint. The aim is for approximately 10 mm of bone resection from the medial acromial facet to the distal clavicle. This can be assessed by measuring it against the width of the shaver.

Closure

See 'Arthroscopic subacromial decompression' (p. 64).

POSTOPERATIVE CARE AND INSTRUCTIONS

See 'Arthroscopic subacromial decompression' (p. 64).

RECOMMENDED REFERENCE

Flatow EL, Duralde XA, Nicholson GP, *et al.* Arthroscopic resection of the distal clavicle with a superior approach. *J Shoulder Elbow Surg* 1995;**4**:41–50.

ROTATOR CUFF REPAIR – OPEN/ ARTHROSCOPIC

PREOPERATIVE PLANNING

Common indications

- Shoulder pain, including night pain
- Loss of function or quality of life
- Traumatic rotator cuff tear
- Failure of conservative management of a chronic rotator cuff tear.

Contraindications

Degenerative changes of the glenohumeral joint – 'rotator cuff arthropathy'.

Consent and risks

- Infection
- Neurovascular injury
- Stiffness
- Failure of the repair
- Recurrence
- Continued weakness/cuff-related pain

Operative planning

Recent radiographs, ultrasound or MRI.

Anaesthesia

Anaesthesia is usually combined general and regional.

Landmarks

- Acromioclavicular joint
- Anterolateral and posterolateral corners of acromion
- Tip of coracoid.

SURGICAL TECHNIQUE – OPEN

Positioning

The patient is in the beach chair position. A small sandbag is put under the shoulder. An arm board can be attached to the side of the table to rest the arm on. The surgical field is prepared and adequately draped.

Incision

Structure at risk

The axillary nerve is approximately 5 cm distal to the lateral acromion and therefore the inferior limit of any incision must not extend beyond this point. This position corresponds to the lower limit of the inferior reflection of the subdeltoid bursa.

An anterosuperior approach is used. An 8 cm incision is made just posterior to the anterior aspect of the ACJ and is directed towards the anterolateral corner of the acromion and down the anterior deltoid raphe. A smaller incision can be performed if an arthroscopic decompression has already been performed such that a mini-open procedure can be undertaken.

Dissection

The deltoid is bluntly split at the anterior raphe (junction of the anterior and middle thirds). The deltoid is detached off the anterior acromion with an osteoperiosteal sleeve. The bursa is split longitudinally. The inferior reflection of the bursa denotes the position of the axillary nerve which can be palpated and avoided thereafter (Fig. 6.6). The coracoacromial ligament is detached from the undersurface of the acromion.

Procedure

Anterior acromioplasty (± ACJ excision) can be carried out as required. The size of the tear is measured and traction sutures are placed through the cuff. The cuff is then mobilized sequentially, initially with blunt dissection, however, a sharp release of the superior capsule and the coracohumeral ligament may be necessary. In massive retracted tears anterior and posterior interval slides may also be necessary. These can also be performed arthroscopically such that only a

mini-open approach need be adopted. The configuration and tension of the mobilized cuff tear is then assessed in order to plan the repair.

A shallow bony trough/footprint is prepared using an osteotome (or burr in a mini open) at the level of tendon insertion. This should be made just lateral to the articular surface. The method of the tendon repair is determined by the operating surgeon.

Single and double row anchor repairs can be undertaken depending on the size of the tear or alternatively a transosseous suture repair can be performed. In the latter method the tendon is repaired with a no. 2 Ethibond Mason Allen suture. In each method the aim is to achieve healing of the tendon to the footprint.

Closure

A good deltoid reconstruction is essential. If the quality of the osteoperiosteal flaps is poor a transosseous deltoid repair, using no. 2 Ethibond, is performed. The deltoid raphe should be closed with 2/0 Vicryl and then 2/0 Vicryl for closure of the subcutaneous tissues and 3/0 Monocryl to skin.

SURGICAL TECHNIQUE – ARTHROSCOPIC

Positioning

The beach chair or lateral positions can be adopted.

Portals

Posterior, anterior, lateral and accessory lateral portals are often required. The superior Neviaser portal can be useful for passing sutures through the cuff, particularly in massive tears.

Procedure

Glenohumeral arthroscopy is performed and any concurrent pathology assessed and treated as necessary. The cuff is then assessed with respect to its size, shape and mobility. The arthroscope is then inserted into the subacromial space and a subacromial decompression (± ACJ excision) is performed as necessary. Any releases are then

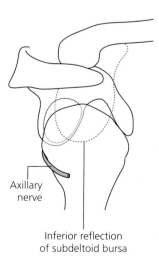

Axillary nerve

Inferior reflection of subdeltoid bursa

Figure 6.6 *The relationship of the subdeltoid bursa to the axillary nerve*

undertaken and the footprint is prepared with the vaporizer and burr.

Various techniques are described for tendon fixation. The type of anchor and whether a single or double row fixation is used remains debatable. However, the principle is to have a large contact area between the tendon and the bone to encourage healing. To achieve this a variety of arthroscopic instruments are required.

The suture anchor is inserted percutaneously or through the superolateral portal, such that the correct bone entry angle is achieved. During anchor placement the choice of viewing portal is often determined by the size of the tear with small or partial tears requiring an intra-articular camera position and larger tears requiring visualization from the subacromial space. The sutures can now be passed using antegrade techniques, using suture passers, or with retrograde techniques where penetrators or suture shuttling instruments are used. When passing sutures a posterior or lateral viewing portal is used depending on the size and location of the tear.

Sutures are placed approximately 1 cm apart. Suture management is critical in rotator cuff repairs as it is easy to confuse or tangle the sutures. To avoid difficulties only two sutures should be used per portal and if a cannula is not used then sutures must be passed through the same portal together to avoid interposing soft tissue when tying knots. Knot tying is done under direct vision in the subacromial space. For large and massive tears, side to side convergence sutures can be used to reduce the size of tear (Fig. 6.7). The final construct can be viewed from both the subacromial space and the glenohumeral joint to ensure footprint reconstruction.

Closure

Sutures are only used with cannula portals, otherwise Steri-Strips suffice.

Postoperative care and instructions

- Small and medium tears:
  - Sling for 6 weeks
  - Passive/active assisted exercises to 30° external rotation (if no subscapularis tear) and elevation to 90° for first 6 weeks

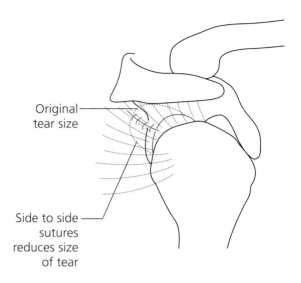

Figure 6.7 *Side to side sutures used to reduce the size of a rotator cuff tear*

  - Passive overhead elevation at 6 weeks with further increase in external rotation as able
  - Active exercises once range is normal and strengthening at 12 weeks.
- Large/massive tears:
  - Immobilize in sling (± abduction pillow) sling for 6 weeks
  - Passive/active assisted exercises elevation to 90° and external rotation to 0° in the presence of a subscapularis repair, otherwise 30° for first 6 weeks
  - Passive overhead elevation at 6 weeks with further increase in external rotation as able
  - Active exercises at 12 weeks and strengthening at 16 weeks.

These regimens can be modified depending on the surgeon's choice.

RECOMMENDED REFERENCE

Sano H, Yamashita T, Wakabayashi I, *et al.* Stress distribution in the supraspinatus tendon after repair – suture anchors versus transosseous fixation. *Am J Sports Med* 2007;**35**:542–46.

ACROMIOCLAVICULAR JOINT RECONSTRUCTION – MODIFIED WEAVER–DUNN

PREOPERATIVE PLANNING

Indications

- Chronic type IV–VI ACJ dislocation
- Chronic type III in the young, athletic, manual worker, dominant side (surgery on Grade III AC joint dislocation is more controversial than conservative treatment and is very much surgeon dependent).

Contraindications

Unreliable patient (important due to postoperative restrictions).

Consent and risks

- Infection
- Neurovascular injury
- Stiffness
- Failure of the procedure or recurrence

Operative planning

Radiographs – anteroposterior, 30° cephalic, axillary ± stress views – are required.

Anaesthesia and positioning

Anaesthesia is usually general, regional or combined. Where general anaesthesia is used alone, local anaesthetic is recommended for postoperative pain relief.

The patient is placed in the beach chair position. A small sandbag is put under the shoulder. An arm board can be attached to the side of the table to rest the arm on. The surgical field is prepared and adequately draped.

Landmarks

- ACJ
- Anterolateral corner of the acromion
- Tip of coracoid

SURGICAL TECHNIQUE

The technique will vary depending on whether an acute or chronic injury is being addressed. Acute injuries do not require a ligament transfer procedure as part of the reconstruction. Chronic injuries are best managed with a biological reconstruction which is supplemented by another fixation device until healing has occurred approximately 3 months post repair.

Approach

A strap incision, 1 cm medial to the ACJ, and extending down to the coracoid.

Procedure

The delto-trapezoidal fascia is incised longitudinally along the distal clavicle with an extension across the superior acromioclavicular capsule/ligament and further laterally over the anterior acromion. The deltoid fibres are elevated off the clavicle and, at the acromion, an osteoperiosteal flap is raised to aid later repair. The coracoacromial ligament is defined by sweeping bluntly laterally with a swab. It is then detached from the acromion with a sliver of bone. It is then mobilized down to the coracoid and a whipstitch applied to the ligament with no. 2 Ethibond. The distal 1 cm of the clavicle is excised obliquely with an oscillating saw. The bone fragment is retained for later autologous bone graft.

The clavicle is reduced to its anatomical position by reducing the arm back up to the clavicle and by further reducing the clavicle downwards and forwards. This position must be maintained prior to the ligament transfer. This can be achieved by a number of techniques, including a Bosworth screw, three strands of PDS cord (Johnson and Johnson) looped around the coracoid and clavicle or, with a TightRope reconstruction device (Arthrex Inc; Naples, FL, USA).

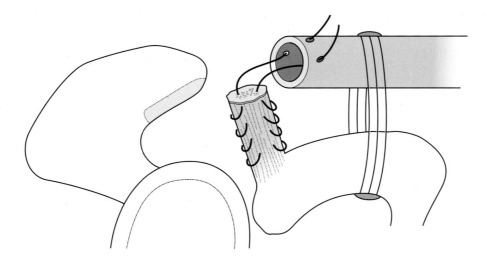

Figure 6.8 *Acromioclavicular joint reconstruction*

Once held in the reduced position two 2 mm drill holes are then made in the superior cortex of clavicle. The bony fragment of the acromioclavicular ligament is passed into the intramedullary canal and the two sutures are passed through the holes, tensioned and tied (Fig. 6.8). An autograft from the resected distal clavicle is then used to graft any redundant space around the transferred ligament.

In acute cases (<3–4 weeks post injury) the coracoclavicular ligaments and superior acromioclavicular capsule/ligament can be repaired and then supplemented with one of the stabilizing techniques described above. A Weaver–Dunn ligament transfer is not required.

Closure

A good delto-trapezoidal reconstruction is essential. If the quality of the anterior acromial osteoperiosteal flap is poor a transosseous repair using No. 2 Ethibond is performed and in cases with significant superior migration of the clavicle any redundant delto-trapezoidal fascia can undergo a 'double-breasted' repair with 1 Vicryl adding further superior support to the reconstruction; 2/0 Vicryl is used for closure of the subcutaneous tissues and 3/0 Monocryl is used for skin.

POSTOPERATIVE CARE AND INSTRUCTIONS

- Six weeks in a sling with passive, and active assisted, forward elevation to 90° and external rotation to 30°
- Progress to active shoulder movement, below shoulder height, from 6 weeks with passive stretching above shoulder height at 10 weeks
- Strengthening at 12 weeks (if a Bosworth screw is used shoulder movement must be restricted to below shoulder height until the screw is removed at 3 months).

RECOMMENDED REFERENCES

Fraser-Moodie JA, Shortt NL, Robinson CM. Injuries to the acromioclavicular joint. *J Bone Joint Surg Br* 2008;**90**:697–707.

Weaver JK, Dunn HK. Treatment of acromioclavicular injuries. *J Bone Joint Surg Am* 1972;**54**:1187–93.

SHOULDER STABILIZATION – OPEN

PREOPERATIVE PLANNING

Primary indication

- Recurrent instability: traumatic structural (type I) and atraumatic structural (type II)
- Relative indication: acute traumatic dislocation.

Contraindications

- Muscle patterning instability (type III)
- If used in isolation in the presence of a large glenoid bone defect
- Unsuitable for anaesthesia.

Consent and risks

- Infection
- Stiffness, particularly loss of external rotation
- Recurrence
- Subscapularis detachment.
- Neurovascular injury

Operative planning

Recent radiographs and CT/MRI arthrogram should be available to the surgeon. Examination under anaesthetic ± diagnostic arthroscopy should be performed prior to the procedure.

SURGICAL TECHNIQUE – ANTEROINFERIOR STABILIZATION

Anaesthesia and positioning

Anaesthesia is usually general, regional or combined. Where general anaesthesia is used alone, local anaesthetic is recommended postoperatively to aid pain relief.

The patient is placed in the beach chair position. A small sandbag is put under the medial scapula of the operated shoulder (this helps to externally rotate the shoulder and 'open' the anterior shoulder joint). An arm board can be attached to the side of the table to rest the arm

on. The surgical field is prepared and adequately draped.

Examination under anaesthesia

The humeral head is translated anteriorly and posteriorly, the direction noted and its excursion is graded:
- 1 – minimal
- 2 – to the edge of the labrum
- 3 – dislocates.

Landmarks

- Tip of the coracoid
- Axillary fold.

Incision

The skin incision runs in the deltopectoral groove, from the coracoid to the axillary fold (with the arm adducted and internally rotated).

Superficial dissection

Structure at risk

- Cephalic vein

The subcutaneous tissue is reflected with sharp and electrocautery dissection, exposing the deltopectoral interval which is marked by a fatty streak and the cephalic vein. The fascia overlying the interval is divided and the cephalic vein lateralized with the deltoid muscle. The deltoid and pectoralis major are then defined with sharp and electrocautery dissection.

Deep dissection

Structure at risk

- Musculocutaneous nerve – in danger from excessive traction

A retractor can be placed over the coracoid process to enhance the exposure and the clavipectoral fascia is then split vertically starting just lateral to the coracoid. This exposes the conjoint tendon. If required, the lateral third of the conjoint tendon can be divided to allow better exposure (by not detaching the coracoid or the tendon fully, the musculocutaneous nerve is protected from excessive traction). A self-retainer is placed between the coracoid/conjoint tendon medially and the deltoid muscle laterally.

The arm is externally rotated to expose the subscapularis muscle. The upper two-thirds of the subscapularis can then be tenotomized approximately 1 cm from its insertion in the lesser tuberosity and dissected free of the underlying capsule. This plane is more easily found inferiorly and becomes easier as the dissection progresses medially. Alternatively, the subscapularis can be split horizontally and retracted, exposing the underlying capsule.

Procedure

The capsulorrhaphy must now be undertaken. This can be performed either laterally or medially. It is the authors' preference to perform this medially as we feel it gives a more accurate anatomical reconstruction and a more reproducible elimination of the axillary pouch.

To achieve a large inferior capsular shift the capsule must be dissected off all of its muscular attachments inferiorly and, indeed, postero-inferiorly in cases of marked laxity. This is best achieved with McIndoe scissors. A bone lever can then be placed inferior to the humeral neck thus protecting the axillary nerve. Depending on the degree of laxity the capsulorrhaphy can involve either a vertical capsular incision or, in cases of greater laxity, a medially based 'T'.

The capsule is split vertically 7–10 mm from the glenoid rim, with a further horizontal incision made midway along the capsule as necessary (Fig. 6.9). Two stay sutures are placed to mark the superior and inferior apices of the flaps. A Fakuda retractor is used to displace the humeral head posteriorly such that the anterior labrum is exposed. The presence of a Bankart lesion, and the degree of capsule–labral disruption, can now be visualized.

The anterior glenoid neck is decorticated using a narrow osteotome or burr and anchors are used to reattach the anterior labrum to the decorticated area of the glenoid neck. The capsular flaps are overlapped so that the inferior flap is taken superiorly and medially such that it is sutured to the medial capsule. A double-breasted suture technique using 1 Vicryl should be used. The superior flap is then sutured inferiorly **taking care not to medialize the flap** otherwise external rotation will be restricted. The rotator interval is then closed (Fig. 6.10).

During the repair, the arm should be held in 30° of external rotation and abduction so that the repair is not over tightened thus causing

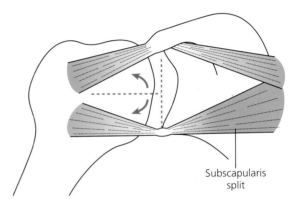

Figure 6.9 *The medial 'T'-shaped capsular incision*

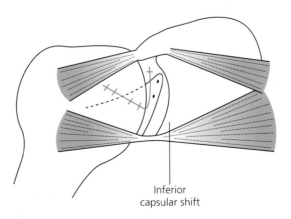

Figure 6.10 *Medially based inferior capsular shift*

postoperative stiffness. Adequate stability and a good passive range of motion should be confirmed before the wounds are closed.

If a large, engaging Hill–Sachs lesion is present a bone block procedure (Bristow–Latarjet or iliac crest bone graft) will be required to increase the depth of the glenoid to prevent recurrent dislocation. A soft tissue procedure alone will not be adequate to restore stability.

Closure

If previously tenotomized, the subscapularis should be repaired with no. 2 Ethibond. Thereafter, a layered closure using 2/0 Vicryl for the subcutaneous tissues and 3/0 Monocryl to skin is used.

SURGICAL TECHNIQUE – POSTERIOR STABILIZATION

Cases of posterior instability will warrant a posterior reconstructive procedure.

Anaesthesia and positioning

Anaesthesia is usually general, regional or combined. The patient is positioned in the prone position.

Incision

A 15 cm posterior vertical incision which extends over the spine of the scapula in the plane of the ACJ gives good access to posterior structures of the shoulder.

Dissection

Structures at risk

The posterior circumflex humeral artery and axillary nerve run together in the quadrilateral space, below teres minor. It is therefore safe provided that the correct plane of dissection is used.

Posteriorly, the deltoid has a tendinous insertion on to the posterior spine of the scapula. This can be incised and reflected inferiorly giving good access to the underlying infraspinatus and teres minor tendons. More laterally an osteoperiosteal flap should be raised off the posterior lateral corner of the acromion with, if necessary, a further extension down the posterior deltoid raphe.

The interval between the infraspinatus and teres minor can be developed by blunt dissection exposing the posterior capsule.

Procedure

The procedure for the repair of a posterior labral injury and /or capsular laxity is similar to that described for an anteriorly based injury. A medial or laterally based capsulorrhaphy can be performed although we favour the former for the reasons described earlier.

Closure

The infraspinatus and teres minor do not need formal closure; however, meticulous repair of the deltoid should be undertaken. Thereafter 2/0 Vicryl to superficial tissues and 3/0 Monocryl to skin is advocated.

POSTOPERATIVE CARE AND INSTRUCTIONS

A polysling with body belt is used for the first 4 weeks. At 4 weeks, the body belt is removed and pendular exercises started. At 6 weeks passive stretching exercises are undertaken aiming for full elevation but only half the external rotation of the contralateral side by 3 months. Strengthening exercises are begun at 6 weeks. Contact sports must be avoided for 6–9 months.

RECOMMENDED REFERENCES

Itoi E, Hattakeyama Y, Kido T, et al. A new method of immobilisation after traumatic anterior dislocation of the shoulder: a preliminary study. *J Shoulder Elbow Surg* 2003;**12**:413–15.

Gill TJ, Micheli LJ, Gebhard F, et al. Bankart repair for anterior instability of the shoulder. Long term outcome. *J Bone Joint Surg Am* 1997;**79**:850.

Lewis A, Kitamura T, Bayley JIL. The classification of shoulder instability; new light through old windows. *Curr Orthop* 2004;**18**:97–108.

Rowe CR, Zarins B, Ciullo JV. Recurrent anterior dislocation of the shoulder after surgical repair. Apparent causes of failure and treatment. *J Bone Joint Surg Am* 1984;**66**:159–68.

te Slaa RL, Wijffels MP, Brand R, *et al*. The prognosis following acute primary glenohumeral dislocation. *J Bone Joint Surg Br* 2004;**86**:58–64.

ANTERIOR REPAIR OF INSTABILITY – ARTHROSCOPIC

PREOPERATIVE PLANNING

For primary indication/contraindications/consent and risks/operative planning, see 'Shoulder stabilization – open' (p. 73).

Anaesthesia and positioning

Anaesthesia is usually general, regional or combined. Where general anaesthesia is used alone, local anaesthetic is recommended post-operatively for pain relief. The patient is in the beach chair or lateral position (see 'Diagnostic shoulder arthroscopy' (p. 60)).

Landmarks

See 'Diagnostic shoulder arthroscopy' (p. 60).

SURGICAL TECHNIQUE

Examination under anaesthesia

As for open stabilization.

Portals

A standard posterior viewing portal is used to assess the labral and capsular pathology.

Using an outside-in technique, an antero-superolateral portal is placed at the junction of the anterior border of the supraspinatus tendon and the upper rotator interval. It should allow a 45° angle of approach to the superior labrum. This will provide both an anterior viewing portal and an accessory portal for SLAP repairs or for suture management. A further anterior portal is placed just above the subscapularis tendon. This is placed such that angle of approach allows accurate suture anchor placement. This can be best assessed using the anterosuperior viewing portal. A clear cannula is recommended for better visualization.

Procedure

Glenohumeral arthroscopy is carried out. The degree of tissue separation and amount of anterior or inferior capsular laxity are assessed. The drive-through sign is noted. This reflects the ease with which the scope is passed between the humeral head and the glenoid and is a sign of significant laxity. The Bankart lesion is released around to the 6 o'clock position on the glenoid, with sharp elevators. A sufficient release is confirmed by grabbing the inferior tissue with a manipulator and elevating it superiorly against the glenoid rim.

The anterior glenoid (2–6 o'clock) is decorticated with a rasp and shaver (ensure that suction is clamped during this stage). An anchor is placed at the 5 o'clock position on the glenoid rim. A suture is passed through the tissue inferiorly using a penetrator or suture shuttle technique. The amount of tissue included in the suture is critical as it will dictate the degree of stability following the repair. To help reduce the labral tissue back to the glenoid rim the knot can be tied with the arm in flexion and internal rotation. Capsular plication (weaving of sutures through the capsule) can also be performed in cases of marked capsular laxity. Further anchors are placed at 4 o'clock and 3 o'clock positions to approximate the labrum and perform a distal to proximal shift of the capsule (Fig. 6.11).

Closure

3/0 Monocryl to cannula portals.

POSTOPERATIVE CARE AND INSTRUCTIONS

See 'Shoulder stabilization – open' (p. 73).

RECOMMENDED REFERENCE

Hobby J, Griffin D, Dunbar M, *et al*. Is arthroscopic surgery for stabilisation for chronic

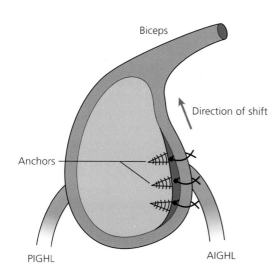

Figure 6.11 *Capsulolabral reconstruction with anterior inferior glenohumeral ligament reconstruction (AIGHL). PIGHL, posterior IGHL.*

shoulder instability as effective as open surgery? A systematic review and meta-analysis of 62 studies including 3044 arthroscopic operations. *J Bone Joint Surg Br* 2007;**89**:1188–96.

TOTAL SHOULDER REPLACEMENT

PREOPERATIVE PLANNING

Common indications

- Osteoarthritis
- Inflammatory arthritis
- Avascular necrosis
- Trauma: four-part proximal humeral fractures
- Postinfective arthritis
- Instability arthropathy
- Cuff tear arthropathy
- Arthritis secondary to glenoid dysplasia or epiphyseal dysplasia.

Contraindications

Active infection.

Consent and risks

- Infection
- Neurovascular injury
- Stiffness
- Aseptic loosening
- Fracture
- Revision

Operative planning

Recent radiographs must be available with CT/MRI/bone scan as required.

Anaesthesia and positioning

Anaesthesia can be general, regional or combined. Where general anaesthesia is used alone, additional local anaesthetic infiltration or patient-controlled anaesthesia is recommended for pain relief. Antibiotics are given at induction.

The patient is placed in the reclining beach chair position and pulled to the side to allow extension and rotation of the arm. A small sandbag is put under the shoulder. The surgical field is prepared and draped.

Landmarks

- Acromioclavicular joint
- Anterolateral/posterolateral corners of acromion
- Coracoid.

SURGICAL TECHNIQUE

Deltopectoral

Incision

From coracoid toward the axillary fold, extending laterally to the anterior arm.

Superficial dissection

Structure at risk

- Cephalic vein

The subcutaneous tissue is reflected with sharp and electrocautery dissection exposing the deltopectoral interval, which is marked by a fatty streak and the cephalic vein. The fascia overlying the interval is divided and the cephalic vein lateralized with the deltoid muscle. In a tight shoulder the pectoralis major tendon can be released at its superior border taking care not to injure the underlying biceps tendon.

Deep dissection

Structures at risk

The axillary and musculocutaneous nerves are in danger from excessive traction.

To enhance the exposure a retractor can be placed over the coracoid process and then the clavi-pectoral fascia is split vertically starting just lateral to the coracoid, extending the incision just lateral to the conjoint tendon and its muscle belly.

To improve external rotation the coraco-humeral ligament should also be released at its coracoid origin. The deltoid is then mobilized from the tissues of the subacromial space and retracted posterolaterally. Provided that the retractors are placed above the inferior subdeltoid bursal reflection the axillary nerve should be safe. If better access is required, as may be the case with a medialized glenoid, the lateral third of the conjoint tendon can be divided to allow better exposure or alternatively a coracoid tip osteotomy can be performed. However, care should be taken not to retract the conjoint tendon excessively as this could put the musculocutaneous nerve at risk. The arm is externally rotated to expose the subscapularis muscle.

The anterior circumflex humeral vessels, which are found at the inferior border of the subscapularis tendon, are then ligated. The axillary nerve can then be exposed so that its position is known and avoided during the remainder of the procedure.

The degree of external rotation that can be achieved should now be assessed. If this is deficient then a subscapularis lengthening procedure may be required. This may involve a layered subscapularis tenotomy or 'Z plasty' and this will need to be planned at this stage. If external rotation is adequate the subscapularis tendon is then tenotomized 1 cm medial to its humeral insertion and raised on stay sutures. This can be taken as one layer with the underlying capsule. In order to lengthen the subscapularis the rotator interval will need to be incised and then the capsule will need to be released from the glenoid neck.

As the capsule is incised an inferior capsular release can be performed, and provided that the axillary nerve has already been identified the nerve should not be at risk. A blunt retractor can be placed inferiorly to protect the nerve and then the humeral head is dislocated anteriorly by applying gentle external rotation to the arm. The LHB tendon should be inspected and tenotomized or tenodesed as necessary.

The head is then prepared by removing any osteophytes so that the true anatomical neck of the humerus is identified. The head can now be prepared for the shoulder replacement; the preparation will vary depending on the implant and whether a resurfacing type prosthesis is to be used. For the purpose of this description, a standard stemmed implant will be used. An oscillating saw is used to resect the humeral head at its anatomical neck. If this has been adequately demarcated during your preparation it can be done freehand otherwise jigs should be used such that the height and version of the resection is appropriate. The resected humeral head is then used as a guide for the size of the subsequent humeral head replacement. With the head resected the remainder of the circumferential glenoid release can be performed and the glenoid inspected.

Once the capsule is released there should be adequate space to approach the glenoid perpendicular to its face such that glenoid preparation can be achieved with the appropriate implant jigs. The process of this preparation will vary according to the implant, however, to assess the true version of the glenoid it is useful to place a narrow retractor down the anterior glenoid neck so that the axis of the glenoid is known prior to definitive glenoid preparation.

The humerus is now prepared using sequentially sized rasps and when the appropriate size is established a trial prosthesis can be constructed and inserted into the humerus. After reducing the implant the surgeon should check the offset, version and soft tissue tension of the trial prosthesis and if satisfactory the definitive prosthesis can be implanted.

Anterosuperior

Incision

An 8 cm incision is started just posterior to the front of the ACJ, directed towards the anterolateral corner of the acromion and down the anterolateral deltoid.

Superficial dissection

Structure at risk

- Axillary nerve – 5 cm below the lateral acromion (below the inferior reflection of the subdeltoid bursa).

The deltoid is bluntly split at the anterior raphe (the junction of anterior middle third of the deltoid). The deltoid is detached off the anterior acromion with an osteoperiosteal sleeve. This is extended medially to the ACJ. The subdeltoid bursa is split longitudinally palpating the inferior bursal reflection which denotes the position of the axillary nerve.

Deep dissection

The coracoacromial ligament is detached from the undersurface of the acromion. Anterior acromioplasty and ACJ excision can be carried out if required.

Procedure

Structure at risk

- Axillary nerve

Blunt soft tissue release is carried out around the cuff. The coracohumeral ligament is released at its coracoid origin. This improves the external rotation. With the arm in external rotation, a bone retractor is inserted on the medial side of the humeral neck, marking the inferior border of the subscapularis muscle. This is detached laterally from its insertion to the lesser tuberosity together with the capsule. Stay sutures are inserted.

If biceps tenodesis is required, a stay suture is placed and the tendon cut. The humeral head is dislocated anteriorly with external rotation and extension. A Bankart skid is placed between the glenoid and the head. Osteophytes are excised. A bone spike is inserted on the medial side of the humeral neck, under the subscapularis to protect the axillary nerve. Humeral and glenoid preparation is then performed as previously described.

Closure

The subscapularis tendon is repaired using no. 2 Ethibond with the arm held in a position of 30° external rotation. This prevents over-tightening of the tendon repair. A deltoid repair is then performed to the anterior acromion if the anterosuperior approach was used. A 2/0 Vicryl to the subcutaneous tissues and 3/0 Monocryl to skin completes the closure.

POSTOPERATIVE CARE AND INSTRUCTIONS

A polysling is used for 6 weeks. Passive and active assisted exercises to 90° of forward elevation and external rotation to 0° for 6 weeks. Full passive movement to re-establish full range thereafter followed by active ranging and strengthening exercises as able.

RECOMMENDED REFERENCES

Boileau P, Walch G. The three-dimensional geometry of the proximal humerus. Implications for surgical technique and prosthetic design. *J Bone Joint Surg Br* 1997;**79**:857–65.

Gartsman GM, Roddey TS, Hammerman SM. Shoulder arthroplasty with or without resurfacing of the glenoid in patients who have osteoarthritis. *J Bone Joint Surg Am* 2000;**82**:26–34.

Neer CS. Replacement arthroplasty for glenohumeral osteoarthritis. *J Bone Joint Surg Am* 1974;**4**:351–9.

Torchia ME, Cofield RH, Settergren CR. Total shoulder arthroplasty with the Neer prosthesis: long-term results. *J Shoulder Elbow Surg* 1997;**6**:495–505.

Viva questions

1. Describe the deltopectoral approach. What structures are at risk?

2. Describe the posterior approach to the shoulder.

3. What are the advantages and disadvantages of the anterosuperior approach?

4. Describe the anatomy of the axillary nerve.

5. Describe the portals in shoulder arthroscopy.

6. What is the pathophysiology of impingement?

7. Describe how you would do an arthroscopic subacromial decompression.

8. What are the indications for ACJ excision?

9. How do you classify cuff tears?

10. What are the indications for rotator cuff repair?

11. What are the complications from rotator cuff repair?

12. Describe your management of ACJ dislocation, including classification.

13. What are the indications for operative stabilization of the shoulder?

14. How would you classify shoulder instability?

15. Would you do open or arthroscopic stabilization?

16. What approach would you use for total shoulder replacement?

17. What are the indications for shoulder replacement?

18. Would you replace the glenoid and why?

19. What are the complications of total shoulder replacement?

20. In what position would you arthrodese a shoulder?

7

Surgery of the elbow

Deborah Higgs and Simon Lambert

	Range of motion	Functional range of motion
Flexion	150°	130°
Extension	0°	30°
Pronation	80°	50°
Supination	80°	50°

Position of arthrodesis

- There is no fixed position of arthrodesis
- Many authors recommend 90°
- There is evidence that 110° is best for activities of daily living but 60° may suit work activities

---

The surgical approaches to the elbow may form a sequence of dissections using segments of, or the whole of, a single utility dorsal approach. If this strategy is followed for the lesser procedures then, should further surgery be required, the risk of vascular compromise of the skin due to multiple incisions is reduced.

ELBOW ARTHROLYSIS

PREOPERATIVE PLANNING

Indications

- Post-traumatic capsular contracture of the ulnohumeral (medial column), radiocapitellar (lateral column), and proximal radioulnar joints (anterior and posterior compartments)
- Degenerative contracture of anterior and posterior compartments
- Intracompartmental adhesiolysis, usually of the radiocapitellar compartment
- In association with intra-articular corrective osteotomy of the distal humerus, proximal ulna, or radial head
- In association with joint replacement arthroplasty of the elbow, including lateral compartment resurfacing and radial head replacement.

Contraindications

- Vascular compromise of the limb
- Infection (generalized or of the limb)
- Compromised skin in the region of the surgical incision
- Inability of the patient to understand the postoperative rehabilitation programme
- Contraindication to regional nerve blockade; previous nerve trauma or palsy (particularly if incomplete nerve lesion) at the elbow or more proximally.

Consent and risks

- Ulnar nerve injury: 10 per cent transient ulnar neuritis; 1 per cent tardy ulnar nerve palsy; <1 per cent acute permanent lesion
- Infection: < 1 per cent

- Heterotopic ossification: 10 per cent
- Recurrence: more common in post-traumatic stiffness syndrome, less common in degenerative or inflammatory contractures
- Failure to achieve desired result (due to surface/topographical articular lesions)
- Need for further surgery, including joint replacement arthroplasty

Operative planning

Anteroposterior and lateral (in flexion and extension) radiographs, less than 6 months old, should be available.

For articular surface lesions a computed tomography (CT) arthrogram is desirable. It should be possible to readily convert from an arthroscopic procedure to an open procedure (see positioning and incision sections).

Anaesthesia and positioning

Anaesthesia is usually general, augmented by infraclavicular regional nerve blockade if not contraindicated (see above). An initial dose of antibiotic is given intravenously. The antibiotic of choice depends on local policy, but a common choice is cefuroxime (1.5 g in the adult). Note: if intraoperative biopsies are to be obtained to diagnose sepsis then the antibiotic is withheld until the biopsy obtained.

The patient is placed in the lateral decubitus position with the operated arm uppermost. Padded lumbar and pelvic supports are used.

A Carter–Brain gutter or well-padded drape support is used to cradle the arm, allowing the forearm to move freely in the vertical position, permitting access to the dorsal aspect and both sides of the elbow, and to the anterior compartment by external rotation of the shoulder (Fig. 7.1). Of note in this position: **the ulnar nerve is always on the side of the elbow facing the feet of the patient** (assuming there has been no previous operation on the ulnar nerve).

A padded narrow tourniquet (inflation to 200 mmHg is usually sufficient) or a S-MART bandage/tourniquet is used. At least 15 cm of the dorsal aspect of the arm is required for ease of

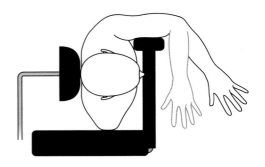

Figure 7.1 *Patient position*

access. The elbow should be sufficiently mobile for appropriate movement intraoperatively. The hand, forearm, and arm to the axilla are prepared with a germicidal solution. Waterproof drapes are used with adhesive edges to provide a seal to the skin. An antibacterial adhesive skin drape is applied.

SURGICAL TECHNIQUE

Arthrolysis can be performed open or arthroscopically.

OPEN ARTHROLYSIS

The choice of approach is governed by which compartment is to be accessed:
- For the lateral side of the anterior and posterior compartments: the lateral column (Morrey) approach. This can be extended proximally into a lateral approach to the humerus, and distally into a Kocher-type approach to the radial head and neck. The anterolateral compartment is readily accessible (see 'Radial head replacement', p. 90)
- For the medial side of the anterior compartment: the direct medial approach anterior to the ulnar nerve (see 'Tennis/golfer's elbow release', p. 93)
- For the anterior compartment alone, e.g. for lengthening of the biceps tendon: the anterior approach. This is a lazy-S incision respecting the flexure crease of the elbow, passing from medial to the tendon of the biceps proximally over the brachial neurovascular bundle, to the

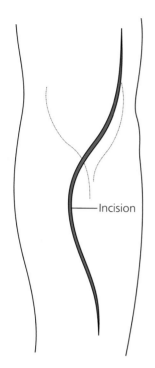

Figure 7.2 *Anterior approach*

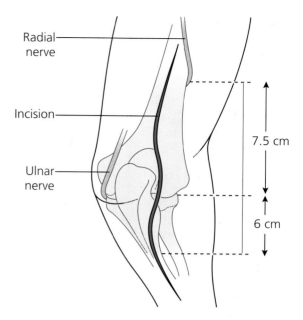

Figure 7.3 *Trans-tricipital approach – skin incision*

medial side of the 'mobile wad' (Henry) distally (Fig. 7.2)

- For the dorsal (olecranon fossa) compartment and ulnar nerve: the dorsal trans-tricipital approach.

TRANS-TRICIPITAL APPROACH

Landmarks

- Midline of the humerus
- Lateral epicondyle
- Radial head
- Tip of the olecranon
- Crest of the proximal ulna.

Incision

The incision is made in a curvilinear fashion towards the tip of the olecranon starting about 7.5 cm proximal to the olecranon, skirting on its lateral side, leaving between 0.5 cm and 1 cm between the incision and the lateral border of the olecranon (to avoid placing the incision on the weightbearing skin of the elbow). The incision is

continued distally parallel to the crest of the ulna (*not* crossing it or on it) for approximately 6 cm (Fig. 7.3).

Superficial dissection

Structure at risk

- Ulnar nerve

The triceps tendon is more correctly an aponeurosis. There is a superficial sheet having a median vertical aponeurotic extension, between the lateral and medial heads of the triceps, which leads to the deep head. This sheet is the guide to the dissection of the triceps.

The lateral and medial musculotendinous boundaries of the triceps are revealed by epifascial dissection in the proximal part of the wound. Minimal epifascial dissection is used distal to the olecranon over the subcutaneous border of the ulna, sufficient only to see the deep antebrachial fascia over anconeus. Medial dissection is continued, sufficient to reveal the ulnar nerve immediately subjacent to the medial border of the triceps about 6–7 cm proximal to the medial epicondyle.

Deep dissection

Structures at risk

- Ulnar nerve

This approach respects the nerve supply to the anconeus (an important contributor to elbow stability): this is a distal branch of the radial nerve which crosses the interval between the distal border of the lateral head of triceps and the proximal border of the anconeus. **Dissection within the lateral head of triceps is to be avoided**. The triceps is split between the nerve and blood supply to the medial head (a segmental branch can occur very distally) and the nerve to the lateral head, both derived from the radial nerve. The deep head nerve supply is more proximal and is out of the surgical field. The ulnar nerve is protected by keeping dissection lateral and then deep to the medial head of the triceps, using the muscular bulk as a protection for the nerve (Fig. 7.4).

It is important to know where the ulnar nerve is if dissection of the medial capsule is likely, but the nerve does not need to be mobilized for simple olecranon fossa debridement, or when the radiocapitellar joint is the only compartment entered.

The ulnar nerve is identified throughout its course, behind the medial condyle, noting the axial vessel and the vena comitans on the deep (articular) surface of the nerve in the cubital sulcus. The fibrous arch between the two bony origins of the flexor carpi ulnaris (FCU) is incised, the incision being carried into the muscle for about 2 cm (Fig. 7.4), marking and protecting the nerve branch to the FCU, which arises proximal to the elbow, and allowing ready displacement of the nerve from the cubital sulcus without tension.

Proximal dissection

The triceps aponeurosis is incised in the midline and undermined to define the vertical sheet between the two superficial heads of the triceps.

The dissection is then taken down the lateral side of this sheet, i.e. in the intervascular/interneural plane to the deep head of the triceps. The superficial heads are parted for about 6 cm, uncovering the filmy layer between them and the deep head. The deep head is then incised (the only muscular incision required in this technique) noting the deep transverse epicondylar vessels under the muscle at the proximal margin of the fat pad in the olecranon fossa. The vessels are cauterized. The fat pad is excised and the olecranon fossa exposed. A posterior capsulectomy is performed and any olecranon osteophytes removed. An Outerbridge–Kashiwagi procedure can now be planned (see below).

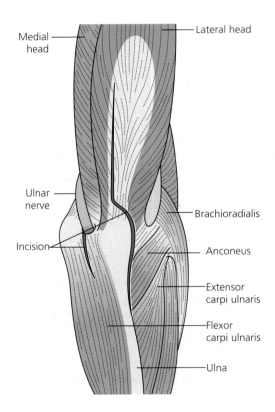

Figure 7.4 *Trans-tricipital approach – deep dissection*

Medial head
Lateral head
Ulnar nerve
Brachioradialis
Incision
Anconeus
Extensor carpi ulnaris
Flexor carpi ulnaris
Ulna

Distal dissection

The antebrachial fascia is incised parallel to and about 1 cm lateral to the crest of the ulna over the anconeus. The dissection is taken under the fascia but outside the anconeus to the crest and then, on bone, down to the supinator crest, the annular ligament and capsule of the proximal radioulnar joint, lifting the anconeus away from the capsule and radial head, but preserving the posterior band of the lateral collateral ligament (to maintain stability in varus strain) (see Fig. 7.4).

This completes the exposure for the olecranon fossa and the posterolateral (radiocapitellar) compartment, permits excision of the radial head if needed, and facilitates adhesiolysis of the ulnohumeral surfaces.

Dissection for the lateral column and anterior compartment: the lateral column and Kocher-type approaches

The attachment of the lateral head of the triceps to the dorsal aspect of the humerus is maintained. Epifascial dissection around the lateral epicondylar ridge and lateral condyle, cauterizing several septal vessels, permits palpation of the entire ridge to the radiocapitellar joint. The common extensor origin is dissected by incision into the apex of the 'axilla' of the musculotendinous fibres, so raising the fibres in an epiperiosteal fashion. The capsule is exposed. The common extensor muscles are split in the interval between the anconeus and extensor carpi ulnaris (ECU), or between the ECU and the extensor digitorum communis (EDC). The former split is safer: the posterior interosseous nerve terminates within the EDC. The dissection is taken down to the radiocapitellar joint capsule by splitting the deeper fibres of the EDC and elevating them from the capsule (Fig. 7.5). The capsule is then incised parallel to the condylar ridge and carried to the annular ligament. This can be incised if the radial head is to be removed (an alternative approach for this resection). An anterior capsulectomy can then be performed while preserving the anterior band of the lateral collateral ligament.

There are now two 'windows': one into the posterior compartment, and one into the anterolateral compartment, through a single skin incision.

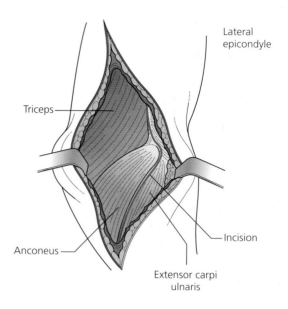

Figure 7.5 *Dissection for lateral column and anterior compartment between the anconeus and the extensor carpi ulnaris*

Supplementary dissection for the anterior compartment using a transhumeral approach (the Outerbridge–Kashiwagi procedure)

An aperture is made through the distal humerus using a high-speed burr, directing the bur radially and proximally: the medial humeral column is thinner and flatter than the lateral column, so the transhumeral opening should be directed radially immediately medial to the lateral column to avoid iatrogenic medial column fracture. The aperture should exit anteriorly immediately behind the tip of the coronoid process (Fig. 7.6).

The diameter of the aperture should be no more than half the transverse diameter of the humerus at this level. The anterior capsule of the radiocapitellar joint, the coronoid tip, and most of the anteromedial capsule can be removed through the aperture, using elbow flexion to bring the capsule into the aperture. It is inadequate for release of the medial capsule and the anterior band of the ulnar collateral ligament should not be incised, to avoid iatrogenic valgus instability.

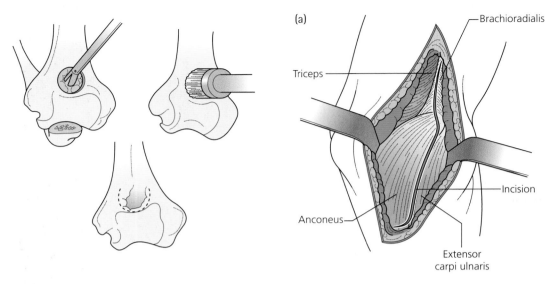

Figure 7.6 *Outerbridge–Kashiwagi procedure*

Figure 7.7a *Incision maintaining lateral head of triceps and anconeus in continuity.*

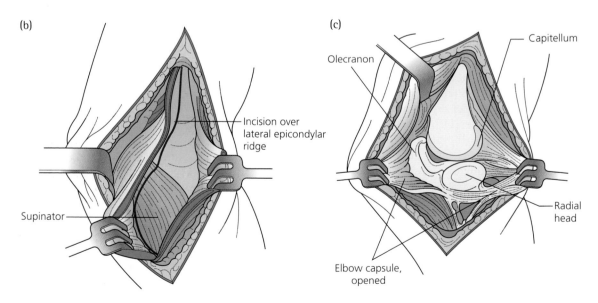

Figure 7.7b *Deep disection showing incision over lateral epicondylar ridge.*

Figure 7.7c *Exposure of radial head.*

Supplementary dissection for massive arthrolysis and capsular release (as for total elbow replacement)

If it is anticipated that this degree of exposure will be needed it is not necessary to perform a separate lateral column exposure: the extensile lateral exposure will permit anterior capsulectomy.

The distal (antebrachial) and proximal (brachial) incisions are linked by incising the lateral capsule, reflecting the posterior band of the lateral collateral ligament, so exposing the radiocapitellar joint. The lateral head of the triceps and the anconeus are thus in continuity, with the remaining capsule deeply attached to the muscle envelope (Fig. 7.7). The radial head can be resected.

Mobilization of the medial head of triceps and medial capsule; dislocation of the elbow joint

A narrow osteotome is used to create a series of osteo-periosteo-fascial shingles (small, superficial shards of bone which remain attached to the tricipital aponeurosis) from the olecranon elevating the medial triceps aponeurotic attachment from the ulna, working from lateral to medial, and distally until the cortical crest of the ulna. The periosteo-antebrachial fascia is then sharply dissected from the crest in continuity with the olecranon shingles. The medial head of the triceps is now in continuity with the medial antebrachial fascia, with a medallion of olecranon bony shingles centrally. As the sleeve is inverted the ulnar nerve is taken out of the cubital sulcus and is protected within a muscular envelope

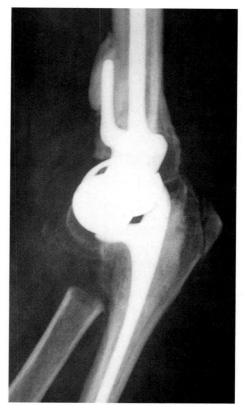

Figure 7.9 *X-ray of total elbow replacement showing the repositioned fragment of olecranon elevated with triceps*

(Fig. 7.8). There are now two longitudinal sleeves of musculotendinous-fascial tissue, exposing the olecranon.

Further medial capsulotomy permits resection of the medial ulnar osteophyte if present and complete dislocation of the elbow for anterior arthrolysis and total elbow replacement (Fig. 7.9).

Technical aspects

Where total capsulectomy has been required in cases such as post-traumatic contracture, heterotopic ossification and myositis ossificans, the collateral ligaments are often released. The elbow is therefore unstable. Fixed splintage is counterproductive. Dynamic splintage is required: a hinged external fixator is indicated if the ligaments cannot be reattached and should be

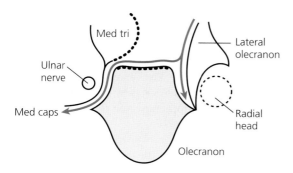

Figure 7.8 *Cross-section showing mobilization of medial head of triceps*

retained for about 8 weeks, before application of a removable hinged brace for a further 4 weeks. If the ligaments can be restored to their optimal tension an external hinged removable brace can be used. Re-fixation of the ligaments to their footprint origins is facilitated by one of the several varieties of anchors that are available. The elbow must be stable enough to permit full-range assisted sagittal motion with gravity eliminated immediately after the operation.

Closure

The olecranon osteo-periosteo-fascial medallion is repaired by transosseous non-absorbable sutures (no. 2 gauge) to the olecranon. A suction drain is placed deep to triceps. The triceps aponeurosis and antebrachial fascia are closed with the elbow flexed at 90° flexion using absorbable braided no. 1 interrupted sutures (continuous suturing reduces the 'give' of the tendon during assisted motion).

- The skin is closed with a dermal supporting absorbable 3/0 suture and an absorbable 4/0 continuous subcuticular suture plus Steri-Strips.
- An occlusive dressing is applied with the elbow in 90° of flexion.
- A bulky wool and crepe bandage dressing is applied in two layers.

ARTHROSCOPIC ARTHROLYSIS

Landmarks

- Lateral epicondyle
- Radial head
- Tip of the olecranon.

Approach

The usual portals (as described in the arthroscopy section, p. 95) are used. In principle the arthroscopic portals respect the same incisions, i.e. the portals are placed in the line of the standard skin incisions to permit extension into an open approach as required.

Using the anteromedial and anterolateral portals, fibrous tissue can be resected from the anterior part of the joint, using a combination of a

full-radius resector and electrocautery. Any loose bodies are removed. The coronoid fossa is re-created, using the resector and a burr for any bony hypertrophy. The coronoid tip is removed if there is evidence of coronoid impingement. The resector is used to strip the capsule proximally, off the distal humerus, for approximately 2.5 cm proximal to the olecranon fossa until the fibres of brachialis come into view proximally. To complete the release a 1 cm capsulotomy of the anterior capsule medial to lateral is required.

Using the direct posterior and posterolateral portals the posterior compartment is debrided similarly. The scope enters through the posterolateral portal and the resector or burr through the direct posterior portal to complete the procedure. Careful release of the contracture, with a full-radius resector, releases the posteromedial and posterolateral gutters. **Beware of the ulnar nerve in close proximity medially.** Manipulation of the elbow is used to achieve maximum extension.

Closure

- A drain is placed in the direct posterior portal and the portals closed with absorbable sutures.
- Occlusive dressings are applied.
- The elbow is splinted in maximum extension.

POSTOPERATIVE CARE AND INSTRUCTIONS

The arm is rested on pillows at chest height for 48 hours. The bandage is reduced at 24 hours and the drain is removed. A Tubigrip bandage is applied. If there is uncertainty about elbow stability a removable extension splint may be applied, to be worn between exercise periods.

Active assisted sagittal full-range motion exercises are performed for 20 minutes four or five times a day. Fist gripping and forearm prosupination are undertaken as comfort permits. Supervised physiotherapy for the neck, shoulder and hand is undertaken.

Active unassisted movement is permitted by 6 weeks and axial weightbearing at about 12 weeks. Passive motion of the elbow may be indicated for recalcitrant/recurrent arthrofibrosis. However, continuous passive motion equipment is difficult to apply accurately, particularly in the unstable joint. A continuous patient-controlled analgesic infusion, or continuous infraclavicular regional anaesthetic infusion are commonly required.

RECOMMENDED REFERENCES

Hertel R, Pisan M, Lambert S, *et al.* Operative management of the stiff elbow: sequential arthrolysis based on a transhumeral approach. *J Shoulder Elbow Surg* 1997;**6**:82–8.

Mansat P, Morrey BF. The column procedure: a limited lateral approach for extrinsic contracture of the elbow. *J Bone Joint Surg Am* 1998;**80**:1603–15.

TOTAL ELBOW REPLACEMENT

PREOPERATIVE PLANNING

Indications

Total elbow replacement is indicated in painful conditions of the elbow which have failed conservative management.

The most frequent underlying conditions are:
- Osteoarthritis
- Inflammatory arthritis and other arthropathies
- Avascular necrosis
- Trauma.

Contraindications

Infection (generalized or of the limb)

Consent and risks

- Nerve paraesthesiae: 11 per cent
- Infection: 7 per cent
- Instability with unlinked implants: 5–20 per cent
- Loosening (semi-constrained): 5 per cent
- Instability (unconstrained): 9 per cent
- Fracture: humerus: 5 per cent; ulna: 5 per cent

Operative planning

Recent radiographs must be available. Availability of the implants must be checked by the surgeon.

Types of replacement

Total elbow arthroplasty

There are two types:
- Unconstrained surface replacements – two-part devices consisting of metal articulating with high-density polyethylene. They do not have a snap-fit, link, or pin connection. Examples are Capitellocondylar and Kudo
- Semi-constrained – two-part or three-part prosthesis that have a metal-to-high-density polyethylene articulation, which may be connected with a locking pin or with a snap-fit device. They have built-in varus and valgus laxity to dissipate forces. Examples are Coonrad Morrey and Discovery.

Anaesthesia and positioning

As for elbow arthrolysis.

SURGICAL TECHNIQUE

Landmarks /incision/dissection

The trans-tricipital approach is used (see 'Elbow arthrolysis', p. 81).

Procedure

Preparation of distal humerus and proximal ulnar

The forearm is rotated laterally to allow exposure of the distal humerus. The radial head and tip of

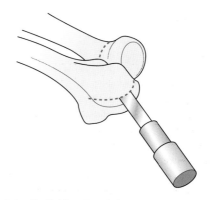

Figure 7.10 *Radial head and tip olecranon excised*

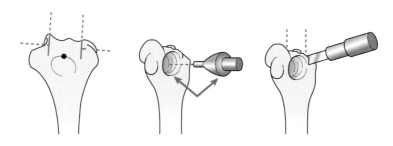

Figure 7.11 *Use of guide, fossa reamer and oscillating saw to prepare the humerus*

olecranon, along a line tangent to the posterior-most portion of the olecranon articulation, are excised with an oscillating saw (Fig. 7.10).

To mark the humeral saw cuts, the olecranon fossa guide is available on the instrument set. To orientate the guide, the shaft of the fossa guide is

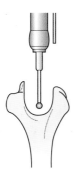

Figure 7.12 *A high-speed burr is used to identify the humeral canal*

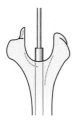

Figure 7.13 *Rasping the humeral canal*

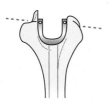

Figure 7.14 *Trial of the humeral component*

aligned with the humeral canal. The medial border should lie along the medial trochlea. The guide should also align with the anatomic internal rotation of the trochlea, which approximates the flat surface posterior and just proximal to the olecranon fossa. Using a fossa reamer, a hole is created and an oscillating saw is used to remove the remains of the trochlea, along the lines previously marked, allowing access to the medullary canal of the humerus (Fig. 7.11).

The canal is identified with a high-speed rotating bur at the proximal aspect of the resection of the olecranon fossa in a proximal direction (Fig. 7.12). Open the medullary canal to a size sufficient to allow a humeral rasp (about 4 mm).

The humeral rasps are now used to prepare the humeral canal (Fig. 7.13). Serial rasps increasing in size are used until cortical resistance is met. If a rasp is unable to be advanced fully, use an implant corresponding to the largest size of rasp which was fully introduced.

The medial and lateral portions of the supracondylar columns **must be preserved** during the preparation of the distal humerus. They act as points of reference to ensure satisfactory orientation and alignment. The trial prosthesis is inserted until the margins of the prosthesis are exactly level with the epicondylar articular surface margin on the capitellar and trochlear sides (Fig. 7.14). Further small pieces of bone are removed with rongeurs or bone nibblers from the distal humerus to aid proper seating of the component.

A high-speed burr is used at an angle of roughly 55° from the vertical in a posterior and distal direction to remove subchondral bone to identify the ulnar medullary canal. Serial rasps are

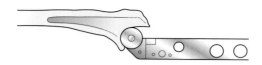

Figure 7.15 *Rasping of the ulnar metaphysic*

introduced into the medullary canal of the ulnar until cortical resistance is met (Fig. 7.15). As with the humerus the size of implant used corresponds with the largest size of rasp fully inserted.

The appropriate rasps are used to shape the proximal ulna as needed.

After the proximal ulna and distal humerus have been prepared, a trial will evaluate the elbow for complete flexion and extension. The medullary canals are cleaned with pulsatile lavage and the canals dried. A cement restrictor is inserted into both canals. A cement gun is used for retrograde insertion of low-viscosity cement into the canals. If the components are cemented separately, the ulnar component is inserted first. The centre of the ulnar component is aligned with the centre of the sigmoid fossa. The humeral component is impacted down to a point that allows articulation of the device and the placement of the axle and the locking clip or interlocking axis pins (if a partially constrained device is used) (Fig. 7.16).

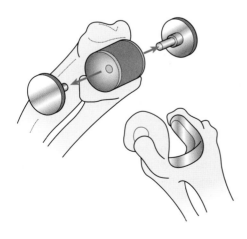

Figure 7.16 *Implanted components*

The arm is held in extension until the cement has cured, and then the humeral device can be articulated with the ulnar component.

Closure

As for elbow arthrolysis.

POSTOPERATIVE CARE AND INSTRUCTIONS

Two further doses of the same antibiotic given on induction are given intravenously. The drain is removed at 24 hours and the compressive dressing removed. Supervised physiotherapy allowing active and gravity extension, active and passive flexion and pronation and supination. The patient is advised against heavy lifting. At 6 weeks, strengthening exercises are begun.

Follow up is recommended at 6 weeks, 6 months and 1 year after surgery. Continuation of follow-up is typically at yearly intervals. The patient should be cautioned to return to clinic if there is pain or functional deterioration.

RECOMMENDED REFERENCES

Bryan RS, Morrey BF. Extensive posterior approach to the elbow joint: a triceps sparing approach. *Clin Orthop Relat Res* 1982;(166): 188–92.

Connor AN. Biomechanics of total elbow arthroplasty. *Semin Arthroplasty* 1998;**9**:25–31.

An KN, Morrey BE. Biomechanics of the elbow. In: Morrey BF, ed. *The Elbow and Its Disorders*, 2nd edn. Philadelphia: WB Saunders, 1993.

Shahane SA, Stanley D. A posterior approach to the elbow joint. *J Bone Joint Surg Br* 1999;**81**:1020–2.

RADIAL HEAD REPLACEMENT

PREOPERATIVE PLANNING

Indications

- Valgus instability (due to medial collateral ligament instability) with type III radial head fractures

- Radial head fracture with distal radioulnar joint instability (Essex–Lopresti injury).

Contraindications

- Vascular compromise of the limb
- Compromised skin in the region of the surgical incision.

Consent and risks

- Nerve injury
- Infection
- Vitallium prosthesis: aseptic loosening, implant impingement, component retrieval difficult
- Silicone replacement: fatigue failure, giant cell synovitis inflammation which may persist after implant removal

Operative planning

Anteroposterior and lateral radiographs, less than 6 months old, should be available. Availability of the implants must be checked by the surgeon:

- Silicone replacement – can be used as a temporary spacer (uncemented)
- Vitallium prosthesis – provides more stability than silicone replacement and does not cause synovitis. Need to be careful not to 'overstuff' the joint as this can lead to pain and loss of extension (cemented or uncemented).

Anaesthesia and positioning

See 'Elbow arthrolysis' (p. 80).

SURGICAL TECHNIQUE

There are two options. The distal dissection for the proximal radioulnar joint as described for the trans-tricipital approach (see 'Elbow arthrolysis', p. 83) or the lateral column approach as described below.

LATERAL APPROACH (MORREY)

Landmarks

The lateral epicondyle, radial head and tip of the olecranon. Palpate the lateral epicondyle and

move the fingers distally until a depression is felt. The radial head lies within a palpable depression distal to the lateral epicondyle. On pronating and supinating the forearm, it can be felt to move.

Incision

The skin incision extends approximately 5 cm proximal to the lateral epicondyle, and continues distally, over the epicondyle, along the anterolateral surface of the forearm for approximately 5 cm (Fig. 7.17).

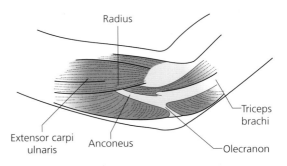

Figure 7.17 *The incision and surface anatomy of the lateral approach to the radial head*

Dissection

Structures at risk

- Radial nerve
- Posterior interosseous nerve (PIN)

The incision is continued through subcutaneous fat and through the fascia between triceps and origins of the extensor carpi radialis longus (ECRL) and brachioradialis. An interval is developed between the triceps posteriorly and the origins of ECRL and brachioradialis anteriorly. In the proximal end of the wound, **the radial nerve must be avoided in the interval between the brachialis and brachioradialis muscles**. The common origin of the extensor muscles is removed from the lateral epicondyle together with a thin flake of bone, using a small osteotome. Reflecting the common origin distally exposes the

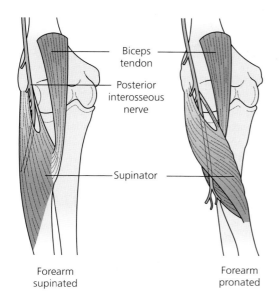

Figure 7.18 *Anatomy of the posterior interosseous nerve*

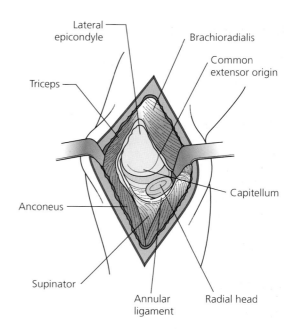

Figure 7.19 *Lateral approach*

radiohumeral joint. The PIN is vulnerable as it enters supinator **and must be protected** (Fig. 7.18).

The origins of the brachioradialis and ECRL muscles are elevated subperiosteally and the capsule incised to expose the lateral aspect of the elbow joint. By incising the capsule anterior to the radial humeral ligamentous complex, (overlying the radial head) in line with the radius, the lateral collateral ligament is avoided. However, the incision must not stray too far anteriorly as the radial nerve runs over the anterolateral portion of the elbow capsule (Fig. 7.19).

The annular ligament is incised longitudinally before transecting the radial neck with an oscillating saw using a radial cutting jig (Fig. 7.20). Exposure distal to the annular ligament risks damaging the PIN and is avoided. The cut surface of the proximal radius should be smooth and even, so that contact between it and the collar of the prosthesis is complete.

The proximal radial medullary canal is prepared with burs or rasps to accept the implant stem. The

radial head trial should be chosen to match the diameter of the articulation surface of the native radial head. If the radial head diameter is between two available sizes, the smaller of the two radial

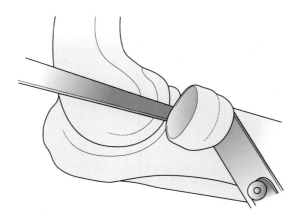

Figure 7.20 *The radial neck cut*

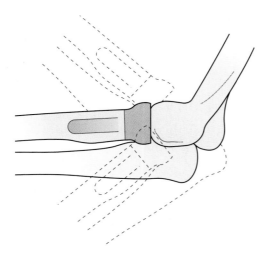

Figure 7.21 *Trial reduction to test range of motion*

heads should be used. A trial is inserted to ensure that contact with the capitellum is satisfactory. To prevent excessive wear of the capitellum from 'overstuffing', the proximal edge of the prosthesis should be level with the lateral edge of the coronoid. The elbow is taken through a range of flexion, extension and rotation (Fig. 7.21). If this is satisfactory, the final prosthesis is inserted.

Closure of lateral approach

The annular ligament is repaired with an absorbable suture. The common extensor origin is reattached to the lateral epicondyle with transosseous sutures. A suction drain is inserted. Superficial closure utilizes absorbable sutures to approximate the subcutaneous fat, then a continuous absorbable subcuticular suture with Steri-Strips. An occlusive dressing is applied and a compression dressing is used around the elbow.

POSTOPERATIVE CARE AND INSTRUCTIONS

Two more doses of the same antibiotic given on induction are given intravenously. The drain and compression dressing are removed at 24 hours. Gentle active mobilization of the elbow is begun under supervision.

Return to work is allowed after around 6 weeks for sedentary jobs, but may be delayed to 3 months or more in active work. Follow-up is recommended at 6 weeks, 6 months and 1 year after surgery. Continuation of follow-up is typically at yearly intervals. The patient should be cautioned to return to clinic if there is pain or functional deterioration.

RECOMMENDED REFERENCE

Ates Y, Atlihan D, Yildirim H. Current concepts in the treatment of fractures of the radial head, the olecranon, and the coronoid. *J Bone Jt Surg Am* 1996;**78**:969

TENNIS/GOLFER'S ELBOW RELEASE

PREOPERATIVE PLANNING

Indications

Tennis/golfer's elbow release is indicated when conservative management has failed.

Patients with tennis elbow have reproducible tenderness at the common extensor origin, with reproduction of symptoms upon resisted wrist extension with the elbow in extension. Non-operative treatment with anti-inflammatories, counterforce bracing and up to three steroid injections to the site of maximal tenderness can achieve success in up to 95 per cent of cases.

In golfers, elbow pain and tenderness are localized to the common flexor origin. Pain is reproduced by resisted forearm pronation and wrist flexion. Non-operative treatment is similar to that for tennis elbow but usually more difficult to treat.

Consent and risks

- Failure
- Nerve injury: 1 per cent
- Infection
- Heterotopic ossification at surgical site: 10 per cent
- Posterolateral instability: if there is excessive debridement of the collateral ligament origins as well as the origins of the extensor muscles from the lateral epicondyle

Operative planning

Recent anteroposterior and lateral radiographs of the elbow should be available to rule out lateral compartment arthrosis (tennis elbow). Calcification may be visible in the flexor origin in longstanding golfer's elbow.

Anaesthesia and positioning

Anaesthesia is usually general, regional or combined. The supine position is used with the arm placed on an arm board. A tourniquet or an S-MART bandage/tourniquet is used.

The elbow should be sufficiently mobile for appropriate movement intraoperatively. The surgical field is prepared with a germicidal solution. Waterproof drapes are used with adhesive edges to provide a seal to the skin.

SURGICAL TECHNIQUE

Extensor origin release (tennis elbow)

Landmark

The lateral epicondyle.

Incision

A 4–5 cm gently curved skin incision is made centred over the lateral epicondyle (Fig. 7.22).

Superficial dissection

The incision is continued through subcutaneous fat and down to fascia. The fascia overlying the posterior edge of the ECRL is incised and elevated to expose the extensor carpi radialis brevis (ECRB), which lies beneath the ECRL. Just

posterior to the ECRL lies the extensor aponeurosis, the anterior edge of which may be abnormal. The ECRL is then dissected sharply off the anterior ridge and displaced anteromedially to expose the ECRB. ECRB is inferior to the origin of the ECRL and deep to the EDC. The border between the ECRB and EDC is often poorly defined.

Deep dissection

Degenerate tissue is excised, taking care not to release any normal looking tendon. The abnormal

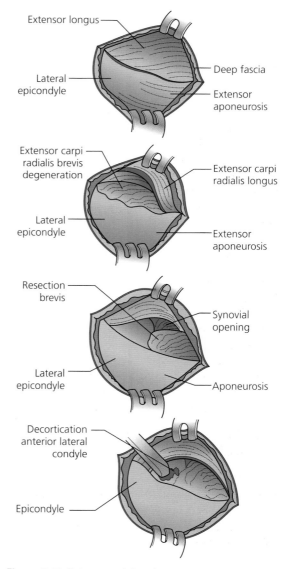

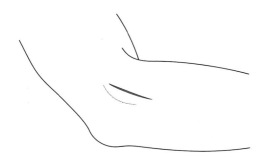

Figure 7.22 *Skin incision*

Figure 7.23 *Extensor origin release*

tissue may appear fibrillated or discoloured and may contain calcium deposits. The anterior lateral condyle is decorticated with an osteotome or bone nibbler to enhance blood supply (Fig. 7.23).

Closure of lateral approach

The defect between the posterior edge of the ECRL and the extensor aponeurosis is repaired with an absorbable suture to restore the normal anatomic position. Superficial closure utilizes absorbable sutures to approximate the subcutaneous fat, then a subcuticular continuous absorbable suture.

An occlusive dressing is applied, followed by a bulky wool and crepe bandage dressing in two layers.

Postoperative care and instructions

Dressings are reduced at 48 hours. Early range-of-motion exercises are begun, followed by strengthening exercises. Strenuous activity is resumed within pain limits at 8–10 weeks and full power should have returned by 3 months. Follow-up is recommended at 6 weeks, with a wound check by the primary care practitioner at 2 weeks.

Flexor origin release (Golfer's elbow)

Landmark

The medial epicondyle.

Incision

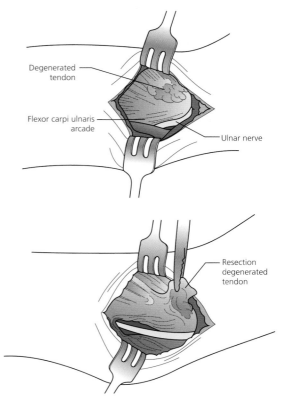

Figure 7.24 *Flexor origin release*

> ### Structures at risk
>
> - Medial antebrachial cutaneous nerve

A 3–4 cm longitudinal skin incision is made just posterior to the medial epicondyle. This avoids sensory branches of the medial antebrachial cutaneous nerve anterior and distal to the medial epicondyle.

Dissection

The incision is continued through subcutaneous fat and down to fascia exposing the common flexor origin. Partial debridement of the flexor carpi radialis (FCR), excising abnormal tissue is usually all that is required (Fig. 7.24). Any normal tissue attached to the medial epicondyle **is left intact**.

Closure of medial approach

The defect in the flexor–pronator origin is closed with absorbable sutures. Superficial closure utilizes absorbable sutures to approximate the subcutaneous fat, then a subcuticular continuous absorbable suture.

An occlusive dressing is applied, followed by a bulky wool and crepe bandage dressing in two layers.

Postoperative care and instructions

Dressings are reduced at 48 hours. Early mobilization of the elbow should be encouraged in all patients.

Follow-up is recommended at 6 weeks, with a wound check by the primary care practitioner at 2 weeks. The patient should be cautioned to return to the clinic if there is pain or functional deterioration.

RECOMMENDED REFERENCES

Stahl S, Kaufman T. The efficacy of an injection of steroids for medial epicondylitis. A prospective study of 60 elbows. *J Bone Joint Surg Am* 1997;**79**:1648–52.

Sevier TL, Wilson JK. Treating lateral epicondylitis. *Sports Med* 1999;**28**:375–80.

ELBOW ARTHROSCOPY

PREOPERATIVE PLANNING

Indications

Elbow arthroscopy is indicated in a variety of painful conditions of the elbow. The most frequent are:
- Debridement for osteoarthritis
- Osteochondritis dissecans of capitellum
- Arthrolysis
- Removal of loose bodies
- Synovectomy or synovial biopsy
- Pyarthrosis
- Radial head resection
- Diagnostic.

Contraindications

- Infection of overlying skin
- Bony or severe fibrous ankylosis.

Consent and risks

- Nerve injury
- Infection: <1 per cent; risk is very low, so prophylactic antibiotics are not recommended

Operative planning

Recent radiographs and, where taken, magnetic resonance (MR) images and MR arthrograms, should be available.

The correct equipment must be available and this should be checked by the surgeon. A 30° 4 mm arthroscope should be used. The water flow should be controlled with an inflow pump.

Anaesthesia and positioning

Anaesthesia is general or combined with regional. The lateral decubitus position is used, the position being maintained by side supports. The tourniquet is applied high around the arm, and the arm placed over a bolster applied to the bed. The elbow should be free to flex to 90° with the hand pointing towards the floor.

The TV monitor is placed on the opposite side of the patient. The surgical field is prepared with a germicidal solution. Waterproof drapes are used with adhesive edges to provide a seal to the skin.

SURGICAL TECHNIQUE

Landmarks

Bone landmarks are outlined with a marker pen:
- Lateral epicondyle
- Radial head
- Tip of the olecranon
- Medial epicondyle.

Portals

The direct lateral portal is located in the soft spot at the centre of the triangle formed by the lateral epicondyle, radial head and tip of the olecranon (Fig. 7.25). This portal traverses the anconeus muscle. The elbow is initially distended through this portal.

The distal anterolateral portal

Structure at risk

- The radial nerve

This portal is usually established first after elbow distension. It is used for instrumentation as well as visualization of the lateral aspect of the radial head. With the elbow flexed to 90° the portal is located 3 cm distal and 1–2 cm anterior to the lateral epicondyle. This should bring the portal just anterior and proximal to the radiocapitellar articulation. The skin incision is made with a no. 11 blade and a haemostat used to bluntly dissect down to the joint capsule.

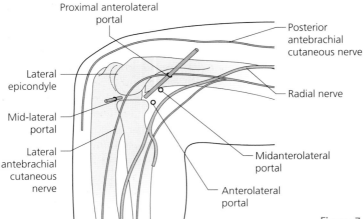

Figure 7.25 *Lateral elbow arthroscopy portals*

This portal traverses the extensor carpi radialis brevis muscle. A blunt trocar is used to enter the joint with the portal driven toward the centre of the trochlea. The elbow joint **must be distended prior to and kept at 90° flexion, during trocar insertion** since extension brings the radial nerve closer to the joint (3–7 mm).

The proximal anterolateral portal

This is located 2 cm proximal and 1 cm anterior to the lateral epicondyle. It is further from the radial nerve than other anterolateral portals. It allows for excellent views of the anterior radiohumeral and ulnohumeral joints as well as the anterior capsular margin.

The anteromedial portal

Structure at risk

• Median nerve

Some surgeons prefer to establish this portal first. The elbow should be flexed to 90° as the portal is established. It is situated 2 cm anterior and 2 cm distal to the medial epicondyle. It must be placed **under direct vision**: the median nerve lies 1–2 cm anterior and lateral to this portal.

The proximal anteromedial portal

Structures at risk

• Median nerve

• Ulnar nerve
• Medial brachial cutaneous nerve
• Medial antebrachial cutaneous nerve
• Brachial artery

This portal allows visualization of the anterior elbow including the anterior joint capsule, medial condyle, coronoid process, trochlea, capitellum and radial head. The joint should already be distended with fluid and the ulnar nerve identified before establishing this portal. The portal is established using a longitudinal skin stab incision and blunt dissection 2 cm proximal to the medial epicondyle and immediately anterior to the intermuscular septum. The trochar is inserted over the anterior surface of the humerus aiming towards the radial head. Contact is maintained with the anterior surface of the humerus **to avoid neurovascular damage**. The ulnar nerve lies 4 mm from the portal. The median nerve lies 7–20 mm from portal with the elbow in flexion.

The posterolateral portal

Structures at risk

The posterior antebrachial or lateral brachial nerves can be damaged with deep incisions.

This is 3 cm proximal to the olecranon tip and just lateral to the border of the triceps tendon.

The direct posterior portal

Structure at risk

The ulnar nerve, if placed too medially.

This is 3 cm proximal to the olecranon tip and 2 cm medial to the posterolateral portal. It is **established under direct vision** with the arthroscope in the direct lateral portal (Fig. 7.26).

Procedure

A systematic approach is essential if pathology is not to be missed. About 15–25 mL of fluid is instilled into the joint, to distend the capsule, through the direct lateral portal using an 18G needle. Backflow of fluid confirms correct placement. The anterolateral portal is established (see above) and the arthroscope and cannula inserted. The capsule medial to the articulation is examined first. Medial laxity can be assessed by supinating the forearm and applying valgus stress to the elbow in varying degrees of flexion. Flexing and extending the elbow allows the trochlear to be viewed. The radioulnar articulation is observed as the forearm is rotated and, for coronoid impingement, as the elbow is fully flexed.

The anteromedial portal is established under direct vision and the arthroscope introduced to view the radioulnar and radiocapitellar articulations plus the annular ligament. Extending the elbow reveals more of the capitellum and forearm rotation exposes more of the radial head. The anterolateral gutter and capsule should also be examined.

Next, the direct lateral portal is established. Via this portal, the radial head (concave) is viewed, articulating with the capitellum (convex). The articulation between the olecranon and the trochlea is also well seen.

Finally, through the posterolateral portal, the olecranon fossa, olecranon tip and posterior trochlea are examined. Loose bodies and osteophytes are sought, particularly on the olecranon tip.

Specific instruments can be used for removal of loose bodies or debridement.

Closure

Non-absorbable suture is used to close the skin defects. Occlusive dressings are applied. Wool and crepe bandage pressure dressing is used.

POSTOPERATIVE CARE AND INSTRUCTIONS

The pressure dressing is removed at 48 hours. The patient mobilizes the elbow fully following a diagnostic arthroscopy.

RECOMMENDED REFERENCE

O'Driscoll SW, Morrey BF. Arthroscopy of the elbow. *J Bone Jt Surg Am* 1992;**74**:84–94.

ELBOW ASPIRATION/INJECTION

Indications

- Inflammatory arthritis and other arthropathies
- Suspected infection
- Haemarthrosis.

Consent and risks

- Nerve injury: 1 per cent
- Infection: 1–2 per cent in osteoarthritis, 5 per cent in rheumatoid arthritis

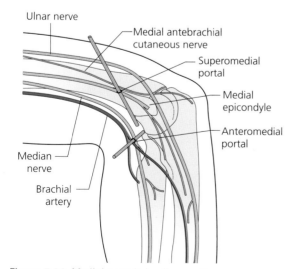

Figure 7.26 *Medial portals in elbow arthroscopy*

Ulnar nerve

Medial antebrachial cutaneous nerve

Superomedial portal

Medial epicondyle

Anteromedial portal

Median nerve

Brachial artery

Approach

The elbow can be entered either ulnarly or radially, but the radial approach is preferred in order to avoid ulnar nerve injury

Landmarks

Radial head, lateral epicondyle, and tip of the olecranon (anconeus triangle) (Fig. 7.27).

Procedure

Structure at risk

• Radial nerve

The skin is prepared with a germicidal solution. Prior to needle insertion, the elbow is flexed and the forearm pronated to protect the radial nerve. An 18G needle is inserted into the joint, through the soft spot at the centre of the anconeus triangle. With this approach the needle will penetrate only the anconeus and joint capsule.

If the needle hits bone, it should be withdrawn slightly and redirected at a slightly different angle. If performing an injection, it is wise to aspirate first to ensure the needle is not in a blood vessel.

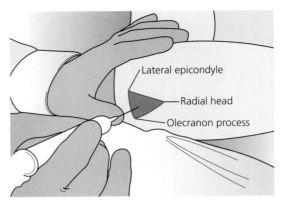

Figure 7.27 *Landmarks for elbow aspiration*

POSTOPERATIVE CARE AND INSTRUCTIONS

An occlusive dressing is applied. Mobilization of the joint depends on the underlying reason for aspiration/injection.

RECOMMENDED REFERENCE

Holdsworth BJ, Clement DA, Rothwell PN. Fractures of the radial head – the benefit of aspiration: a prospective controlled trial. *Injury* 1987;**18**:44–7.

Viva questions

1. How do you approach diagnosing and the treatment of a painful elbow?

2. What are the indications, benefits and drawbacks for total elbow replacement?

3. How do you further investigate an elbow replacement shown to be loose on X-ray?

4. What are the treatment options for a 50-year-old man with symptomatic osteoarthritis of the elbow?

5. Describe the anatomy of the ulnar nerve around the elbow.

6. Describe the anatomy of the posterior interosseous nerve around the elbow.

7. What complications do you warn the patient about prior to elbow replacement? What are their incidences?

8. What are the indications for arthrolysis?

9. What is your postoperative management post arthrolysis?

10. Which approach do you use for total elbow replacement?

11. What factors influence whether you use a semi-constrained or resurfacing type total elbow replacement?

12. What are the contraindications to total elbow replacement?

13. How would you manage someone after total elbow replacement?

14. Which nerves can be injured in elbow surgery?

15. What factors contribute to loosening in total elbow replacement?

16. Describe the portals used in elbow arthroscopy.

17. What structures are at risk from each portal?

18. What are the advantages/disadvantages of radial head replacement versus radial head excision?

19. What approach would you use for a radial head replacement?

20. What are the complications associated with radial head replacement?

8

Surgery of the wrist

James Donaldson and Nicholas Goddard

Wrist	Range of motion
Dorsiflexion	80°
Palmarflexion	90°
Radial deviation	20°
Ulnar deviation	35°
Pronation	75°
Supination	80°

Position of arthrodesis

- Dorsiflexion: 10–20° (neutral in rheumatoid)
- Ulnar deviation: 0–5°

WRIST ARTHROSCOPY

PREOPERATIVE PLANNING

Indications

- Triangular fibrocartilage complex (TFCC; 'the meniscus of the wrist') repair or debridement
- Carpal instability – diagnostic or arthroscopic assistance in reduction and treatment
- Distal radius or scaphoid fractures – reduce fracture and treat associated TFCC tears
- Chondral lesions
- Dorsal ganglion excision
- Bone excision procedures – loose body removal, radial styloidectomy, excision of the distal ulna

- Kienbock's disease – lunate excision or debridement of head of capitate
- Synovectomy or synovial biopsy, adhesion release, etc.

Contraindications

- Infection of overlying skin
- Lack of proper instrumentation

Consent and risks

- Nerve injury: 1–2 per cent
- Infection: <1 per cent; deep infection/septic arthritis (0.04 per cent); prophylactic antibiotics not recommended.
- Haematoma: 0.2 per cent
- Tendon injury: 0.15 per cent
- Chronic regional pain syndrome: 0.5 per cent
- Compartment syndrome of the forearm associated with fluid extravasation: 0.01 per cent

Operative planning

Recent radiographs ± magnetic resonance (MR) images should be available. The proper equipment must be available; usually 2.5–3.0 mm scope and any specific, procedure-dependent equipment.

Anaesthesia and positioning

Anaesthesia is general with a supine position and the shoulder abducted, placing the arm on a hand table. Finger traps are applied to the index and long fingers and tied to a drip-stand. The elbow is flexed to 90° and up to 4.5 kg of counter-traction applied to the arm (depends on sex and weight).

The dorsal wrist veins are marked out before exsanguination and inflating the tourniquet. Gravity-assisted inflow of irrigation fluid is used.

SURGICAL TECHNIQUE

Landmarks

- Bony
  - Second and third carpometacarpal joints
  - Distal radioulnar joint (DRUJ)
  - Lister's tubercle
  - Radial styloid in the anatomical snuff box
  - Neck of the capitate
- Tendinous
  - Extensor carpi ulnaris
  - Extensor pollicis longus
  - Extensor digitorum communis.

Approach

The portals are named according to the wrist compartments on either side of them. The commonly used portals are all on the dorsal surface of the wrist. Before their creation, they should be drawn on prior to fluid injection and wrist distension.

A minimum of two portals are used; the most common ones used are portal 3–4 for the arthroscope and portal 4–5 or portal 6/R for the instruments (Fig. 8.1).
- The 1–2 portal is between the extensor carpi radialis brevis (ECRB) and the abductor pollicis longus (APL).

Structures at risk

- The radial artery and dorsal branch of the radial nerve – restrict the portal to the dorsal and proximal part of the snuff box to reduce the risk.

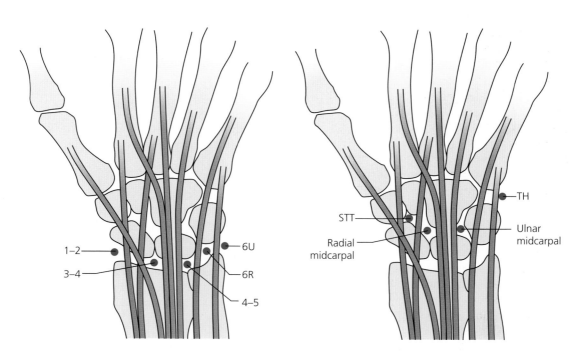

Figure 8.1 *Radiocarpal and mid-carpal portals*

- The 3–4 portal is between the extensor carpi radialis longus (ECRL) and the extensor pollicis longus (EPL), 1 cm distal to Lister's tubercle. This is commonly the first portal marked in place and the site for injection of saline into the wrist in order to distend the capsule. The scope is then inserted in line with the dorsal radial slope.
- The 4–5 portal is between extensor digitorum communis (EDC) and extensor digiti minimi (EDM), 1 cm distal to the DRUJ line.
- The 6/R portal is radial to the extensor carpi ulnaris (ECU) at the level of the ulnar styloid.
- The 6/U portal is ulnar to the ECU at the level of the ulnar styloid.

Structure at risk

- Dorsal ulnar cutaneous nerve

- The mid-carpal portal is in the scaphocapitate interval, 1 cm ulnarwards and 1 cm distal to 3–4 portal.

Saline (± adrenaline) are injected, to distend the capsule, using an 18G needle at an arthroscopic portal site. This is usually done at the 3–4 portal and with the wrist pronated and in ulnar deviation. The needle is removed and the skin incised. Blunt dissection is used to penetrate the capsule: a small haemostat is easiest to use. The cannula and blunt obturator are inserted, and inflow irrigation established.

Procedure

This is dependent on the indication. As always, an organized pattern ensures identification of pathology and normal structures within the wrist.

Closure

Steri-Strips are sufficient to close the skin defects and a compression bandage is then applied.

POSTOPERATIVE CARE AND INSTRUCTIONS

The patient is usually advised to mobilize according to comfort; this may depend on the specific pathology treated.

RECOMMENDED REFERENCES

Nagle DA, Benson LS. Wrist arthroscopy indications and results. *Arthroscopy* 1992;**8**:198.
Warhold LG, Ruth RM. Complications of wrist arthroscopy and how to prevent them. *Hand Clin* 1995;**11**:81.
Whipple TL, Marotta JJ, Powell III JH. Techniques of wrist arthroscopy. *Arthroscopy* 1986;**2**:244.

WRIST ARTHRODESIS

PREOPERATIVE PLANNING

Indications

- Post-traumatic arthritis
- Joint destruction secondary to infection or tumour resection
- Rheumatoid arthritis
- Failed arthroplasty or limited fusion
- Scapholunate advanced collapse (SLAC) or scaphoid non-union advanced collapse (SNAC) wrist
- Spastic flexion contracture
- Kienbock's disease.

Contraindications

- Skeletal immaturity
- Elderly patients or sedentary lifestyle, where a replacement may be more appropriate.

Consent and risks

- Subsequent re-operation: metalwork removal for painful hardware (15 per cent); or non-union (2 per cent with AO plate fixation), with or without hardware failure (common)
- Complex regional pain syndrome (CRPS) and persistent pain: up to 10 per cent
- Nerve damage and neuroma formation: 1 per cent
- DRUJ pain: 1–3 per cent
- Carpal tunnel syndrome: 2–4 per cent

- Infection: 1–2 per cent; local wound complications: 4 per cent
- Extensor tenosynovitis: 5–7 per cent
- Ulnar abutment: 1–2 per cent
- Intrinsic muscle contracture: 3–5 per cent

Operative planning

The surgeon must decide between full and partial wrist fusion (both described below). Consider need for bone grafting – autologous bone from the distal radius or iliac crest is usually sufficient, unless there is severe bone loss. Ulnocarpal impaction may necessitate radial lengthening at the same time.

Position of fusion is: 10–20° of dorsiflexion and 0–5° of ulna deviation allows for maximum grip strength. In rheumatoid arthritis, a more neutral position may be preferred. In bilateral wrist fusions, both wrists are fixed in neutral, allowing maximal function. The equipment must be available – an AO, titanium, precontoured, wrist fusion dynamic compression plate (Synthes) is commonly used (Fig. 8.2).

The advantages of using a dynamic compression plate (DCP) are:
- Good stability, less need for bone grafting and good fusion rates
- Different sizes – straight, short carpal bend, long carpal bend. All have tapered edges and are filled with recessed screw heads (2.7 mm screws in distal four holes; 3.5 mm holes in proximal four holes).

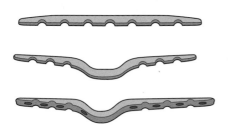

Figure 8.2 *AO wrist fusion plates*

Anaesthesia and positioning

Anaesthesia is general and the supine position is used; a hand table, tourniquet and image intensifier are required.

SURGICAL TECHNIQUE – FULL FUSION

Landmarks

- Styloid process
- Lister's tubercle
- DRUJ
- Third metacarpal.

Incision

A dorsal approach is used: a longitudinal incision in line with the distal radius and the third metacarpal, centred on the DRUJ (Fig. 8.3).

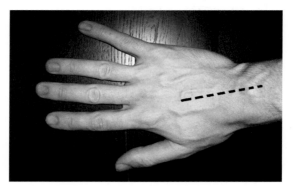

Figure 8.3 *Dorsal incision for wrist arthrodesis*

Dissection

Structures at risk

- Dorsal veins and superficial nerves – these should be identified and protected
- Posterior interosseous nerve – see below

Full-thickness skin flaps are developed medially and laterally. The extensor retinaculum is incised, using a straight incision on the radial border of the fourth compartment. The approach continues between the EPL (third compartment), which is retracted radially, and the EDC (fourth compartment) which is retracted ulnarly. Once the EPL is retracted, Lister's tubercle is excised (using an osteotome or bone nibblers) to allow flat plate apposition.

The posterior interosseous nerve is identified as it enters the fourth compartment just proximal to the extensor retinaculum and a 2 cm segment is excised. The ECRB tendon may need to be released off the third metacarpal for plate apposition. An H-shaped capsulotomy is created to access the wrist joint (Fig. 8.4).

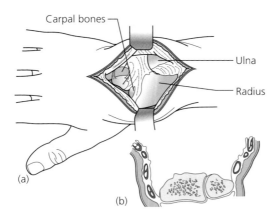

Figure 8.4 *(a) Approach to the wrist joint. (b) Axial view showing the approach between the third and fourth compartments*

Procedure

The articular surfaces are denuded of cartilage using rongeurs and burrs, exposing cancellous bone in the radioscaphoid and radiolunate joints, and the intercarpal joints (scaphocapitate, lunocapitate and triquetrohamate). Any gaps are filled with cancellous bone harvested from the excised bone and distal radial metaphysis as necessary.

The precontoured plate is applied and bony edges are contoured as necessary to allow good apposition. The distal end of the plate should reach the mid-shaft of the third (or occasionally second) metacarpal. The most distal screw hole is drilled with a 2 mm drill, in the dorsal to volar direction, in the middle of the metacarpal.

Following measurement and tapping, a 2.7 mm screw is inserted. The two remaining metacarpal screws are inserted in a similar manner. The wrist fusion is compressed with a 3.5 mm screw, on compression mode, in the second most distal hole in the radius. The remaining three proximal radial screws are inserted with the usual method. Often a screw is inserted into the capitate through the remaining hole. Any remaining defects are filled with bone graft and a check radiograph (Fig. 8.5) is obtained.

Closure

The capsule is approximated, as far as possible, with Vicryl. The extensor retinaculum is closed with Vicryl over the plate but under the extensor tendons. Vicryl is also used to suture the fat, and an appropriate suture closes the skin. A volar plaster slab is applied.

SURGICAL TECHNIQUE – PARTIAL FUSION

The 'four corner' fusion (capitate–hamate–triquetrum–lunate fusion) is indicated in SLAC

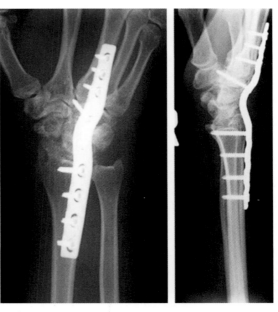

Figure 8.5 *Radiographic and intraoperative views of the AO wrist fusion plate*

wrist, SNAC wrist or mid-carpal instability. The landmarks, basic approach and structures at risk are similar to those of full wrist fusion.

Incision

A 'lazy S incision', slightly ulnar-sided, is made on the dorsum of the wrist.

Dissection

The extensor retinaculum is incised on the ulnar side of the fourth compartment. The posterior interosseous nerve is resected and an H-shaped capsulotomy is used as in full fusion or, alternatively, a radially based oblique flap can be created for exposure of the joint (Fig. 8.6).

Procedure

If radioscaphoid arthrosis is present, the scaphoid is excised, preserving the bone to be taken for later use as cancellous graft. If unstable, the lunate can be reduced to neutral position using a K-wire as a joystick; equally the capitate, hamate, triquetrum and lunate may be stabilized with volar placed K-wires. A Spider Limited Wrist Fusion (KMI) plate (Fig. 8.7) may be used as follows:

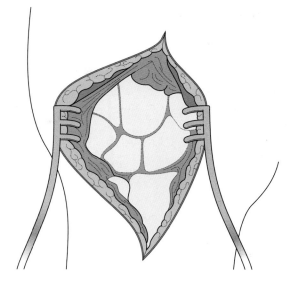

Figure 8.6 *Exposure of the carpal bones*

- A reamer is used to create a trough on the four bones, which are reamed to a depth so as not to cause impingement dorsally
- The articular surfaces are removed with rongeur or bone nibbler
- Cancellous bone is used to pack the cavity

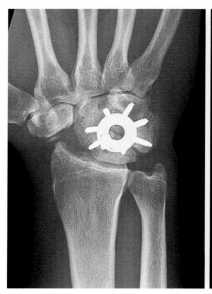
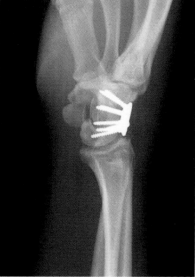

Figure 8.7 *A spider plate*

- Two screws are placed in each bone under image intensifier control.

Other fixation methods include K-wires, staples or headless screws.

Closure

See 'Surgical technique – full fusion' (above).

POSTOPERATIVE CARE AND INSTRUCTIONS

- The volar slab is removed at 2 weeks (it can be left longer if the bone quality is poor). A removable slab is required for the following 3 weeks in the case of partial fusion.
- Hand therapy and finger exercises are commenced 1 week after surgery.
- Union is usually achieved by 3 months.

RECOMMENDED REFERENCES

Barbier O, Saels P, Rombouts JJ, et al. Long-term functional results of wrist arthrodesis in rheumatoid arthritis. *J Hand Surg Br* 1999;**24**:27.

Chung K, Watt A, Kotsis S. A prospective outcomes study of four-corner wrist arthrodesis using a circular limited wrist fusion plate for stage II scapholunate advanced collapse wrist deformity. *Plastic and Recon Surg* 2006;**118**:433–42.

Haddad RJ, Riordan DC. Arthrodesis of the wrist: a surgical technique. *J Bone Joint Surg Am* 1967;**49**:950.

Watson H, Goodman M, Johnson T. Limited wrist arthrodesis. Part II Intercarpal and radiocarpal combinations. *J Hand Surg Am* 1981;**6**:223–33.

Zachary SV, Stern PJ. Complications following AO/ASIF wrist arthrodesis. *J Hand Surg Am* 1995;**20**:339–44.

DE QUERVAIN'S DECOMPRESSION

PREOPERATIVE PLANNING

Indications

- Stenosing tenosynovitis of the APL and extensor pollicis brevis (EPB) in the first dorsal compartment

- Failed conservative treatment (injection, thumb spica: success rate up to 70–80 per cent).

Contraindication

Infection of overlying skin.

Consent and risks

- Nerve injury and/or neuroma formation: superficial radial nerve branches (2 per cent)
- Failure of symptomatic relief: 5 per cent
- Tendon instability, subluxation or adherence: <1 per cent

Operative planning

Awareness of potential anatomical variations in the first dorsal compartment is important (Fig. 8.8).

Anaesthesia and positioning

The authors prefer general anaesthesia. The supine position is used with a hand table and tourniquet. Local anaesthesia can be used as an alternative ± tourniquet.

SURGICAL TECHNIQUE

Landmarks

- Bony: radial styloid, scaphoid tubercle, Lister's tubercle
- Tendinous – APL and EPB – lie over the lateral aspect of the distal radius. They represent the radial border of the anatomical snuffbox.

Incision

One of the following three skin incisions may be used:
- **Transverse**: 2 cm incision over the first dorsal compartment, 1 cm proximal to tip of radial styloid. Higher risk of nerve injury
- **Oblique**: from dorsal to volar – allows for extension distally

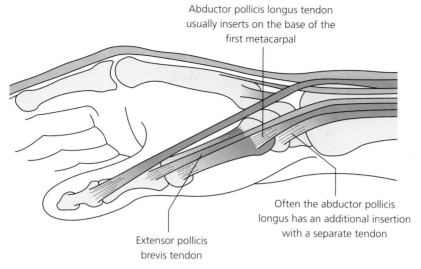

Figure 8.8 *First dorsal compartment anatomy*

- **Longitudinal**: better exposure but creates a longer area in which skin may potentially tether to cutaneous nerves and tendons.

Dissection

Structures at risk

- Branches of superficial radial nerve – protected by using blunt dissection
- Superficial veins

Sharp dissection follows the line of the chosen incision through dermis but not into superficial fat. Blunt longitudinal dissection is now used through the fat, whichever skin incision was selected, identifying and protecting branches of the superficial radial nerve, usually deep to superficial veins.

Procedure

The tendons are identified proximally within the incision and the first dorsal compartment opened with a longitudinal incision (Fig. 8.9) on the dorsal side, leaving a flap of palmar sheath to prevent subluxation.

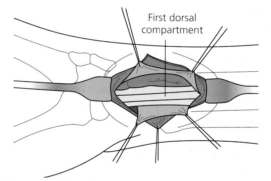

Figure 8.9 *First dorsal compartment*

The APL and EPB are lifted out of their groove with a tendon hook. If they cannot be easily freed, septae, 'aberrant' tendons and separate compartments are sought.

If the procedure is done under local anaesthesia, the tendons are replaced and the patient asked to move their thumb to demonstrate adequate decompression and independent movement. Instability is checked for and corrected, if necessary, by loosely opposing the edges of the tendon sheath.

Closure

The tourniquet is released and haemostasis achieved. The skin is closed with a subcuticular suture. Pressure dressing is applied to the area and a thumb spica may be applied to control postoperative pain and swelling (authors' preference).

POSTOPERATIVE CARE AND INSTRUCTIONS

The pressure dressing is removed after 48 hours. Thumb and hand movements are initiated and increased according to comfort. The thumb spica is removed at 2 weeks.

RECOMMENDED REFERENCES

Harvey FJ, Harvey PM, Horsley MW. De Quervain's disease: surgical or nonsurgical treatment. *J Hand Surg Am* 1990;**15**:83.

Witt J, Pess G, Gelberman RH. Treatment of De Quervain tenosynovitis: a prospective study of the results of injection of steroids and immobilization in a splint. *J Bone Joint Surg Am* 1991;**73**:219.

Kay NR. De Quervain's disease: changing pathology or changing perception? *J Hand Surg Br* 2000;**25**:65.

Giles K. Anatomical variations affecting the surgery of De Quervain's disease. *J Bone Joint Surg Br* 1960;**42**:352–55.

Littler JW, Freedman DM, Malerich MM. Compartment reconstruction for de Quervain's disease. *J Hand Surg Am* 2002;**27**:242.

EXCISION OF THE DISTAL ULNA (DARRACH PROCEDURE)

PREOPERATIVE PLANNING

Indications

- Pain relief following DRUJ disruption and incongruity – commonly for symptomatic malunion of Colles fractures in elderly patients (younger patients may do better with a Sauvé–Kapandji or hemi-resection arthroplasty procedure)
- Rheumatoid disease
- Salvage operation following other failed DRUJ procedures.

Contraindications

- Young and high-demand patients
- Congruent DRUJ.

Consent and risks

- Outcomes vary depending on primary pathology and operative indication
- Decreased grip strength is expected and found in nearly all following the procedure
- Pain, instability and subluxation of the ECU over the ulnar stump: 5–40 per cent
- Radioulnar impingement: convergence – 60 per cent radiographically but symptomatic in 5–10 per cent

SURGICAL TECHNIQUE

Incision and dissection

Structures at risk

- Dorsal sensory branch of ulnar nerve
- Ulnar artery and nerve

A common approach (Fig. 8.10) is a longitudinal incision along the subcutaneous border of the ulna through the interval between the ECU and the

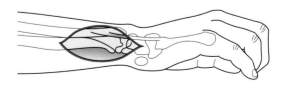

Figure 8.10 *Approach to the distal ulna*

flexor carpi ulnaris (FCU). The authors prefer an incision between the fifth and sixth compartments. The periosteum is incised longitudinally and reflected off the distal ulna; Hohmann retractors are then carefully placed around the ulna.

Procedure

The dissection is followed by resection of 1–2 cm of the distal ulna. Aim for minimal amount of bone resection that eliminates radioulnar contact at the sigmoid notch. A common error is too great a bone resection leaving an unstable and troublesome protrusion of the distal ulna.

It is important to leave soft tissue attachments and the TFCC at the ulnar styloid (Fig. 8.11). This can be achieved by subperiosteal dissection of the ulna styloid or preserving the styloid itself. Remnants of the TFCC are opposed to the capsule and radius. Ensure full rotation is achieved before closure.

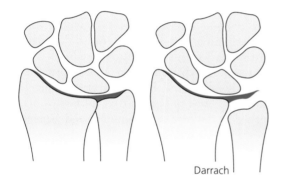

Figure 8.11 *Resection and soft tissue preservation in the Darrach procedure*

Closure

Haemostasis is achieved followed by closure in layers with Vicryl. Subcuticular or interrupted sutures are preferred for skin closure.

POSTOPERATIVE CARE AND INSTRUCTIONS

A volar slab is used for 2 weeks, followed by early active exercises.

RECOMMENDED REFERENCES

Darrach W. Partial excision of lower shaft of ulna for deformity following Colles fracture. *Ann Surg* 1913;**57**:764–65.

Peterson MS, Adams BD. Biomechanical evaluation of distal radioulnar reconstructions. *J Hand Surg Am* 1991;**18**:338.

ULNAR SHORTENING

PREOPERATIVE PLANNING

Indications

Ulna positive variance:
- Acquired:
  - Distal radial fracture
  - Essex-Lopresti type injury
  - Traumatic distal radial growth arrest
  - Resection of the radial head
- Congenital:
  - Idiopathic ulnar impaction syndrome
  - Madelung deformity (often in conjunction with other procedures).
  - Development of degenerative changes in the TFCC, DRUJ, ulnar head and articular surfaces of the lunate and triquetrum owing to ulnar abutment.

Contraindications

- Advanced osteoarthritis (OA) or significant malalignment of the DRUJ
- Relative contraindications – smokers (higher incidence of delayed and non-union) or non-compliant patient.

Consent and risks

- Non-union and delayed union: 0–4 per cent with oblique cuts; 8–15 per cent with transverse cuts
- Prominent metalwork and tendonitis from hardware irritation necessitating removal: up to 55 per cent
- Nerve damage, commonly dorsal sensory branch of the ulnar nerve: 1–2 per cent

- CRPS (Chronic Regional Pain Syndrome): up to 5 per cent
- Reduced grip strength: variable depending on the primary pathology.

Operative planning

Radiograph (90° shoulder abduction/90° elbow flexion) of the wrist is required to estimate amount of ulnar positive variance. The measurement should indicate the length of excision required to achieve a final ulnar variance of neutral or −1 mm.

Anaesthesia and positioning

Anaesthesia can be general or with an axillary block; a tourniquet is applied. The supine position, with a hand table and image intensifier, is used.

SURGICAL TECHNIQUE

Incision

Structures at risk

- The dorsal sensory branch of the ulnar nerve is present at the distal extent of the incision. Its transection should be avoided to prevent painful neuroma formation

A longitudinal incision over the subcutaneous border of the ulna is started distally 3–4 cm from the ulnar styloid and continued proximally for 10 cm.

Dissection

Dissection is simply continued straight down to the ulna, between the ECU and FCU. Sub-periosteal dissection exposes the ulna (Fig. 8.12).

Procedure

A six-hole, 3.5 mm DCP is held against the ulna (a dorsal side position can be easier but a volar position reduces the prominence of the metalwork) with the distal end just proximal to

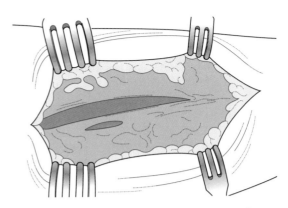

Figure 8.12 *Approach between the extensor carpi ulnaris and flexor carpi ulnaris*

the sigmoid notch of the ulna. The two distal screws are inserted in the standard fashion. The osteotomy site is marked at the middle of the plate with a longitudinal diathermy mark for rotational orientation. The most distal screw is loosened and the second screw is removed, allowing the plate to be swung out of the way by hinging on the distal screw.

An oblique osteotomy is fashioned from a proximal ulna to a distal radial direction. Continuous saline irrigation reduces heat production (and non-union rate); the distal osteotomy is created first. After measuring the thickness of bone to be removed, a free saw blade is placed in the first osteotomy cut and a parallel osteotomy is cut proximally removing the required amount of bone. The osteotomy is reduced and the plate swung around onto the ulna. The first screw is tightened and the second screw is replaced. The remaining screws are inserted using the dynamic compression technique (Fig. 8.13). An inter-fragmentary screw, at 90° to the plate, can also be used.

Closure

A standard closure of the skin in layers is undertaken. A below elbow cast is applied.

POSTOPERATIVE CARE AND INSTRUCTIONS

The cast is left on for 4–6 weeks then a thermoplastic splint used until the osteotomy has

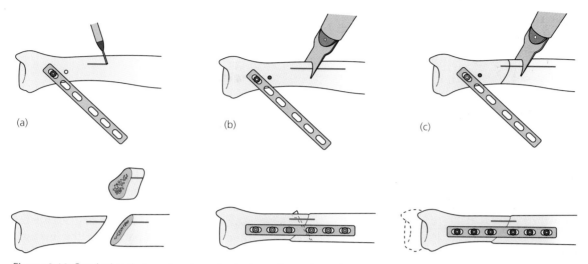

Figure 8.13 *Surgical technique for ulnar shortening using a dynamic compression plate*

united. Strenuous activities are avoided until evidence of bony union is seen.

RECOMMENDED REFERENCES

Chen NC, Wolfe SW. Ulna shortening osteotomy using a compression device. *J Hand Surg Am* 2003;**28**:88.

Chun S, Palmer AK. The ulnar impaction syndrome: follow up note of ulnar shortening osteotomy. *J Hand Surg Am* 1993;**18**:46–53.

Rayhack JM, Gasser SI, Latta LL, *et al.* Precision oblique osteotomy for shortening of the ulna. *J Hand Surg Am* 1993;**18**:908–19.

GANGLION EXCISION AT THE WRIST

The commonest site for a wrist ganglion is on the dorsum of the wrist arising from the scapholunate ligament; the second commonest site is volar, arising from the scapho-trapezoid joint.

PREOPERATIVE PLANNING

Indications

- Symptomatic:
  - Pain (often worse with repeated use)
  - Enlarging
  - Feeling of abnormal sensation or weakness
- Cosmesis
- Failed aspiration (success rate 35–50 per cent with needle aspiration and immobilization for 3 weeks).

Contraindications

Uncertain diagnosis, e.g. potential malignant lesion.

Consent and risks

- Numbness and scar sensitivity: 15–28 per cent
- Recurrence: variable depending on location; 5–20 per cent
- Nerve injury and neuroma formation: superficial branch of radial nerve in dorsal ganglia: 2–5 per cent; palmar cutaneous branch of median nerve in volar ganglia: 1–2 per cent
- Vascular injury: 4–5 per cent radial artery injury requiring repair with volar ganglia
- Stiffness: rare
- Scapholunate instability: rare

Anaesthesia and positioning

General anaesthesia is preferred as it is associated with lower recurrence rates than local anaesthesia. A tourniquet is applied and the forearm and hand positioned on a hand table.

SURGICAL TECHNIQUE – DORSAL GANGLION OF THE SCAPHOLUNATE LIGAMENT

Consideration is first given to using arthroscopic techniques. These involve less surgical dissection and scarring allowing more rapid return to activities. They also allow identification and management of any other intra-articular wrist pathology. Potential risks include damage to tendons if not visualized adequately and higher recurrence rates than open procedures.

Incision

Structures at risk

- Dorsal sensory branches of radial nerve – these must be identified and protected.

A transverse incision of appropriate length is created over the ganglion (Fig. 8.14).

Dissection

The extensor retinaculum overlying the ganglion is incised. The EPL and ECRB tendons are retracted radially and EDC tendons retracted ulnarly, exposing the ganglion.

Procedure

Structures at risk

- The scapholunate ligament: see below
- Terminal branches of the posterior interosseous nerve: see below

The ganglion and its stalk are mobilized with sharp and blunt dissection down to the joint capsule. The capsule is opened along the border of the radius and proximal pole of the scaphoid. Care must be taken to visualize and excise the stalk from the superficial portion of the ligament without cutting the scapholunate ligament (Fig. 8.15) and causing scapholunate instability.

Some authors advocate identification and cauterization of terminal branches of the posterior interosseous nerve as it runs past the fourth dorsal compartment, to reduce the incidence of neuroma.

Closure

The joint capsule is left open and haemostasis achieved after tourniquet release. Vicryl is used to close the retinaculum and subcuticular suture to close the skin. A volar splint is applied.

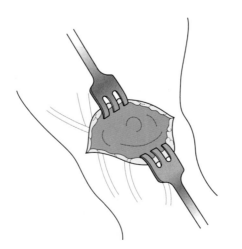

Figure 8.14 *Skin incision for dorsal ganglion excision*

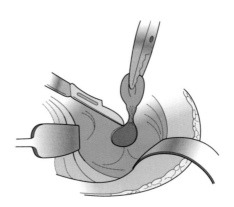

Figure 8.15 *Excision of the ganglion and its stalk from the scapholunate ligament*

SURGICAL TECHNIQUE – GANGLION OF THE SCAPHO-TRAPEZOIDAL JOINT

Incision

Structure at risk

- The palmar cutaneous branch of the median nerve

A longitudinal incision is created over the ganglion.

Dissection and procedure

Structure at risk

- The radial artery: identification and mobilization is vital (may course through the ganglion).

The artery is retracted radially and the ganglion dissected down its stalk to its origin (usually the scapho-trapezoidal joint). The ganglion is excised with a small portion of surrounding capsule.

POSTOPERATIVE CARE AND INSTRUCTIONS

Immobilization of the wrist is continued for 2 weeks then range of movement exercises are initiated.

RECOMMENDED REFERENCES

Luchetti R, Badia A, Alfarano M, *et al.* Arthroscopic resection of dorsal wrist ganglia and treatment of recurrences. *J Hand Surg Br* 2000;**25**:38.

Mehdian H, McKee M. Scapholunate instability following dorsal wrist ganglion excision. *Iowa Orthop J* 2005;**25**:203–6.

Nelson CL, Sawmiller S, Phalen GS. Ganglions of the wrist and hand. *J Bone Joint Surg Am* 1972;**54**:1459.

Viva questions

1. How many dorsal compartments are found at the wrist and what are their contents?

2. Which nerve and artery are at risk during surgical release of the first dorsal compartment?

3. What is the optimal position for wrist arthrodesis?

4. Between which dorsal wrist compartments do you classically approach through to access the wrist joint?

5. What is a 'four corner' fusion?

6. Name and describe the common wrist arthroscopy portals?

7. Dorsal wrist ganglions usually arise from which ligament?

8. What is the recurrence rate following excision of a volar wrist ganglion?

9. Describe the radiographic features of a wrist with scapholunate advanced collapse.

10. What is the non-union rate in total wrist fusions?

11. What are the main functional disadvantages with the Darrach procedure?

12. What alternatives are there to the Darrach procedure in younger and higher-demand patients?

13. What is chronic regional pain syndrome? What is the incidence after wrist or hand procedures?

14. When should an ulnar shortening osteotomy not be performed?

15. What is the most significant factor influencing the rate of non-union in an ulnar shortening osteotomy?

16. What is the significance of the posterior interosseous nerve in wrist procedures?

17. Where is the posterior interosseous nerve identified at the wrist?

9

Surgery of the hand

Norbert Kang, Robert Pearl and Lauren Ovens

DUPUYTREN'S SURGERY

PREOPERATIVE PLANNING

Indications

Patients are ready for Dupuytren's surgery if they have a flexion deformity that is interfering with their activities of daily living. Using the 'table-top test' (i.e. inability to get the hand flat on the table) or specific degrees of flexion deformity (e.g. =30° at the proximal interphalangeal [PIP] joint) as an indication for surgery is unhelpful as they may over- or underestimate the need for surgery.

Operative planning

It is vital to record the range of movement, vascularity and sensation in the digits preoperatively so that a comparison can be made postoperatively.

There are three common procedures:
- Fasciotomy (either open or needle) or segmental fasciotomy
- Fasciectomy
- Dermofasciectomy.

FASCIOTOMY

This is a procedure to divide rather than excise the Dupuytren's cord tissue. It can be done under direct vision (open fasciotomy), percutaneously (needle fasciotomy) or by excising a short segment of cord tissue – also under direct vision (segmental fasciotomy).

Indications

- Discrete Dupuytren's cord
- Metacarpophalangeal (MCP) joint flexion deformity
- Patient unwilling or unsuitable for major operative procedure
- Needle fasciotomy can be performed under local anaesthesia and is particularly useful for patients who wish to avoid or are unsuitable for general anaesthesia.

Contraindications

- Diffuse Dupuytren's disease
- PIP joint flexion deformity – there is a significant risk of neurovascular injury
- Patient unable or unwilling to comply with indefinite night-splintage with the digit in full extension.

Consent and risks

Injury to the neurovascular bundle (reduced with open/segmental fasciotomy).

Anaesthesia and positioning

Local anaesthesia, upper limb blockade or general anaesthesia can be used. The arm should be placed supine on an arm table or arm board. It is helpful to use a tourniquet for open and segmental fasciotomy; no tourniquet is required for needle fasciotomy.

Surgical technique

Landmarks

The cord to be divided is palpated and marked.

Needle fasciotomy

A green hub (21G) hypodermic needle is passed through the skin into the cord. Only the first 2–3 mm of the tip are inserted under the skin. The tip of the needle is then used like a knife (Fig. 9.1). Small sweeping movements are made with the needle tip to divide the cord tissue. Simultaneously, the digit is pushed into extension. If successful, a tearing sound is often heard as the divided cord tissue is torn in half allowing the finger to extend. The skin over the cord often tears open for a few millimeters as well.

Open fasciotomy

The skin is opened formally, through a longitudinal incision made over the course of the cord tissue. The incision is made sufficiently long to allow direct visualization of the cord and adjacent structures. The cord tissues are divided with a scalpel while forcibly extending the digit. If successful, the cord tissues are torn in half allowing the finger to extend.

Segmental fasciotomy

The procedure is the same as open fasciotomy but, in addition, a short segment (approximately 1 cm) of cord tissue is excised in the belief that this reduces the risk of recurrence.

Closure

After needle fasciotomy, the puncture wounds are allowed to heal by secondary intention. For open and segmental fasciotomy, the skin is closed with absorbable sutures (e.g. 5/0 Vicryl rapide).

Postoperative care and instructions

All patients undergoing fasciotomy should be allowed to mobilize their digits freely after treatment. However, all patients will need to wear a splint at night indefinitely to keep the treated digit in full extension. Otherwise, the flexion deformity will recur within a few weeks.

FASCIECTOMY

Indications

Any degree of involvement with Dupuytren's contracture including recurrent disease and MCP, PIP and distal interphalangeal (DIP) joint flexion deformity.

Contraindications

- Diffuse Dupuytren's disease with extensive skin involvement (pits and fixed skin over cords)
- Multiple previous fasciectomies with subsequent recurrence of flexion deformities

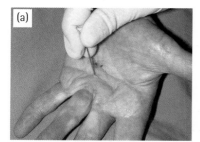 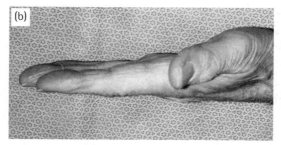

Figure 9.1 *Needle fasciotomy: (a) needling of fascia and (b) postoperative appearance*

- Patient with severe Dupuytren's diathesis (multi-digit involvement, radial disease, bilateral, family history and plantar involvement or Peyronie's disease)
- Patient unwilling or unable to comply with hand therapy postoperatively
- Heavy smoker and unwilling to stop smoking preoperatively.

Consent and risks

- 'White finger' due to injury to the vascular supply followed by necrosis of the finger
- Paraesthesia or anaesthesia due to injury to the nerve supply (10 per cent risk if redo procedure)
- Infection
- Skin flap necrosis
- Loss of flexion
- Recurrence of Dupuytren's followed by recurrence of the flexion deformity

Anaesthesia and positioning

Fasciectomy can be performed under local anaesthesia (maximum of two digits), upper limb blockade or general anaesthesia. The arm should be held supine on an arm table with a lead hand. All surgery should be carried out under tourniquet with loupe magnification.

SURGICAL TECHNIQUE

Landmarks

A straight line incision is marked over the midline on the volar aspect of the affected digit beginning at the distal finger crease. This is extended proximally to the mid-palmar crease. A further transverse incision is marked across the palm following the line of the mid-palmar crease. The length and position of the transverse incision is determined by the position and number of digits which are being treated (Fig. 9.2).

Incision

The transverse incision is created before proceeding into the digits. All incisions should be full thickness.

Dissection

Structures at risk

- Neurovascular bundles
- Skin edges of the flaps

Thin skin flaps should be developed above the cords. Particular care must be taken to avoid

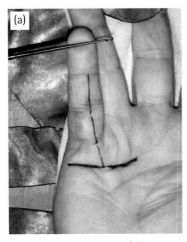 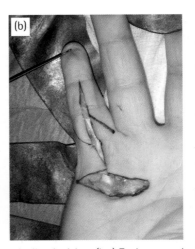 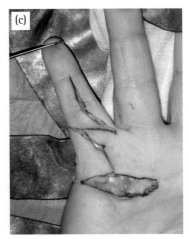

Figure 9.2 *Fasciectomy. (a) Skoog's straight line incision. (b,c) Z-plasty marked out and performed*

button-holing the skin when there is significant pitting or skin involvement. Ensure that the skin flaps are thick enough to be viable (ideally just thicker than sub-dermal) but thin enough so that not too much cord tissue is left in the hand (to avoid recurrence).

For fingers with significant flexion deformities due to a pretendinous cord, it is often helpful to carry out a fasciotomy after opening the palm. This allows the finger to be extended and simplifies access to the rest of the digit.

Procedure

Structure at risk

• Neurovascular bundles

Any longitudinal cord tissue should now be excised, leaving the transverse fibres of the palmar aponeurosis in place where possible. The neurovascular bundles should be visualized in the palm on either side of the flexor tendon. **The rest of the dissection is directed at freeing the neurovascular bundles from the cord tissue** on both sides of the finger by a combination of blunt and sharp dissection. Once both bundles have been skeletonized as far as the DIP joint, any soft tissues remaining between the skin and the tendon sheath can be excised and discarded.

Any remaining flexion deformity must now be assessed (e.g. from a boutonnière deformity at the PIP joint, volar plate contracture, shortening of the flexor sheath or volar skin shortage). In many cases, it is due to a combination of all of these factors. Boutonnière deformities respond well to splintage in full extension for 1 week. Volar plate contractures require either passive manipulation of the PIP joint or sharp release of the volar plate/check-rein ligaments.

'White fingers' need to be detected. The tourniquet **must be released before beginning closure** to check perfusion of the digit and carry out haemostasis. If the finger fails to perfuse, then both vessels need to be visualized to ensure that they are in continuity. You only need one intact artery to perfuse the digit. If the vessels are intact but the digit is still white, the digit is allowed to

flex to its former position for 5–10 minutes. If this fails, the surgeon can try bathing the vessels in a few drops of verapamil (2.5 mg/mL) or glyceryl trinitrate (5 mg/mL). It is important to tell the anaesthetist before doing this. If the vessels have been divided, they will need to be repaired by someone experienced in microvascular techniques.

Closure

Treatment of any skin shortage in the digit requires closure of the skin with a Z-plasty. The ideal Z-plasty for closure has a 30° angle and is as large as possible. It is not necessary to locate the transverse limb of the Z-plasty at the flexor creases – this simply makes planning difficult. Often, only one Z-plasty is required to allow sufficient lengthening of the volar incision to allow comfortable closure. The skin of the finger is closed with interrupted or continuous absorbable sutures (e.g. 5/0 Vicryl rapide).

The transverse palmar incision should be left open. If the maximum width of this incision does not exceed 1.5 cm it will heal by secondary intention within 2 weeks. Leaving the palm open also simplifies closure of the hand and reduces the risk of a haematoma by allowing free drainage from the dissected areas.

Postoperative care and instructions

All patients undergoing fasciectomy should be allowed to mobilize their digits freely after treatment unless they have a significant boutonnière deformity and/or needed significant manipulation/release of the PIP joint intraoperatively. This latter group of patients should be splinted continuously in full extension for 1 week. Thereafter, all patients must use a splint at night for 3 months to keep the treated digit(s) in full extension.

DERMOFASCIECTOMY

This is a fasciectomy with excision of the proximal digital skin. The aim is to excise all the soft tissues except the tendon/tendon sheath and the neurovascular bundles on the volar side of the proximal part of the finger. The resulting defect is then resurfaced with a full-thickness skin graft. The aim is to remove any tissue that may result in subsequent recurrence of a longitudinal cord volar to the axis of flexion of the digit.

Indications

As for fasciectomy (p. 115) but with added indications:
• Recurrent disease
• Severe diathesis
• Extensive skin involvement.

Contraindications

• Inexperienced surgeon
• Patient unwilling or unable to comply with hand therapy postoperatively
• Heavy smoker and unwilling to stop smoking preoperatively.

Consent and risks

As for fasciectomy and:
• Loss of the full-thickness graft
• Loss of flexion
• Infection
• Scarring at the donor site for the skin graft

Anaesthesia and positioning

Dermofasciectomy can be performed after infiltration of local anaesthetic (single digit only), upper limb blockade and general anaesthesia. The arm should be placed supine on an arm table with a lead hand.

Surgical technique

As for fasciectomy (p. 116). The neurovascular bundles must be freed from all the soft tissues and skeletonized from the palm to the fingertip. After excising all the soft tissues between the skin and the tendon sheath, the skin on the volar side of the **proximal segment** of the finger is also excised down to the mid-lateral line (Fig. 9.3).

Correction of the flexion deformity is now checked as for a fasciectomy (p. 116). Haemostasis and perfusion of the digit are also now checked as

for a fasciectomy (p. 116). Then a full-thickness graft of appropriate size is harvested from the forearm or groin and secured to the finger with 4/0 or 5/0 Vicryl rapide. The authors' preferred approach is to anchor the four corners of the graft and then secure all the edges of the graft with a continuous over and over suture of 5/0 Vicryl rapide. The middle of the graft is then secured to the tendon sheath with two or three quilting sutures of 5/0 Vicryl rapide to reduce the tendency for the graft to slide around. This improves the take of the graft and reduces haematoma formation.

Postoperative care and instructions

The hand should be splinted with the digits in full extension for 1 week continuously. The splint and

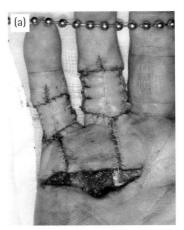

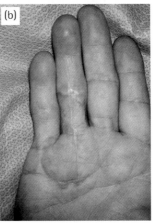

Figure 9.3 *(a) Dermofasciectomy of little and ring fingers and (b) 3 months postoperatively with healed graft*

dressings are then removed and the graft is checked. If it is pink and secure, then the patient can begin to mobilize the digit with the assistance of a hand therapist. Patients will still need to **splint the digit at night for 3 months** in full extension.

RECOMMENDED REFERENCES

Hall PN, Fitzgerald A, Sterne GD, *et al*. Skin replacement in Dupuytren's disease. *J Hand Surg Br* 1997;**22**:193–7.

Hueston JT. Recurrent Dupuytren's contracture. *Plast Reconstr Surg* 1963;**31**:66–9.

McFarlane RM. Patterns of the diseased fascia in the fingers in Dupuytren's contracture. Displacement of the neurovascular bundle. *Plast Reconstr Surg* 1974;**54**:31–44.

van Rijssen AL, Werker PM. Percutaneous needle fasciotomy in Dupuytren's disease. *J Hand Surg Br* 2006;**31**:498–501.

SYNOVIAL CYST TREATMENT

PREOPERATIVE PLANNING

Long-term follow-up of ganglia has now demonstrated that the majority of ganglia should be treated non-surgically in the first instance because 50 per cent of ganglia will resolve spontaneously within a few years and the morbidity of surgical excision is significant. This does not mean that ganglia should never be treated but patients should be informed appropriately and over-enthusiastic reliance on surgical excision should be avoided. In specific cases, simultaneous treatment of the underlying pathology (e.g. arthrodesis of a DIP joint for osteoarthritis) will remove the ganglion and the cause for the ganglion.

Indications

- Pain (may be caused by underlying pathology)
- Impaired function (if a ganglion is large enough it may catch on clothing)
- Cosmesis. This is probably the most common reason for patients to seek help.

Contraindications

There are no absolute contraindications for treating a ganglion.

Consent and risks

- Bleeding
- Infection
- Recurrence
- Joint instability
- Stiffness
- Troublesome scars

Anaesthesia and positioning

This depends on the site of the ganglion and the preference of the patient. Anaesthesia is unnecessary for aspiration of a ganglion. For excision of a ganglion in the digit, most cases can be treated under local anaesthesia. However, excision of a ganglion at the wrist should be treated under regional block or general anaesthesia as the dissection is often involved. A tourniquet should be used in all cases.

SURGICAL TECHNIQUE

Aspiration of ganglia

The largest gauge needle compatible with comfort for the patient is attached to a 2 mL syringe – typically, a blue hub (23G) needle. The needle is plunged into the ganglion with one swift movement and aspiration begun immediately. If the contents will not enter the syringe, the needle is extracted and the contents manually expressed through the small puncture hole. Injecting a small amount of Adcortyl (5 mg) into the ganglion/adjacent tissues reduces post-treatment inflammation and discomfort.

Flexor sheath ganglia

Landmarks and incision

Typically, the ganglion arises from the A2 pulley at the level of the proximal finger crease. A transverse incision, directly over the ganglion, is used.

Dissection and procedure

The ganglion is excised *en bloc* with (if necessary) a small cuff of the flexor sheath.

Closure

The skin is approximated with interrupted 5/0 Vicryl rapide sutures. A light dressing is applied, which will not impede movement and allows immediate mobilization.

Mucous cysts

Landmarks and incision

Typically, the ganglion arises dorsally from the joint capsule of the DIP joint. As it enlarges, it emerges on either the ulnar or radial side of the finger in the interval between the terminal extensor tendon and the collateral ligament of the joint (Fig. 9.4). The skin over the mucous cyst is often very thin. Therefore, attempts to separate the skin from the ganglion wall are frequently fruitless. The surgeon can decide to either excise the skin with the ganglion or simply make a longitudinal incision over the ganglion knowing that it will burst.

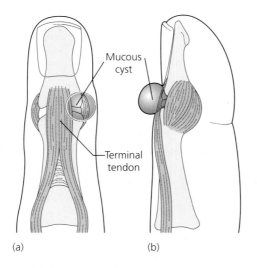

Mucous cyst

Terminal tendon

(a)   (b)

Figure 9.4 *A mucous cyst*

Dissection and procedure

Whether or not an ellipse of skin was excised with the ganglion, excision of the rest of the ganglion wall is often an academic exercise because the remnant is usually so flimsy. Excise whatever remains of the ganglion wall (piecemeal if necessary) down to the DIP joint. Any obvious osteophytes should also be removed with a bone nibbler as this improves cosmesis.

Closure

The skin is closed with interrupted 5/0 Vicryl rapide sutures. If an overly large ellipse of skin has been excised, it will be difficult to close the skin directly. The options then are to use a small split-thickness skin graft or a local flap – converting an operation of dubious value (excising a mucous cyst) into an operation with a multitude of potential complications! If the defect is very small and no important structures are exposed, then allowing the wound to heal by secondary intention may be acceptable. The finger is dressed lightly, which allows immediate mobilization.

POSTOPERATIVE CARE AND INSTRUCTIONS

The hand is elevated to reduce pain and swelling. Any bulky dressings are removed after 48–72 hours. The hand/finger is mobilized, with the help of a hand therapist, as quickly as possible.

RECOMMENDED REFERENCES

Dias JJ, Dhukaram V, Kumar P. The natural history of untreated dorsal wrist ganglia and patient reported outcome 6 years after intervention. *J Hand Surg Eur Vol* 2007;**32**:502–8.

Green DP, Hotchkiss RN, Pederson WC (eds). *Green's Operative Hand Surgery* (5th edn). Edinburgh: Elsevier, 2005.

ARTHRODESIS IN THE HAND

PREOPERATIVE PLANNING

Indications

An arthrodesis is a very reasonable salvage treatment for certain joints and for certain situations, which can restore pain-free form and function in one operative step. Indications include:
• Pain
• Instability
• Deformity
• Failed arthroplasty
• Joints where arthroplasty is not desirable/possible

Certain joints respond well to arthrodesis because of the functional requirements of the hand. Others do less well (see operative planning – below).

Contraindications

• Poor skin cover over the joint
• Active infection in the upper limb – inserting metalwork should be avoided
• Non-compliant patient – the joint needs to be immobilized for 8 weeks after surgery to allow bony union
• Smoking is a contraindication because of poor wound healing.

Consent and risks

• Damage to any of the adjacent structures (e.g. tendons, neurovascular bundles, damage to the nail bed in DIP joint fusion)
• Infection
• Malunion
• Non-union (up to 10 per cent – especially the DIP joint)
• Stiffness of adjacent joints and fingers
• Flexor and/or extensor adhesions.

Operative planning

Distal interphalangeal joint

Patients do very well after arthrodesis of these joints because joint replacements do very badly

here and the loss of range of movement at the DIP joint has little effect on overall hand function. DIP joint arthrodesis is a particularly useful treatment for rupture of the flexor digitorum profundus (FDP) tendon, chronic mallet deformity or painful arthritis of the DIP joint (with or without deformity) and chronic mucous cyst.

Proximal interphalangeal joint

Arthrodesis of the PIP joints results in significant impairment of hand function but is still a reasonable option to deal with chronic pain and instability, especially for the little and ring fingers. This is because PIP joint replacements do particularly badly in the little and ring fingers.

Interphalangeal (IP) joint of the thumb

The IP joint of the thumb responds very well to arthrodesis.

Metacarpophalangeal joint

The MCP joints of the fingers should not be arthrodesed as this results in very significant impairment of function. In contrast, arthrodesis of the MCP joint of the thumb is an excellent procedure which significantly enhances hand function.

Carpometacarpal (CMC) joint

The first CMC joint should not be fused, as this will result in very significant impairment of hand function. The second and third CMC joints normally behave as if they are fused, therefore, arthrodesis of these joints is seldom necessary. The fourth and fifth CMC joints are surprisingly mobile in normal hands. Nevertheless, arthrodesis is a reasonable solution to problems of chronic pain and instability (typically after trauma).

Anaesthesia and positioning

Local anaesthetic digital block with finger tourniquet is suitable for IP joint, DIP joint or PIP joint arthrodesis. Regional block or general anaesthesia with arm tourniquet is suitable for arthrodesis of the thumb MCP joint or CMC joints.

SURGICAL TECHNIQUE

Several different techniques are available for arthrodesis of a joint (e.g. K-wires, interosseous wires, screws, plates and staples). Different methods of fixation are more or less suitable for particular joints and in particular situations. Regardless of the technique, the usefulness of the arthrodesis is determined by the final position of the bones after fusion (Table 9.1). Also, the arthrodesed digit will be shorter by the amount of bone that needs to be removed to allow the arthrodesis to be performed.

Landmarks and incisions

- DIP and thumb IP joint – an 'H' or 'Y' incision over dorsum of joint or a mid-lateral incision for plating (Fig. 9.5).
- PIP joint – longitudinal incision over dorsum of joint.
- Thumb MCP joint – longitudinal incision over dorsum of joint.
- CMC or intercarpal arthrodesis – longitudinal incisions over the dorsum of the relevant joint.

Fusion techniques

This depends on the joint. Image intensifier control (preferably using a mini-C-arm) is absolutely essential to ensure that any metalwork goes in the right place.

Distal interphalangeal joint

The terminal extensor tendon is detached from the base of the distal phalanx, exposing the joint. The collateral ligaments are excised and the volar plate detached from the base of the distal phalanx. This allows the joint to be disarticulated completely. The joint surfaces are removed with a saw or bone nibbler to expose the cancellous bone

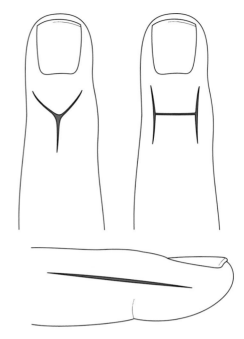

Figure 9.5 *Incisions for access to DIP joint*

and create matching surfaces, ensuring that there are two flat surfaces with the correct angulation (i.e. 0–10°). For fixation, 90–90° wiring is probably the easiest technique. Tension band wiring is also acceptable but technically more difficult to do (Fig. 9.6). Other acceptable alternatives include a Lister loop (although the K-wire needs to be removed at 8 weeks), Herbert or cannulated screw fixation and plating.

Table 9.1 Arthrodesis positions in the hand

	Thumb	Index	Middle	Ring	Little
DIP joint	*N/A*	*0–10°*	*0–10°*	*0–10°*	*0–10°*
PIP joint	*N/A*	*30°*	*30–40°*	*40–50°*	*50°*
IP joint	*0–20°*	*N/A*	*N/A*	*N/A*	*N/A*
MCP joint	*0°*	*Do not fuse*	*Do not fuse*	*Do not fuse*	*Do not fuse*
CMC joint	*Do not fuse*	*0°*	*0°*	*0°*	*0°*

N/A, not applicable.

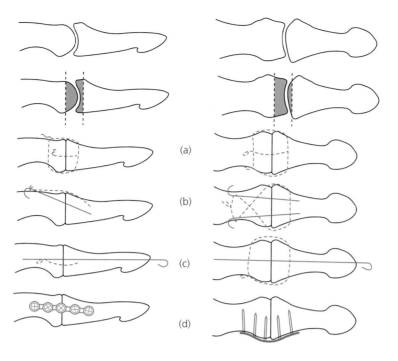

Figure 9.6 *Methods of distal interphalangeal (DIP) joint fusion. (a) '90–90' wiring. Two interosseous wires of 0.35 to 0.45 gauge dental wire passed at 90° to each other. (b) Tension band wiring using two 1.1 mm K-wires and a 0.35–0.45 gauge dental wire. (c) Lister loop with a single 1.1 mm K-wire and a 0.35–0.45 gauge dental wire. The K-wire must be removed at 4 weeks. (d) Plating of the DIP joint with a mini-plate (the most difficult technique)*

Proximal interphalangeal joint

A longitudinal split in the extensor tendon or a Chamay approach (distally based 'V' shaped incision in the central slip; Fig. 9.7) can be used to expose the PIP joint. The joint is disarticulated by excising the collaterals and detaching the volar plate. The joint surfaces are removed with a saw or a bone nibbler to create two flat surfaces with the correct angulation (Table 9.1).

As for the DIP joint, there is no preferred method for fixation. Any of the techniques which are used for the DIP joint are also suitable for the PIP joint. The authors' preference is to use a tension band technique.

Metacarpophalangeal joint of the thumb

The joint is exposed through a longitudinal split in the extensor tendon and disarticulated by excising the collateral ligaments and detaching the volar plate. The joint surfaces are excised. The authors' preference for arthrodesis of the thumb MCP joint is a tension band wire technique.

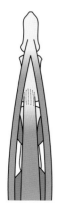
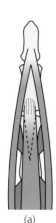
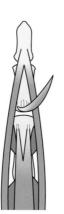
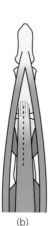
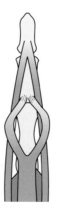

(a)   (b)

Figure 9.7
(a) Chamay approach.
(b) Longitudinal split

Carpometacarpal joint

The extensor tendons are retracted from over the CMC joints and soft tissue excised to expose the specific joint. The image intensifier confirms that the correct joint has been identified. The joint surfaces are excised and bone graft is inserted. The graft is harvested from the distal radius. Bone substitute (e.g. hydroxyapatite) can also be used. The joint is secured with an oblique K-wire passed through the base of the respective metacarpal and the corresponding trapezoid, capitate or hamate. The wire is buried and removed after 8 weeks.

Closure

The extensor tendons are repaired with 4/0 or 5/0 PDS interrupted or continuous sutures. The tourniquet is released and haemostasis achieved with bipolar diathermy. The wound is washed out with saline and closed with interrupted absorbable 4/0 or 5/0 Monocryl sutures and a subcuticular 5/0 Monocryl or 4/0/5/0 Vicryl rapide suture.

Interrupted, non-absorbable sutures on the dorsum of the hand and fingers should be avoided as they leave very unsightly suture marks.

Postoperative care and instructions

A light dressing is used and removed after 48–72 hours to allow active mobilization of the joints on either side of the treated joint. A splint must be used to immobilize the joint for 8 weeks.

- Scars are massaged from 2 weeks onwards. Coban elastic bandage is applied to reduce swelling at about 2 weeks post-surgery.

RECOMMENDED REFERENCES

Allende BT, Engelem JC. Tension band arthrodesis in the finger joints. *J Hand Surg Am* 1980;**5**:269–71.

Green DP, Hotchkiss RN, Pederson WC (eds). *Green's Operative Hand Surgery* (5th edn). Edinburgh: Elsevier, 2005.

Lister G. Intraosseous wiring of the digital skeleton. *J Hand Surg Am* 1978;**3**:427–35.

Pechlaner S, Hussl H, Kerschbaumer F. *Atlas of Hand Surgery*. Stuttgart: Thieme, 2000.

Sennwald G, Segmuller G. The metacarpophalangeal arthrodesis of the thumb according to the tension-band principle: indications and technique. *Ann Chir Main* 1983;**2**:38–45.

ARTHROPLASTY IN THE HAND

PREOPERATIVE PLANNING

The decision to operate **must not be made on the basis of the X-ray appearances alone**. However, function is not always the only consideration. Although it is generally not a good idea to perform an arthroplasty in patients who have good function, some patients still ask for surgery to 'improve' the appearance of their hands.

Indications

- Painful or stiff joints unresponsive to medical treatment
- Deformity and/or loss of range of movement affecting activities of daily living
- Failure of conservative measures. Before this can be said, patients must have had an adequate trial of:
  - Regular non-steroidal anti-inflammatory drugs (NSAIDs) and splintage
  - Steroid injections (administer at least one or two of these)
  - Using home or work aids
  - Appropriate alterations to their home or work circumstances
- To 'improve' the appearance of the hand
- MCP joint in preference to PIP joint
- Index or middle finger PIP joints

Contraindications

- Absent or poor flexor or extensor tendon function
- Absent or poor nerve function (e.g. peripheral neuropathy)
- Patients with significant vascular compromise (e.g. scleroderma, Raynaud's phenomenon)
- Patients with poor skin cover over the joint
- Patient unwilling or unable to comply with postoperative hand therapy

- Heavy smoker and unwilling to stop preoperatively
- DIP joint – an arthrodesis is recommended
- PIP joint of ring and little fingers – joint instability is often worse in these digits.

Consent and risks

- Flexor tendon/neurovascular injury
- Instability (only for PIP joint arthroplasty)
- Recurrent deformity (affects one-third of arthroplasties)
- Dislocation, loosening or fracture of the implant (implant failure affects one-third of implants)
- Infection necessitating removal of implant
- Loss of range of movement
- Ongoing pain
- Dislocation, fracture or extrusion of the implant (7–15 per cent).
- Silicone synovitis

Operative planning

The choice is between a replacement arthroplasty or a resurfacing/interposition arthroplasty. A replacement arthroplasty excises the joint completely and replaces it with an artificial or autologous joint (usually taken from the foot). Artificial joints do better in older/lower-demand patients. A resurfacing/interposition arthroplasty is less destructive and tries to restore the normal shape of the joint using either autologous or artificial materials and is more suitable for young or active patients.

In general, replacement arthroplasty works best for the MCP joints and not the PIP joints. If PIP joint arthroplasty must be considered, then this is best done in the index and middle fingers only. DIP joint arthroplasty is rarely successful. These patients are better served by an arthrodesis.

Many types of artificial material have been described for replacement arthroplasty. The only material that has withstood the test of time is silicone, e.g. Swanson's implant (Fig. 9.8). The technique for insertion is described here.

Anaesthesia and positioning

Local, regional or general anaesthesia can be used. The position is supine with the hand on an arm table.

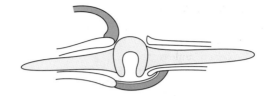

Figure 9.8 *Swanson's implant in place*

SURGICAL TECHNIQUE

Metacarpophalangeal joint

Landmarks and incision

A longitudinal incision (straight or curvilinear) is made over the dorsum of the joint. Any curvature in the incision is usually towards the radial side. This makes it easier to access and reef the radial saggital bands of the extensor hood. Reefing of the extensor hood allows ulnar subluxation of the extensors to be corrected in rheumatoid arthritis.

Dissection

The skin and subcutaneous fat are widely degloved over the joint to expose the extensor tendons and the saggital bands. The sagittal bands are divided longitudinally on the radial side, leaving a minimum 2–3 mm fringe along the edge of the extensor tendon: this allows the bands to be reefed at a later stage. The extensor mechanism is now freed from the underlying capsule and retracted ulnarly. The joint capsule is often flimsy in these patients and it is often easiest to simply excise it. After excising the capsule and any associated synovial tissue, any remnants of the collateral ligaments can also be excised.

Procedure

The volar plate must be freed from the neck of the metacarpal to allow the base of the proximal phalanx to come into correct alignment with the metacarpal. The metacarpal head is now excised with an oscillating saw. In the rheumatoid patient, the metacarpal head is often excised with a slight radial tilt to help correct any ulnar drift. The amount of bone excised is determined by the need to accommodate intrinsic muscle tightness: the tighter the intrinsics, the more bone that needs to be excised (up to a limit – excessive shortening is best avoided). The base of the proximal phalanx is not excised unless there is severe deformity. However, any osteophytes must be removed with bone nibblers since these may interfere with flexion.

The base of the proximal phalanx is now pierced with an awl. This opening is enlarged and the medullary cavities of the proximal phalanx and metacarpal are now reamed by hand using progressively larger reamers. Sizers are used to determine the correct size of Swanson's implant which should be used. In general, the largest implant that fits should be selected. The implant fits when the long stem fits snugly in the metacarpal and the short stem fits snugly in the proximal phalanx. There should be no compression of the mid-section with the fingers in extension. Generally, size 3 or 4 implants are used for the MCP joints.

The sizer is removed and the wound is washed out with saline. The appropriate permanent implant is inserted using a 'no touch' technique. The implants are usually supplied with stainless steel 'grommets'. These should not be used.

Closure

It is not necessary to formally repair the collateral ligaments – scar tissue forms rapidly around the implant and confers some stability to the joint. The sagittal bands are repaired with 4/0 or 5/0 PDS and are reefed as necessary if there is significant subluxation of the extensor tendons into the ulnar gutters.

The skin is then closed with absorbable sutures. The author recommends using interrupted 5/0 Monocryl for the dermis (to approximate the wound edges) then a running subcuticular 5/0 Monocryl suture for final closure.

PROXIMAL INTERPHALANGEAL JOINT

Landmarks and incision

A longitudinal incision (straight or curvilinear) is made over the dorsum of the joint.

Dissection

After the incision is made, the skin and subcutaneous fat are widely degloved over the joint to expose the extensor tendon and the lateral bands. To reach the joint, the central slip of the extensor tendon can be split longitudinally or a Chamay approach used (see Fig. 9.7). It is important to preserve the central slip insertion whichever method is used.

As with the MCP joint, the capsule of the PIP joint is usually very flimsy and excised together with any associated synovium. If possible, the collateral ligaments and volar plate are preserved to maintain the stability of the joint. However, sometimes these structures are grossly damaged and it is necessary to excise/detach them to restore the correct alignment of the proximal and middle phalanges.

Procedure

Structure at risk

- Flexor tendon

The head of the proximal phalanx is now excised, at neutral, using an oscillating saw. Care is taken not to damage the flexor tendon on the volar side of the joint. The base of the middle phalanx is not normally resected except in severe deformity. However, osteophytes must be nibbled away as these may interfere with flexion. Sizing and reaming of the middle and proximal phalanges is performed in the same way as for the MCP joint. For the PIP joint **a size 1 or 2 implant is usually used**.

Closure

The longitudinal split in the extensor tendon or the Chamay flap is repaired with a continuous 4/0 or 5/0 PDS suture. In all other respects, closure is the same as described for MCJ arthroplasty.

POSTOPERATIVE CARE AND INSTRUCTIONS

- **MCP joint**: Patients are placed in a resting splint or bulky bandage for 3–5 days. This is then replaced with alternate-day flexion (MCP joints at 70–90°) and then extension (MCP joint at neutral) splints for 24-hour periods. After 4 weeks these splints are worn at night only and the patient mobilizes the hand during the day with protective splinting only.

- **PIP joint**: The digit is placed in a T-bar splint. This keeps the PIP joint in full extension and the MCP joint flexed at 60° for 6 weeks at night and at rest. During the day, the patient is encouraged to begin immediate, regular, active mobilization of the PIP joint out of the splint.

The emphasis in therapy for both MCP and PIP joint arthroplasty is early, supervised, active and passive movement.

RECOMMENDED REFERENCES

Swanson AB. Silicone rubber implants for replacement of arthritic or destroyed joint in the hand. *Surg Clin North Am* 1968;**48**:1113–27.

Swanson AB. Flexible implant arthroplasty for arthritic finger joints: rationale, technique and results of treatment. *J Bone Joint Surg Am* 1972;**54**:435–7.

Takigawa S, Meletiou S, Sauerbier M, *et al.* Long-term assessment of Swanson implant arthroplasty in the proximal interphalangeal joint of the hand. *J Hand Surg Am* 2004;**29**:785–95.

EXTENSOR TENDON REPAIR

PREOPERATIVE PLANNING

Injuries to the extensor apparatus of the hand are common and non-surgical intervention is often the best form of treatment for some of the commoner injuries – especially in the finger. The key to a successful outcome is recognition of the specific injury and selection of the appropriate form of surgical repair, splintage and/or early mobilization required to deal with the particular problem. Treatment differs depending on the zone of injury (Fig. 9.9; Table 9.2) and whether the patient presents early (within a few days) or late (weeks or months later). In all cases, appropriate hand therapy and splintage is more important than any surgery in restoring full function.

Indications and operative planning

- **Zone 1 – a mallet deformity**. If it is open, the wound should be washed out as the DIP joint is

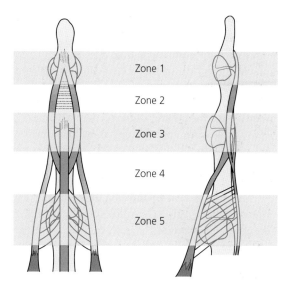

Figure 9.9 *The zones of the extensor tendon*

Table 9.2 Anatomy of the extensor tendon

Zone	Description of tendon anatomy
1	The terminal tendon formed from the convergence of the two lateral bands
2	Lateral bands held together by the triangular ligament
3	Insertion of the central slip into the proximal phalanx
4	Central slip and intrinsic tendons
5	Extensor hood
6	Over the metacarpals
7	Over the wrist
8	In the forearm

often opened as well. The skin is then closed (converting an open mallet injury into a closed mallet injury) but the extensor tendon should not be repaired. Surgical repair is usually fruitless and leaves sutures close to the skin where they often extrude. If 12 weeks of dedicated and consistent splintage fails, then the patient should either accept the position or consider arthrodesis of the DIP joint. An avulsion fracture of the insertion of the terminal extensor tendon also results in a mallet deformity. **This fracture does not need surgical fixation** regardless of the size of the fragment and the appearances on an X-ray.

- **Zone 2** – injuries to the extensor apparatus in zone 2 result in a mallet deformity and are treated as for injuries in zone 1.
- **Zone 3** – injury to the central slip results in a boutonnière deformity and is often a late presentation. If this is an open injury and the damage to the central slip is recognized acutely, then it is worth considering surgical reinsertion of the central slip. The lack of soft tissue for reattachment means a mini-Mitek bone anchor or a 'washing-line' will need to be used to suture the tendon to the bone (see below for details of the surgical technique). Even if the central slip is reinserted surgically, the patient will need the same splintage and hand therapy postoperatively as for a closed injury. Therefore, there is a strong argument for not doing anything other than closing the skin as in zones 1 and 2. If the presentation is delayed or chronic, the PIP joint is statically splinted in full extension for 3 weeks followed by treatment with a Capener (dynamic) splint for another 3 weeks. Only if this fails should surgery be considered to reinsert/reef the central slip and/or to mobilize the lateral bands which will have slipped volar to the axis of movement of the PIP joint.
- **Zone 4** – injuries in zone 4 behave like injuries in zone 3. However, there is now sufficient tendon material to consider surgical repair using interrupted horizontal mattress sutures of 4/0 PDS.
- **Zone 5** – injuries in zone 5 result in an extensor lag which can be very debilitating. Patients usually do very well after surgical repair of the tendons in this zone followed by early active mobilization (see below for mobilization regimen).
- **Zones 6–8** – in these zones, the extensor tendons are more rounded, making a surgical repair much easier.

Contraindications

- Active infection – the repair will rupture and the tendon will become adherent
- Skeletal instability – unstable fractures must be fixed at the same time as any tendon repair
- Fixed joints

- Delayed presentation (more than 6–8 weeks) of extensor ruptures in zone 6, 7 and 8 can rarely be repaired primarily because the tendon ends will have retracted and shortened
- Attrition ruptures – tendon grafts or transfers are required and may or may not be possible
- Smoker
- Poor social or psychological circumstances. Patients who do not understand their injury and cannot/do not comply with the hand therapy that is required after a tendon injury seldom regain full function of the affected part. This often includes very young children
- If there is 20 per cent (or less) division or loss of the extensor apparatus at any level then the skin should be closed and the tendon injury ignored.

Consent and risks

- Scars: it is often necessary to extend the wounds to gain access to the tendon ends
- Splintage and physiotherapy: the patient will not have full use of the affected hand for 8–10 weeks. This may have significant economic consequences. The importance of compliance with the postoperative physiotherapy must be stressed
- Infection
- Rupture: 5 per cent
- Adhesions: a particular problem if there is an underlying fracture.
- Bowstringing: in zone 7 injuries

Anaesthesia and positioning

For finger injuries up to zone 5, a ring block is sufficient. For more proximal injuries, in zones 6–8, a general anaesthesia or regional block is used. Positioning is supine with an arm table and a tourniquet appropriate to the part affected.

SURGICAL TECHNIQUE

Landmarks and incisions

If there is a skin laceration over the injured extensor tendon then it can be incorporated into any incision after suitable debridement of the wound edges. Incisions are extended proximally and distally as needed to gain access to the tendon ends. This is particularly necessary in zones 6, 7 and 8 where the proximal ends may have retracted a considerable distance.

'Zig-zag' or 'lazy-S' incisions are preferred as these heal better when making long incisions over the dorsum of the hand and wrist.

Dissection

Structures at risk

- Edges of the skin flaps
- Dorsal veins and nerves

Skin and subcutaneous fat are incised and then skin flaps are elevated. These can be retracted with skin hooks or held in place with 'stay' sutures. The dorsal veins and nerves are always preserved where possible.

The extensor tendons are identified and care is taken to preserve the paratenon.

Procedure

- **Zones 1 and 2** – the tendon injury is treated non-operatively.
- **Zone 3** – where appropriate, the central slip can be reinserted using a mini-Mitek anchor or a 'washing-line' (Fig. 9.10). Two mini-Miteks are inserted into the base of the middle phalanx.

The PIP joint is fully extended and the central slip secured with the two strands of suture. Alternatively, a 0.35–0.45 gauge dental wire is inserted across the base of the middle phalanx. The wire is formed into a loop close to the bone, leaving enough of a gap to allow the passage of multiple sutures under the wire. The whole wire now acts as a suture anchor allowing multiple sutures to be passed into the central slip and under the 'washing line'.

- **Zones 4 and 5** – the extensor tendon is flat, so horizontal mattress sutures using 5/0 or 4/0 PDS are best for the repair. The repair is augmented with a continuous, over and over suture of 5/0 PDS to keep the tendon ends tidy (Fig. 9.11). In zone 5, any lacerations to the sagittal bands must be repaired with 5/0 PDS to prevent the extensor tendon subluxing into the radial or ulnar gutters.
- **Zones 6–8** – the ends of the tendon are minimally trimmed and repaired with a modified Kessler core suture, using a 3/0 or 4/0 PDS. If necessary, the core suture can be further augmented with a single horizontal mattress suture of 4/0 PDS. A continuous epitendinous suture is then placed around the circumference of the repair using 5/0 or 6/0 PDS (Fig. 9.12).

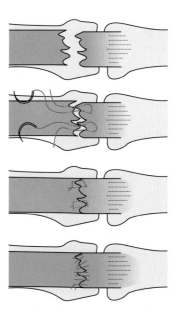

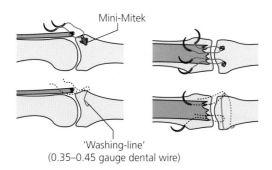

Figure 9.10. *Reinserting the central slip with mini-Mite anchors or a 'washing line'*

Figure 9.11 *Repair of an extensor tendon in zones 4 and 5*

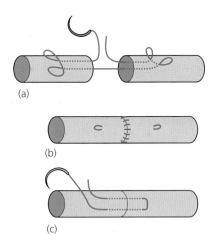

(a)

(b)

(c)

Figure 9.12 *Zones 6–8 extensor tendon repair. (a) Kessler stitch, (b) epitendinous suture and (c) augmentation with a horizontal mattress suture*

This also augments the repair and helps to keep the tendon ends tidy. A round-bodied needle is preferred for both core and epitendinous sutures to reduce the chance of cutting the core suture accidentally.

If a primary repair of the extensor tendon cannot be performed (e.g. delayed presentation or loss of tendon substance) an interposition tendon graft or tendon transfer must be used, e.g. with palmaris longus tendon. A Pulvertaft weave (Fig. 9.13) must be used to secure the tendon graft to the ends of the tendon as this is strong enough to allow early mobilization.

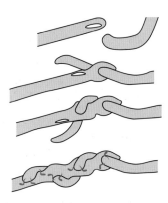

Figure 9.13 *A Pulvertaft weave*

In Zone 7, free excursion of the repaired extensor tendon is confirmed under the retinaculum. If necessary, the retinaculum is divided to allow free movement of the tendon but preserving as much of it intact as possible prevents later bowstringing.

The repair is now tested by passively flexing and extending the finger. There must be no gaping of the repair and it must glide freely through the full excursion of the tendon.

Closure

The tourniquet is released and haemostasis achieved. The wound is washed out with saline and closed with interrupted absorbable 4/0 or 5/0 Monocryl sutures and a subcuticular 5/0 Monocryl suture. Interrupted, non-absorbable sutures are avoided on the dorsum of the hand and fingers as this leaves very unsightly suture marks.

Mepitel is applied to the wound together with dressing gauze and Velband before placing the hand and forearm in a volar slab plaster of Paris with the fingers in full extension. The plaster should be set before the patient comes off the operating table.

POSTOPERATIVE CARE AND INSTRUCTIONS

The authors use the Norwich regimen for injuries in zones 5–7. The plaster of Paris is replaced with a thermoplastic splint the day after surgery. Passive and active extension is commenced straight away, protected in the splint for 4 weeks. For a further 4 weeks, the patient removes the splint for active extension and active flexion of the IP joint/MCP joint, but wears it at all other times.

For central slip injuries (zones 3 to 4) the finger is placed in a cylinder splint (PIP joint static in extension, DIP joint free) for 3 weeks and then 3 further weeks in a Capener splint.

RECOMMENDED REFERENCES

Abouna JM, Brown H. The treatment of mallet finger. The results in a series of 148 consecutive cases and a review of the literature. *Br J Surg* 1968;**55**:653.

Lange RH, Engber WD. Hyperextension mallet finger. *Orthopedics* 1983;**6**:1426.

Newport ML, Williams CD. Biomechanical characteristics of extensor tendon suture techniques. *J Hand Surg Am* 1992;**17**:111.

Newport ML, Pollack GR, Williams CD. Biomechanical characteristics of suture techniques in extensor zone IV. *J Hand Surg Am* 1995;**20**:650–6.

Stuart D. Duration of splinting after repair of extensor tendons in the hand. A clinical study. *J Bone Joint Surg Br* 1965;**47**:72.

Sylaidis P, Youatt M, Logan A. Early active mobilization for extensor tendon injuries. The Norwich regime. *J Hand Surg Br* 1997;**22**:594.

Wehbé MA, Schneider L. Mallet fractures. *J Bone Joint Surg Am* 1984;**66**:658.

FLEXOR TENDON REPAIR

PREOPERATIVE PLANNING

Indications and operative planning

- **Zone 1** – the technique for flexor repair in zone 1 depends on how close to the insertion the FDP has been divided. If the tendon is divided close to the bone (e.g. FDP avulsion) then it may be necessary to use a suture anchor such as a mini-Mitek to secure the tendon end.
- **Zone 2** – proximal zone 1 and zone 2 repairs of the FDP tendon are similar. The aim is to repair the tendon but to avoid any bulkiness at the repair site to allow the tendon to glide within the flexor sheath. If the repair is done badly it will be too bulky and may trigger, rupture or jam in position unless the flexor sheath is opened. Special care must be taken with repairs of FDS in this zone (see below).
- **Zone 3** – zone 3 repairs are easier to perform because there is no tight flexor sheath to contend with and the tendon ends are larger. Distal zone 3 repairs may catch on the A1 pulley, which may need to be divided.
- **Zones 4–5** – repairs in these zones are the same as repairs of the extensor tendons in zones 6–8.
- **Complete division** – primary repair of a flexor tendon rupture should be performed as soon as possible. Unlike the extensor tendons, surgical intervention of some form is always necessary when the flexor tendons have been divided.
- **Timing of repair** – there is good evidence that the outcome of primary repair is superior when carried out as quickly as possible (within 72 hours). There is a particular urgency in carrying out a repair of the flexor tendons (as compared with extensor tendons) because the flexor pulleys will eventually collapse/fill with scar tissue after 3–4 weeks. Any tendon repair will then need to reconstruct the pulleys as well, making surgery more complicated than necessary.
- **Particular tendons** – the flexor muscle bellies (especially flexor pollicis longus – FPL) have a tendency to shorten quickly. This may make primary repair of a tendon impossible. The ring and middle fingers are particularly prone to avulsion injuries of the FDP tendon. Repair of combined injuries of flexor digitorum superficialis (FDS)/FDP tendons in the little and ring fingers are particularly prone to formation of adhesions. Therefore, consideration should be given to repairing just the FDP tendon in these digits.
- **Zone of injury** – as for extensor tendons, the surgical technique for repair of flexor tendons varies depending on the zone of injury (Fig. 9.14).

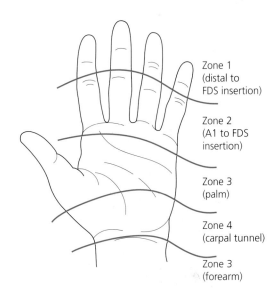

Figure 9.14 *The zones of flexor tendon injury. FDS, flexor digitorum superficialis*

- **Partial division of flexor tendons** – there is good evidence that inserting sutures into a tendon results in necrosis of the tendon substance. Therefore, the use of sutures should be avoided for any partial tendon injury involving less than 50 per cent of the diameter of the tendon. Instead, we recommend trimming the edges of the tendon laceration to prevent triggering (if any is present) followed by supervised mobilization in a splint as for a complete flexor tendon division for the next 8 weeks.

Contraindications

- Active infection
- Skeletal instability
- Fixed joints
- Delayed presentation (more than 3–4 weeks) can rarely be repaired primarily as the tendon ends will have retracted and shortened and the flexor pulleys will have collapsed.
- Attrition ruptures
- Smoker
- Poor social or psychological circumstances
- Partial tendon rupture of less than 50 per cent should not be repaired
- Delayed presentation.

Consent and risks

- Scars: it is often necessary to extend the wounds to gain access to the tendon ends
- Splintage and physiotherapy: patients will not have full use of the affected hand for 12 weeks. The importance of compliance with the postoperative physiotherapy must be stressed
- Infection
- Adhesions: a particular problem when there is an underlying fracture. Overall, there is a 5 per cent tenolysis rate
- Rupture: zone 2 finger flexors – 5 per cent, FPL repair – 12 per cent
- Bowstringing: may not be evident for some years after the original event. It may occur if it proves necessary to divide the flexor sheath completely in order to repair the tendons. A subsequent pulley reconstruction will then be required
- Neuroma formation

Anaesthesia and positioning

For isolated FDP injuries, it is often possible to perform a repair under digital nerve block with a finger tourniquet. For FPL, FDS and more proximal flexor injuries, general anaesthesia or a regional block is necessary because of the need for an arm tourniquet. The arm is positioned in the supine position with an arm table.

SURGICAL TECHNIQUE

Landmarks and incisions

The Bruner (zigzag) incision (Fig. 9.15) is preferred. If there is a laceration then it can be incorporated into the incision after suitable debridement of the wound edges. Bruner incisions are marked out and the skin and fat are incised down to the level of the flexor sheath using a no. 15 scalpel blade and/or tenotomy scissors.

Dissection

Structures at risk

- Edges of the skin flaps
- Neurovascular bundles

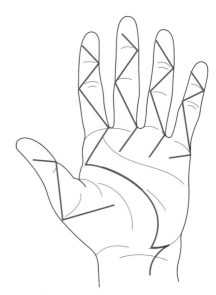

Figure 9.15 *Suggested Bruner incisions to approach the flexors*

The flaps can be retracted with skin hooks or held in place with 'stay' sutures. A 'window' is opened in the flexor sheath by creating zigzag flaps. Ideally, the window should be as small as possible and should be positioned only between the annular pulleys to allow maximum preservation of the pulley system.

If the flexor sheath is opened with zigzag flaps it is usually possible to repair the sheath with a slightly larger diameter by approximating the tips of the flaps. This will allow any reconstructed pulley system to accommodate a more bulky, less than perfect, tendon repair.

Procedure

Tendon retrieval

If a tendon has been fully divided, flexion of the finger or thumb normally delivers the distal end into the wound. If the proximal end of the tendon has retracted it can sometimes be retrieved by passing a small curved artery clip into the flexor sheath. If this proves impossible, then the palm of the hand must be opened and the tendons pushed up into the finger with forceps. If the laceration is in the wrist or palm, it may be necessary to extend incisions even more proximally to find the tendon ends. Once retrieved, a 20G (blue-hub) needle can be passed through the tendon ends to prevent them from retracting again until the repair is complete.

Tendon suture technique

Zone 1 – If there is a very short stump of tendon (<1 cm), then it is possible to repair the tendon by inserting 4/0 or 5/0 PDS sutures as a half-Kessler proximally and horizontal mattress distally. Multiple sutures can be inserted to increase the strength of the repair since there is no concern about the bulk of the repair getting caught in the flexor sheath. When the tendon is avulsed and/or there is a fracture of the distal phalanx, then alternative methods of fixation must be considered, e.g. suture the tendon to the remnants of the periosteum or use a suture anchor such as two mini-Miteks. If there is a fracture, then mini-plate fixation is the best option to repair the fracture, using the plate as a suture anchor.

Flexor digitorum superficialis distal to the metacarpophalangeal joint

If the FDS is injured where it is beginning to flatten out or after it has split into its two terminal slips, then horizontal mattress sutures must be used to repair the tendon because there will not be enough tendon substance for a modified Kessler core suture. Each terminal slip must be repaired separately. If there is room for it, an epitendinous suture using 5/0 or 6/0 PDS can be used to tidy the ends of the repair. Note that in combined FDS/FDP injuries of the little and ring fingers there is an argument for **not repairing the FDS** tendon to avoid creating two bulky tendon repairs, both of which will be unable to glide in the flexor sheath.

FDP, FPL and FDS proximal to the metacarpophalangeal joint

The tendon ends are approximated and held in position by transfixing them with a 20G needle. The ends of the tendon are minimally trimmed and the back wall of the repair is begun with a continuous 5/0 or 6/0 PDS over and over suture. A modified Kessler core suture is now inserted using 4/0 or 3/0 PDS, taking particular care to bury the knot. The core suture can now be augmented with a single horizontal mattress suture using 4/0 PDS. The anterior part of the epitendinous suture is then completed (Fig. 9.16). The core suture should always be over-tightened to prevent gaping when early active mobilization is started postoperatively. A round-bodied needle should also be used to reduce the risk of cutting the core suture accidentally. There must be no gaping of the repair and it must glide freely through the full excursion of the tendon when the repair is complete. Any pulleys restricting the glide of the tendon should be divided in a zigzag fashion or excised altogether.

Closure

All wounds are washed out with saline and closed with interrupted absorbable 4/0 or 5/0 Vicryl rapide sutures. Unlike the dorsum of the hand, suture marks are not so much of a problem on the volar side because of the thicker epidermis. Therefore, subcuticular sutures do not have to be used.

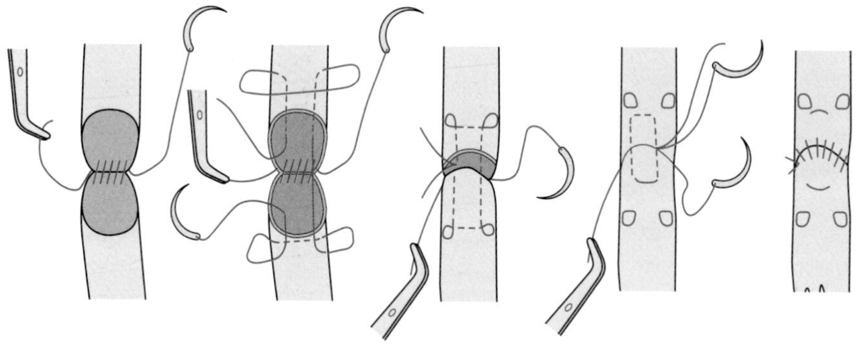

(a)   (b)   (c)   (d)   (e)

Figure 9.16a–e *Steps in the repair of flexor tendons*

Mepitel, dressing gauze and Velband bandage are applied and the hand and forearm are placed in a dorsal plaster of Paris with the fingers flexed at 90° at the MCP joint and the wrist in neutral. The plaster should be set before the patient comes off the operating table.

POSTOPERATIVE CARE AND INSTRUCTIONS

Early active mobilization begins on day 1 following the Belfast regimen. The plaster of Paris is replaced with a thermoplastic splint the following day. Full passive flexion is commenced in all digits. The repaired tendon is allowed to commence immediate, controlled, active flexion and extension.

All exercises are performed in the splint for the first 4 weeks. After 4 weeks, the patient can remove the splint, but only to do exercises. At all other times, the splint remains in place. No passive extension is permitted for 8 weeks.

RECOMMENDED REFERENCES

Kessler I, Nissim F. Primary repair without immobilization of flexor tendon division within the digital sheath. *Acta Orthop Scand* 1969;**40**:587–601.

Kleinert HE, Kutz JE, Ashbell TS, *et al.* Primary repair of lacerated flexor tendons in 'No Man's Land'. Proceedings, American Society for Surgery of the Hand. *J Bone Joint Surg Am* 1967;**49**:577.

Silfverskiold KL, Anderson CH. Two new methods of tendon repair: an in vitro evaluation of tensile strength and gap formation. *J Hand Surg Am* 1993;**18**:58–65.

Sirotakova M, Elliott D. Early active mobilization of primary repairs of the flexor pollicis longus tendon with two Kessler two strand core sutures and a strengthened circumferential suture. *J Hand Surg Br* 2004;**29**:531–5.

Small JO, Brennan MD, Colville J. Early active mobilisation following flexor tendon repair on Zone 2. *J Hand Surg Br* 1989;**14**:383–91.

TENDON TRANSFERS

PREOPERATIVE PLANNING

Tendon transfers are useful to restore hand function in patients where a primary tendon repair is difficult or impossible. The essence of a good transfer is to keep it simple and to plan carefully. The authors recommend listing all functions (absent and present) to allow formulation of a plan. An example is given in Table 9.3.

Indications

- **Nerve palsies** – Tendon transfers are particularly useful for **isolated nerve palsies**. For a transfer to be possible, the hand or upper limb must

Table 9.3 Planning for an anterior interosseous nerve injury

Tendons present	Tendons absent	Suggested options
All extensors + brachioradialis (BR)	Flexor pollicis longus (FPL)	FDS from ring to FPL
		BR to FPL
		Arthrodesis interphalangeal joint
Pronator teres	FDP to index	Suture FDP middle to FDP index
Flexor carpi ulnaris (FCU)	Pronator quadratus	Do not replace
Flexor digitorum profundus (FDP) to little, ring and middle		
Flexor digitorum superficialis (FDS)		
Flexor carpi radialis (FCR)		

have sufficient numbers of functioning tendons which can be used for the transfer without adversely affecting overall hand function. Therefore, patients with a global loss of nerve function (e.g. cerebral palsy) will always do less well.
- **Delayed presentation of tendon rupture** – Tendon transfers may be necessary to restore function even in delayed presentations because of shortening of the muscle bellies after rupture.

Contraindications

- If the joint which the tendon is intended to move is not fully supple
- If the part of the hand/upper limb which is to be moved by the tendon is not fully sensate
- If the tissue bed through which the transfer will pass is poorly vascularized and/or heavily scarred (e.g. under a skin graft)
- If the transfer results in loss of an essential function
- If the power of the transferred muscle is less than 5 (Medical Research Council [MRC] grade). This is because any transferred muscle loses at least 1 grade after the transfer
- If the amplitude of the transferred muscle is not similar to the muscle that it is replacing. For example, finger flexors have an excursion of about 70 mm. Wrist extensors/flexors have an excursion of only 30–40 mm. This is not a good match

- Before 9–12 months have elapsed after any motor nerve repair. If motor recovery has not occurred by this time, then it is very unlikely to occur and a tendon transfer is justified
- Where other procedures would be more beneficial, e.g. for delayed presentation of an FDP laceration or avulsion, a tendon graft or an arthrodesis of the DIP joint may be the preferred options. Similarly, a flexor rupture in zones 1 and 2 for patients with rheumatoid arthritis is usually best treated with a tendon graft.

Consent and risks

- Donor site morbidity: patients may experience weakness or some loss of function after harvest of a tendon. For example, after harvest of the extensor indicis proprius (EIP), patients may experience an extensor lag at the index finger MCP joint
- Additional scarring: after harvest of the tendons/grafts
- Rupture: this is a particular risk if a Pulvertaft repair has not been used for the tenorrhaphy and/or when an interposition, free tendon graft has been used to lengthen any donor tendon (resulting in two tendon repairs)
- Patients must be warned of the prolonged rehabilitation that must be followed after any tendon transfer (8–12 weeks) during which they will be unable to use their hand normally

- Infection
- Neuroma: the superficial branch of the radial nerve is a particular problem because of its propensity to neuroma formation
- Recurvatum deformity (essentially a swan-neck posture) due to hyperextension of the PIP joint after harvest of the FDS in patients with hyperextensible joints
- Damage to adjacent tendons or pulleys
- Imbalance of the transfer, i.e. too tight or too loose
- Tendon imbalance due to spontaneous recovery of normal functions if the tendon transfers were performed too early (i.e. before 9–12 months after repair of a motor nerve)

Anaesthesia and positioning

Most transfers are performed under general or regional anaesthesia. Patients should be supine, and the arm should be placed on a hand table. Use of an arm tourniquet is essential.

SURGICAL TECHNIQUES

Over many years, hand surgeons have developed standard combinations of transfers to deal with specific nerve palsies.

- For a high radial/posterior interosseous palsy:
  - Palmaris longus (PL) to extensor pollicis longus (EPL) to restore thumb extension
  - Flexor carpi radialis (FCR) or flexor carpi ulnaris (FCU) to extensor digitorum communis (EDC) to restore finger extension. For posterior interosseous palsy, FDS from ring or middle finger to EDC is preferred instead
  - Pronator teres (PT) to extensor carpi radialis longus or brevis (ECRL/ECRB) to restore wrist extension
- For a low median palsy:
  - FDS from ring finger or EIP or abductor digit minimi (ADM) (Huber) to abductor pollicis brevis (APB). Palmaris longus can also be used to improve abduction
  - Loss of the lumbricals may result in clawing of the index and middle fingers. The best solution is a dynamic transfer using FDS from the ring finger split into two slips inserted

into the A2 pulleys of index and middle fingers (i.e. a Zancolli lasso)
- For a high median palsy:
  - FDS from ring finger or EIP or ADM to APB for an opponensplasty as in a low median palsy
  - The FDP from ring or little fingers can be side-to-side sutured to the FDP of index and middle fingers to restore finger flexion
  - BR or FDS from ring or little finger to FPL for thumb flexion
  - If clawing is present, then a Zancolli lasso as for a low median palsy. Alternatively, a PL free tendon graft from the transverse carpal ligament to the radial lateral bands of the index and middle fingers for a static extension block
- For a low ulnar palsy:
  - The best solution for clawing is a Zancolli lasso
  - FDS from the middle or index finger to adductor pollicis for weak adduction
  - EIP to extensor digitorum minimi (EDM) corrects Wartenberg's deformity
- For high ulnar palsy:
  - Suture of FDP middle and index side-to-side to FDP little and ring fingers.
  - FDS from middle or index to adductor pollicis if adduction is weak.

Other technical aspects of tendon transfer

When measuring the length of donor tendon required for transfer, remember that 2–3 cm of tendon are required to perform the Pulvertaft weave. A Pulvertaft weave is one of the keys to a good transfer because the repair is sufficiently strong to allow early mobilization. Getting the correct tension in the transferred tendon is another key point. The joint should be positioned where the transfer will be at its maximum length and the tendon is then sutured under maximum tension. Unfortunately, this is not always possible if the donor tendon is too short. Therefore, it is important to carry out a tenodesis test to ensure that an overly tight transfer has been avoided. That said, all repairs should be 'over-tensioned' on the table to allow for a small amount of subsequent 'stretching' of the tendon.

Closure

All wounds are closed in layers with absorbable sutures using interrupted 4/0 or 5/0 Monocryl to dermis and 4/0 or 5/0 Vicryl rapide as a subcuticular stitch. Mepitel, dressing, gauze and Velband bandage are applied as needed and the hand and forearm are placed in a resting volar plaster. The plaster should be set before the patient wakes up.

POSTOPERATIVE CARE AND INSTRUCTIONS

After 24–48 hours, the plaster is removed and the patient can be placed in an appropriate thermoplastic resting splint which can be removed by the patient and therapist to allow early mobilization to begin. The precise rehabilitation regimen depends on the tendons which have been transferred. However, in all cases, one of the keys to a successful outcome is the ability to begin early active mobilization. In order for this to happen, any tenorrhaphy must be sufficiently strong to allow this mobilization to occur.

RECOMMENDED REFERENCE

Green DP, Hotchkiss RN, Pederson WC (eds). *Green's Operative Hand Surgery* (5th edn). Edinburgh: Elsevier, 2005.

SOFT TISSUE RECONSTRUCTION

PREOPERATIVE PLANNING

For the purposes of this handbook, the focus is on three areas:
- The operative correction of aberrant scarring
- The use of split thickness skin grafts
- The use of full thickness skin grafts

Indications

- Primary wound closure cannot be achieved
- Primary wound closure can be achieved but may result in functional impairment
- Allowing a wound to heal by secondary intention will result in functional impairment. For example, leaving tendons exposed which would result in their desiccation and necrosis
- There is aberrant scarring. Examples include: webbed volar scars from poorly placed incisions, burns or other traumatic scarring (Fig. 9.17).

Contraindications

- Active infection. **Beta-haemolytic streptococci**, in particular, will dissolve any graft. Other bacteria will reduce the likelihood of the graft taking and can result in a patchy take

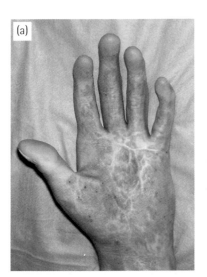
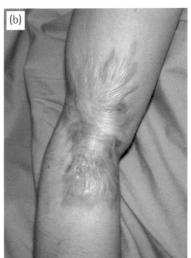
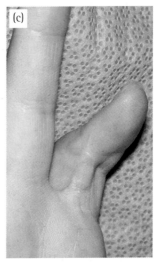

Figure 9.17 *Soft tissue reconstruction needed for (a) skin loss after sepsis, (b) burns or (c) a poor volar scar*

- Smoking. Expect a 40 per cent increase in wound healing complications in any patient who smokes
- Long term steroid use. Particularly in rheumatoid arthritis (relative contraindication)
- Peripheral vascular disease or similar e.g. Buerger disease, scleroderma or severe Raynaud
- Previous radiotherapy to the hand
- Recipient site unsuitable. Grafts will not take on bare bone or tendon unless these areas are very small (<5 mm diameter) in which case the grafts can survive by 'bridging'
- Donor site problems.

Consent and risks

- Scarring: particularly with split skin grafting which leaves large, unsightly scars
- Infection
- Flap necrosis: this is nearly always the result of technical error (e.g. flaps too narrow, closure too tight) but may also be a consequence of infection
- Graft loss
- Prolonged healing: a split skin graft (SSG) donor site may take months (or even years) to heal if the patient and donor site are poorly selected

Operative planning

There are three main techniques to master:
- **The Z-plasty**: an operation which involves the transposition of two triangular skin flaps of equal dimension to lengthen a scar or change its direction. There is a risk of necrosis of the flaps if they are poorly designed.
- **Split thickness skin grafts**: if an SSG is used, it is often a temporary biological dressing rather than for definitive skin cover.
- **Full thickness skin grafts (FTG)**: these can be used for definitive skin cover anywhere on the hand **except the pulps of the fingers and thumb**.

Anaesthesia and positioning

The form of anaesthesia depends on the size of graft that needs to be harvested and the area

where it is needed. Local anaesthesia is suitable for harvesting small grafts and for surgery to the digits. However, patients may be more grateful for a general anaesthetic when harvesting large grafts and operating on multiple areas (e.g. harvest a FTG from the groin for use in the hand) and on the palm of the hand. The hand is placed in the supine position on an arm table. A tourniquet is essential for any surgery involving the use of flaps or grafts in the hand.

SURGICAL TECHNIQUE

Z-plasty is used when there is a need to change the direction and/or length of a scar. The best example of its use is to correct a webbed volar scar. Z-plasty can also be used to lengthen a scar after Dupuytren's fasciectomy (see Fig. 9.2, p. 116).

Landmarks and incisions

In most cases, a 30° or 60° angle is used for the flap design. A 60° angle achieves more lengthening of the scar but a 30° angle is often easier to transpose. The width of the base of the flap in relation to its length is important in determining flap survival. The longer and narrower the flap, the less likely it is to survive. The flaps are marked out as shown in Figure 9.2 (p. 116).

It is a myth that the limbs of the Z-plasty must be aligned to fall in the skin creases – skin creases exist because the fingers flex. When the fingers cease to flex, the creases disappear. The Z-plasty is best placed where it is needed.

Superficial dissection

The flaps are raised with a small amount of subcutaneous fat to ensure that the subdermal plexus is uninjured. When raising the flaps, the underlying anatomy must be considered. For example, it is very easy to divide the neurovascular bundle when raising the Z-plasty flaps after a Dupuytren's fasciectomy.

Procedure

- The first stage is to raise one flap and transpose it across the scar. This ensures that the design is right for the second flap before you commit yourself to raising it.

- If the design is right then the two flaps should automatically transpose themselves across the scar when the finger straightens.
- The flaps are tacked into the correct corners and any dog-ears ignored. (These will flatten in a few weeks anyway.)

Closure

Interrupted or continuous, absorbable, 4/0 or 5/0 Vicryl rapide sutures are used for closure. **Do not use non-absorbable sutures** in the hand. There is no difference in wound healing after skin closure using absorbable and non-absorbable sutures in the hand. Patients find it very painful to have non-absorbable sutures removed so avoid using them.

Split thickness skin grafts

A small SSG (<3 cm × 3 cm) can be harvested with a hand-held knife. However, ideally, a powered dermatome should be used to harvest all SSGs (Fig. 9.18).

Landmarks and incisions

The first decision is the amount of SSG needed. This is best worked out in terms of the length and width of the defect which needs to be covered. A marginally larger area than you think you will need should always be taken (approximately 1 cm beyond is about right). It is easy to trim the SSG down to size but harvesting more graft is always a problem. Ensure the correct settings are selected

on the hand knife or dermatome. Typically, the SSG should be between 0.2 mm and 0.4 mm thick. The thicker the SSG, the less it will contract, but the longer it will take for the donor site to heal and the more obvious the donor site scar.

Harvesting

Liquid paraffin is applied to the skin and the knife. This acts as a lubricant and prevents the blade from catching on the skin. If the blade catches rather than cuts, it will tear the SSG or result in holes where you do not want them. It is also critically important to ensure that the skin at the donor site is under tension. The best way to do this is to have an assistant who can squeeze the thigh or arm while you concentrate on harvesting the skin. A rapid sawing motion is used to harvest the skin with a hand-knife, keeping the blade flat with respect to the skin and not pressing too hard or the graft thickness will increase. If a powered dermatome is used, the machine does the sawing for you. The aim is to harvest in one smooth action.

Meshing the skin increases the area which can be covered with a given size of SSG. It also increases the take rate by allowing free drainage of haematoma and seroma. It is possible to mesh skin by hand but using a skin mesher is quicker and neater. However, once it has taken, meshed skin contracts even more than a sheet graft. An alternative is to perforate it with multiple stabs using a no. 15 blade to allow haematoma and seroma to ooze through.

The donor site is dressed with Mefix adhesive dressing applied directly to the wound. Gauze,

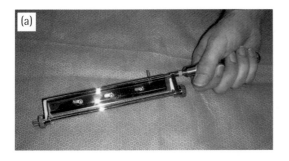
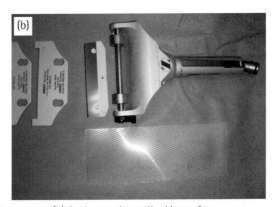

Figure 9.18 *A Watson hand knife (a) and an air-powered dermatome (b) for harvesting split skin grafts*

Velband and crepe are applied over this to absorb any exudate.

Grafting

The SSG is applied shiny side down onto a prepared wound bed and secured with absorbable 4/0 or 5/0 Vicryl rapide either as interrupted or continuous sutures. The same sutures are used to 'quilt' the SSG onto the wound bed to reduce shearing movements, improve contact with the wound bed and improve haemostasis under the graft. The SSG is dressed with Jelonet and a layer of gauze. A bulky bandage (Velband and crepe) is applied and the hand immobilized with a plaster of Paris. The graft should be reviewed in 2–3 days.

Full thickness graft

The best donor sites for a FTG are the groin and post-auricular sulcus because these areas are well hidden. However, skin taken from these sites has a poor colour match with the skin of the hand. Therefore, a FTG applied to the hand will always be obvious as a dark area with a different texture. In males, a FTG from the groin is also likely to be hairy resulting in obvious problems when applied to any part of the hand unless a concerted effort is made to remove the hair follicles before the FTG is used.

Landmarks and incisions

An assessment of the area of FTG needed is made, using a piece of paper as a template. The template is transferred to the donor site to mark out a similar area of skin. If harvesting a FTG for a case of Dupuytren's dermofasciectomy, multiple small pieces of FTG may be needed (Fig. 9.19).

Harvesting

The outlines of the pieces of skin that you intend to take are scored with a no. 15 scalpel blade. This ensures that you do not lose the outline of the individual pieces of skin. Lift up one corner of the ellipse that you intend to raise and grip this with an artery clip. This saves your hand from getting tired and allows the graft to be held firmly over your index finger while harvesting the graft. Fat should be removed from the graft as it is harvested. This avoids the need to de-fat the graft after it has been detached from the donor site.

The donor site is now closed with a couple of interrupted 4/0 Monocryl sutures and completed with a continuous over and over suture of 4/0 Monocryl into the dermis locked at both ends with a buried knot. Once the dermal suture is knotted the suture simply continues with a 4/0 Monocryl subcuticular suture.

Grafting

Any remaining fat on the graft is removed using a pair of tenotomy scissors. This is a very tedious but very important step. The more fat there is on your FTG, the less likely it is to take. The FTG is secured to the recipient site with a couple of interrupted 4/0 or 5/0 Vicryl rapide sutures. Securing the grafting is completed with a continuous over and over suture at the edge, using 4/0 or 5/0 rapide. It is important to add quilting sutures to the centre of the graft to prevent haematoma formation and shearing movements. Copious quantities of Vaseline ointment are now spread onto the graft and a Jelonet and gauze dressing is applied. The graft should be reviewed in 5–7 days.

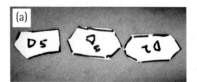 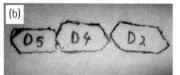 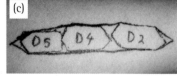

Figure 9.19 *(a) Templating, (b) marking and (c) planning incision for multiple full thickness grafts for Dupuytren's dermofasciectomy*

POSTOPERATIVE CARE AND INSTRUCTIONS

- Z-plasty: the patient can mobilize their hand immediately unless a graft was also used. Even if the last 2–3 mm of the tips of the flaps do not survive, the wounds should go onto heal by secondary intention without compromising the final outcome.
- SSG: the graft is left undisturbed for 48–72 hours. If it is pink after that, then it has taken and gentle mobilization can begin. The donor site on the thigh or arm is left undisturbed until 10–14 days have passed and the patient says it is no longer painful. If the dressing is taken off too early, newly formed epithelium will rip off with the dressing. Once a continuous layer of epithelium is present at both recipient and donor sites, the patient applies a thick layer of Vaseline to both areas. The SSG has no glands and will quickly dry out, crust, flake and crack if not protected in this way.
- FTG: the hand is immobilized for 1 week in a plaster of Paris to further minimize shearing forces that would interfere with graft take. At 5–7 days, all the dressings are removed and the graft inspected. If graft take is complete, then copious quantities of Vaseline ointment must be applied daily for the next 3 months by which time the glands in the graft will have started to function and it can self-moisturize.

RECOMMENDED REFERENCES

McGregor AD, McGregor IA. *Fundamental Techniques of Plastic Surgery and Their Surgical Applications*, 10th edn. Edinburgh: Churchill Livingstone, 2000

Thorne CH, Bartlett SP, Beasley RW, *et al.* (eds). *Grabb and Smith's Plastic Surgery*, 5th edition. New York: Lippincott-Raven, 1997.

TRIGGER FINGER SURGERY

PREOPERATIVE PLANNING

The diagnosis of triggering is normally easy to make but overt triggering is sometimes absent and the patient only gives a history of pain on flexion of the digit which may be confused with or concurrent with arthritis. Trigger finger is common in patients over the age of 50, diabetics and rheumatoid patients. Where overt triggering is absent but pain is present, the use of steroid injections is particularly efficacious.

Indications

- Persistent triggering (not relieved by steroid injections).
- Acutely locked finger.

Contraindications

- Presence of infection
- Triggering in a patient with rheumatoid arthritis (RA). A rheumatoid patient with triggering needs steroid injections or a synovectomy. Release of the A1 pulley in RA patients may make ulnar drift worse by creating further changes in the alignment of the tendons.

Consent and risks

- Infection
- Injury to the tendon and neurovascular bundles
- Recurrence
- Stiffness/loss of flexion

Anaesthesia and positioning

Local anaesthesia is used with the patient supine, the arm on an arm table and a tourniquet applied.

SURGICAL TECHNIQUE

Landmarks and incision

The proximal border of the A1 pulley lies at the neck of the corresponding metacarpal (Fig. 9.20), roughly at the level of the mid-palmar crease. A 1.5 cm long, transverse, incision is made in the crease over the corresponding metacarpal.

Surgical dissection

Blunt dissection is performed through the subcutaneous fat and palmar fascia, using tenotomy scissors, to expose the flexor sheath. It is rarely necessary to visualize the neurovascular bundles running parallel to the flexor tendons: in any case, these should be protected by the retractors.

The proximal edge of the A1 pulley is identified and the pulley is then divided longitudinally with a scalpel taking particular care to stay over the midline of the tendon to avoid the risk of damage to the neurovascular bundles.

The patient is then asked to flex and extend the digit several times to test for any residual triggering. The arm tourniquet is released, the wound washed out with saline and haemostasis achieved.

Closure

Skin closure is with interrupted absorbable sutures. A bulky dressing is applied to the hand for 24–48 hours. This can then be de-bulked by the patient to allow the fingers to flex freely.

POSTOPERATIVE CARE AND INSTRUCTIONS

Active mobilization of the hand is commenced immediately. The bulky dressing should be taken down after 24–48 hours to facilitate this.

RECOMMENDED REFERENCES

Doyle JR, Blythe WF. The finger flexor tendon sheath and pulleys: anatomy and reconstruction. In: *AAOS Symposium on Tendon Surgery in the Hand*. St Louis: Mosby, 1975:81–7.
Idler RS. Anatomy and biomechanics of the digital flexor tendons. *Hand Clin* 1985;**1**:3–11.

TRIGGER THUMB SURGERY

PREOPERATIVE PLANNING

Indications

- Persistent triggering not relieved by steroid injections. Administer at least one, sometimes two injections before going ahead with surgery and wait 3 months after each injection to assess outcome
- Locked thumb in an adult
- Locked thumb in a child (usually noticed at <2 years) unresolved for ≥12 months. Thirty per cent of trigger thumbs in infants will resolve within the first year after it is noticed. Flexion contractures do occur but these will correct themselves spontaneously if the triggering resolves or if surgical release is performed before the age of 3.

Contraindication

Presence of infection.

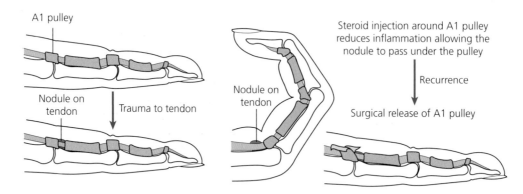

Figure 9.20 *Trigger finger*

Consent and risks

- Infection
- Injury to the tendon and neurovascular bundles
- Recurrence
- Stiffness/loss of range of movement
- Bow-stringing due to accidental division of A1 pulley and oblique pulley (more likely if the A1 pulley is divided through its ulnar attachment)

Anaesthesia and positioning

Local or general (in child) anaesthesia is used with an arm board and tourniquet.

SURGICAL TECHNIQUE

Landmarks, incision and dissection

Structures at risk

- Digital nerves and arteries – these are close to the skin in the thumb
- Ulnar attachments of the A1 pulley – their division may lead to bowstringing of the FPL

In the thumb, the proximal border of the A1 pulley is at the level of the proximal digital skin crease over the MCP joint. A 1–1.5 cm transverse incision is created in the crease. Tenotomy scissors are used for blunt dissection through the subcutaneous fat and palmar fascia to expose the FPL tendon sheath and A1 pulley. The digital nerves and vessels running parallel to the FPL tendon are identified and protected with right-angle retractors The A1 pulley is identified and **the radial attachment of the pulley** is divided completely with a scalpel from proximal to distal.

The thumb is then flexed and extended several times to test for any residual triggering. The arm tourniquet is released and haemostasis is achieved. The wound is washed out with saline.

Closure

The skin is closed with 5/0 Vicryl rapide interrupted or subcuticular sutures. A light bandage should be applied which does not interfere with movements of the thumb.

POSTOPERATIVE CARE AND INSTRUCTIONS

Active mobilization of the hand and thumb is begun immediately after surgery. Heavy use of the hand is avoided for 1–2 weeks.

RECOMMENDED REFERENCE

Ger E, Kupcha P, Ger D. The management of trigger thumb in children. *J Hand Surg Am* 1991;**16**:944–7.

Viva questions

1. Why perform a dermofasciectomy rather than a fasciectomy for Dupuytren's disease?

2. How do you deal with any residual flexion of the digit after excision of all diseased Dupuytren's cord tissue?

3. What are the possible complications of a fasciectomy?

4. Describe a permanent solution for a painful distal interphalangeal joint with mucous cyst in a 50-year-old manual worker.

5. An elderly woman with rheumatoid arthritis comes to you with a painful unstable thumb metacarpophalangeal joint. Describe your management.

6. A man of 30 with a history of psoriatic arthropathy attends your clinic with painful and deformed distal interphalangeal joints affecting all fingers of both hands. How would you treat this?

7. A woman of 40 attends your clinic with a history of an untreated pilon fracture of the PIP joint of her right little finger, dominant hand, 10 years ago. The finger is painful, angulated and has restricted (20–40°) active flexion. What surgical options would you give her?

8. A 50-year-old builder attends your clinic with a painful right index finger carpometacarpal joint. He punched a fellow builder 5 years ago and heard a loud 'click' at the time. Since then, he has experienced increasing movement at the joint associated with pain on lifting heavy objects. What options would you offer him?

9. Describe the management and treatment options for a young manual worker with a painful, stiff, proximal interphalangeal joint after previous trauma with evidence of marked joint deformity on X-ray.

10. A young woman presents with a painless but stiff index finger metacarpophalangeal joint after an infection. What surgical options would you present to her?

11. Describe the surgical management of a manual worker with a laceration in zone 6 and loss of extension of the thumb and index finger of his dominant hand?

12. What is the management of a closed mallet injury in a 16-year-old rugby player?

13. A 60-year-old woman presents with a passively correctible boutonnière deformity of her index and middle fingers of her dominant hand 1 year after a fall in the street. How would you treat this?

14. A 50-year-old lawyer with rheumatoid arthritis has suddenly lost extension of his little and ring fingers of his non-dominant hand. What options can you offer him?

15. How do you manage an isolated division of the flexor digitorum profundus tendon in the little finger of a dominant hand?

16. Describe the operative steps involved in the repair of a combined flexor digitorum superficialis/flexor digitorum profundus tendon injury in zone 2 of the ring finger of a 30-year-old painter and decorator?

17. A patient presents with a tight volar web scar after Dupuytren's fasciectomy. How would you correct this?

18. You have decided to carry out a correction of a congenital camptodactyly of the little finger. The finger is now straight but it is obvious that there is a shortage of skin on the volar side of the finger which contributed to the flexion deformity in the first place. How would you correct this?

19. Describe the risks and pitfalls in the management of trigger finger.

20. Describe your management of an acutely locked trigger thumb.

10

Surgery of the hip

Jonathan Miles and John Skinner

Hip	Range of motion
External rotation	60°
Internal rotation	40°
Flexion	125°
Extension	0°
Adduction	25°
Abduction	45°

Position of arthrodesis

- External rotation 0–10°
- Flexion 20–25°
- Adduction 0–5°

PRIMARY TOTAL HIP ARTHROPLASTY

PREOPERATIVE PLANNING

Indications

Total hip arthroplasty is indicated in painful conditions of the hip that have failed conservative management. These are too numerous to list in this book but the most frequent underlying conditions are:
- Osteoarthritis
- Inflammatory arthritis and other arthropathies
- Avascular necrosis
- Trauma.

Contraindications

- Infection (generalized or of the limb)
- Absolute dysfunction of the abductor complex, including profound neurological disease.

Young age is a relative contraindication, though in the highly symptomatic patient replacement should be discussed with and performed by an appropriately experienced surgeon.

Consent and risks

- Mortality: 0.3 per cent
- Nerve injury: 1 per cent
- Infection: 1–2 per cent in osteoarthritis, 5 per cent in rheumatoid arthritis
- Thromboembolism; deep vein thrombosis: 2 per cent
- Pulmonary embolism: 1 per cent
- Dislocation: 3 per cent
- Heterotopic ossification: 10 per cent (though the majority are asymptomatic)
- Limb length discrepancy: 15 per cent
- Loosening: revision surgery is required for loosening in up to 10 per cent at 15 years
- Component failure: stem fracture, locking mechanism failure in uncemented cups and other failures of components are rare, but recognized, complications

Operative planning

Recent radiographs must be available. Templates should be routinely used to indicate the appropriate site for the femoral neck cut and provide a guide to implant placement and sizing. Availability of the implants must be checked by the surgeon.

Anaesthesia and positioning

Anaesthesia is usually general, regional or combined. An initial dose of antibiotic is given intravenously. The antibiotic of choice depends upon local policy, but a common choice is a second-generation cephalosporin or a combination of gentamicin and flucloxacillin.

The lateral position is used and requires well-fixed supports abutting the lumbar spine posteriorly and the bony pelvis anteriorly (Fig. 10.1). The pelvis should be vertically orientated; if it is not vertical, the operating table can be tilted to properly align the pelvis.

Bony prominences must be carefully padded. The hip should be sufficiently mobile for appropriate movement intraoperatively. The surgical field is prepared with a germicidal solution. Waterproof drapes are used with adhesive edges to provide a seal to the skin. The foot and leg are covered with a stockinette. If a lateral approach is to be used, a sterile 'leg bag' should be used to maintain sterility when the hip is displaced.

SURGICAL TECHNIQUE

The two common approaches are the posterior and lateral approaches.

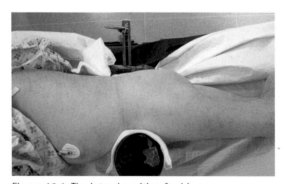

Figure 10.1 *The lateral position for hip surgery*

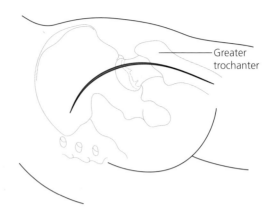

Figure 10.2 *The skin incision for the posterior approach to the hip*

Posterior approach (extensile)

Landmarks

The greater trochanter is palpated, particularly noting the posterior border.

Incision

A 15 cm skin incision is made with its midpoint lying over the posterior half of the greater trochanter (Fig. 10.2). The proximal extent of the incision is curved posteriorly, to lie in the line of the fibres of gluteus maximus. The distal portion lies along the femoral shaft.

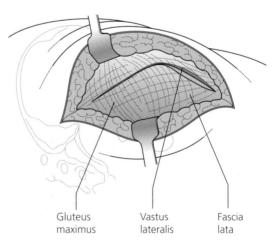

Gluteus maximus   Vastus lateralis   Fascia lata

Figure 10.3 *Dissection of the posterior approach to the hip*

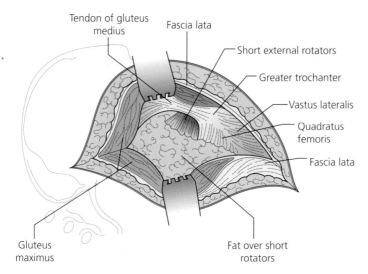

Tendon of gluteus medius

Fascia lata

Short external rotators

Greater trochanter

Vastus lateralis

Quadratus femoris

Fascia lata

Gluteus maximus

Fat over short rotators

Figure 10.4 *Deep dissection of the posterior approach*

Superficial dissection

The incision is continued through subcutaneous fat and down to fascia lata. Beginning distally, the fascia lata is incised in line with the skin incision, overlying the lateral femur. Proximally this continues beyond the greater trochanter, in a posterior direction, to incise in line with the underlying fibres of the gluteus maximus. The fibres of the gluteus maximus are gently split, using diathermy to coagulate the inevitable bleeding vessels. The incision should run from 6 cm to 8 cm above the greater trochanter down to the insertion of the gluteus maximus tendon on the posterior femur (Fig. 10.3).

A self-retaining retractor is inserted, such as a Charnley retractor.

Deep dissection

Structures at risk

- Sciatic nerve: see below
- Inferior gluteal artery: lying below piriformis. If it is cut, immediate supine repositioning of the patient and abdominal approach to tie off the internal iliac artery may be required to arrest the haemorrhage
- Obturator arterial branches: present within quadratus femoris

The trochanteric bursa is now visible, covering the short external rotators and lying below the posterior border of gluteus (Fig. 10.4). This can be swept off the short external rotators, using blunt or sharp dissection.

At this point the sciatic nerve can be visualized. Aggressive dissection around the nerve is not recommended, certainly in primary arthroplasty it is unnecessary and just increases the risk of damaging the epineurial vessels, creating a haematoma and neuropraxia. The sciatic nerve exits the sciatic notch and passes into the posterior thigh overlying the short external rotators.

The sciatic nerve exits below piriformis and lies on the following muscles, running from superior to inferior (Fig. 10.5):

- Gemellus superior
- Obturator internus
- Gemellus inferior
- Quadratus femoris.

The nerve then runs down **underneath** the gluteus maximus' tendon at its femoral insertion.

An assistant now internally rotates the extended hip and flexes the knee, stretching the short external rotators, making them easier to divide. This also increases the distance between the sciatic nerve and the site of division of these short muscles. Strong, non-absorbable, braided stay

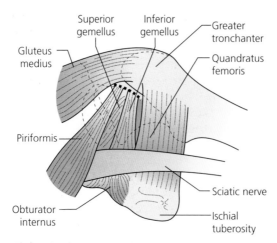

Figure 10.5 *The path of the sciatic nerve over the external rotators of the hip*

sutures (e.g. no. 2 Ethibond) are inserted into the tendons of obturator internus and piriformis, just below their insertion into the femur, i.e. as anteriorly as possible. Visible vessels within the operative field are coagulated: typically these lie on the tendon of piriformis and within the substance of quadratus femoris. The short external rotators, from piriformis down to gemellus inferior, are divided as close to their insertion onto the femur as possible. If further room is required, the division can be carried on further distally. If the quadratus femoris is divided, it should be done around 5 mm away from its insertion into the femur so that a cuff is left to repair it back on to.

The muscles are allowed to 'flop' over the sciatic nerve, providing some protection for it throughout the rest of the operation. This exposes the posterior capsule of the hip joint. To improve visibility, the interval between the superior part of the hip capsule and the gluteus minimus is identified and dissected free with blunt dissection or scissors. This view is maintained by inserting a Hohmann retractor in the interval to displace the gluteus minimus superiorly. The capsule is incised transversely to gain access. The visible portion of capsule can be excised or preserved and later repaired. The visible portion of the acetabular labrum is excised.

Lateral approach

Landmarks

- Central landmark – the greater trochanter
- The anterior superior iliac spine and the femoral shaft are also palpable and act as useful reference points.

Incision

A straight 15 cm incision is created, parallel to the femoral shaft and centred on the anterior half of the greater trochanter (Fig. 10.6).

Superficial dissection

The incision is continued through subcutaneous fat and down to fascia lata. The fascia lata is incised in line with the skin incision overlying the lateral femur (Fig. 10.7). At this point a self-retaining retractor is inserted.

Deep dissection

> **Structures at risk**
>
> Superior gluteal nerve – between the gluteus medius and minimus; this may be as close as 3 cm above the tip of the greater trochanter.

The incision continues in line with the skin incision. This begins proximally within the fibres of the gluteus medius and must be limited to a point 3 cm above the tip of the greater trochanter to avoid damage to the superior gluteal nerve. The

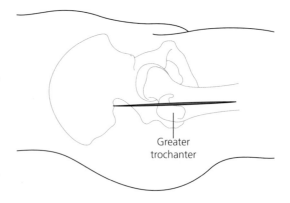

Figure 10.6 *The skin incision for the lateral approach to the hip*

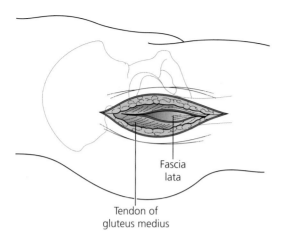

Fascia
lata

Tendon of
gluteus medius

Figure 10.7 *Dissection of the lateral approach to the hip*

incision continues distally, in the line of the fibres of the gluteus medius and across the greater trochanter, entering the vastus lateralis. The fibres of the vastus lateralis overlying the greater trochanter are split.

The incision develops an anterior flap, consisting of the anterior fibres of the gluteus medius and gluteus minimus above the greater trochanter and the anterior fibres of the vastus lateralis lying over and below the greater trochanter. This is elevated off the greater trochanter subperiosteally, with either a scalpel or cutting diathermy. A cuff of gluteus medius is left posteriorly on the greater trochanter, allowing reattachment at the time of closure.

The incision progresses anteriorly, detaching the insertion of the gluteus medius and minimus onto the greater trochanter, to reveal the capsule of the hip. The anterior flap is retracted by placing a Hohmann retractor. The capsule is incised in a T shape, with the downstroke of the T lying in line with the femoral neck and the bar of the T running under the femoral head (Fig. 10.8).

- **Dislocation and retractor positioning** – This must be done gently as excess force can fracture the femur (typically a spiral fracture running from the subtrochanteric region down the shaft). In younger patients, the ligamentum teres can remain intact, preventing full dislocation; if this occurs it can be easily divided with a scalpel. If the dislocation is difficult, further capsule can be excised; remove any more visible labrum and remove any acetabular osteophytes with nibblers or an osteotome. If

the hip can still not be removed with minimal force, division of the femoral neck *in situ* and removal the head with a corkscrew is recommended.

- **Posterior approach dislocation and retraction** – The hip joint can now be dislocated. This is performed by placing the hip in adduction and flexion then internally rotating it, bringing the calf to lie vertically and the foot pointing towards the ceiling. A bone hook can be carefully passed around the femur, at the level of the lesser trochanter, and used to ease the femoral head away from the acetabulum.
- **Lateral approach dislocation and retraction** – The hip can be dislocated with adduction, flexion and external rotation, again with a blunt bone hook around the femoral neck. The leg is then placed in the leg bag, i.e. the foot pointing to the floor, on the opposite side of the operating table.

Procedure

Structures at risk

- Femoral nerve – injudicious placement of anterior retractors may, rarely, damage the femoral nerve
- Sciatic nerve – vulnerable posteriorly
- Obturator arterial branches – large branches are present below the transverse acetabular ligament; cutting them should be avoided

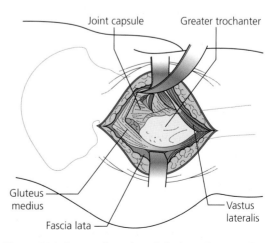

Joint capsule   Greater trochanter

Gluteus
medius

Fascia lata

Vastus
lateralis

Figure 10.8 *Deeper dissection of the lateral approach*

Hohmann retractors are inserted around the superior and inferior aspects of the femoral neck, supporting and stabilizing the proximal femur and exposing the whole of the intertrochanteric line. Any soft tissues along this line are removed until the superior portion of the lesser trochanter is seen.

The planned femoral osteotomy site is marked with an osteotome. A number of hip replacement sets have a specific instrument to aid identification of the right site for this osteotomy; use of a trial prosthesis or a rasp as a guide is recommended in those sets without a neck cutting guide. This is particularly important with collared stems. Templating will have provided a guide to the height above the lesser trochanter that the osteotomy should pass through the calcar (typically, this is around 15 mm above the lesser trochanter). An oscillating saw is used to perform the osteotomy, with the Hohmann retractors protecting the surrounding soft tissues. The cut is made with the saw blade 45° to the femoral shaft and in the plane of the tibia. If the line of the osteotomy passes into the greater trochanter, the osteotomy is stopped before entering the trochanter and a second osteotomy carried vertically down from the piriformis fossa to meet the lateral extent of the first osteotomy (Fig. 10.9). The femoral head is removed and kept in case of its later requirement as graft.

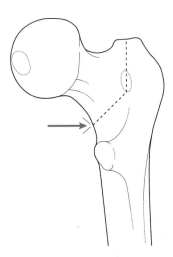

Figure 10.9 *A typical neck cut*

Acetabular preparation

Any soft tissues overhanging the acetabulum around its circumference, including the labrum, are excised. It is vital to obtain a clear view around the whole acetabulum. The transverse acetabular ligament is identified, lying across the inferior boundary of the acetabulum; if it is large this may need careful division, which should be done with the blade directed laterally towards the acetabular roof. Any remaining ligamentum is also excised. Preservation of the transverse acetabular ligament is advocated by some surgeons who use cemented acetabular components: it helps to prevent inferior cement extrusion. If using the posterior approach, sharp Hohmann retractors are placed over the anterior wall, to lever the femur anteriorly, and under the transverse acetabular ligament to expose the whole acetabulum for its preparation. In the lateral approach, the proximal femur is levered posteriorly rather than anteriorly.

Within the acetabulum the medial wall is defined. This is sometimes visible as a flat plate of cortical bone which can be seen inferiorly. If it is not, it is covered in osteophytes or soft tissue, which should be gently removed with an osteotome or curette to reveal the floor. This is an important step as definition of the medial wall allows proper and safe 'medialization', providing maximum cover of the cup when it is inserted.

Sharp, hemispherical, cheese-grater reamers are now used to remove the remaining acetabular cartilage and expose subchondral bone. Beginning with the smallest reamer, reaming is directed medially and stopped regularly to ascertain the depth of reaming. The desired depth is up to, but not through the true medial wall (the flat cortical bone of the quadrilateral plate). The acetabulum is enlarged with increasing sizes of reamers, not increasing the depth but just the width. This is performed in the desired alignment of the acetabular component to be inserted. The appropriate alignment is **45° from the horizontal and 15–20° of anteversion** (Fig. 10.10). The aim is creation of a hemisphere, removing all cartilage but preserving as much subchondral bone as possible.

If the acetabular component to be used is of uncemented design, a trial is inserted at the correct angle to assess the coverage and stability.

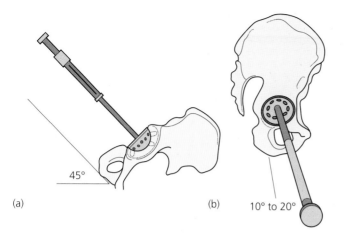

(a)

(b)   10° to 20°

45°

Figure 10.10 *Acetabular reaming (a) 45° from vertical and (b) 10°–20° of anteversion*

The cemented implants also have trials, allowing for a cement mantle. At this point any excess osteophytes around the acetabulum (that may lead to impingement) are often apparent. These can be removed with nibblers or an osteotome. The component is inserted using the appropriate technique. It is worthwhile to ensure that the pelvis has remained vertical, as any malposition of the patient will transfer into improper angulation of the implant, with consequent risk of instability.

Technical points in uncemented cup insertion

- The uncemented cup relies on a secure fit to confer initial stability.
- In the press-fit technique an implant 1–2 mm larger than the last reamer is used. This can be augmented with screws as necessary.
- The line-to-line technique uses an implant of the same size as the last reamer and relies on augmentation with screws to obtain fixation.
- If fixation is not solid and stable, even after screws have been used a switch to a cemented cup is recommended.
- Screws holes are aligned to coincide with the safe zone, described below. Pilot holes should be drilled, their depth ascertained with an angled depth gauge and screws inserted with a universally jointed screwdriver and a screw holder to control the direction.
- Screw augmentation, if to be used, should be done with care and awareness of the safe

quadrants. These are defined by a first line passing inferiorly from the anterior superior iliac spine, through the centre of the acetabulum and a second line perpendicular to the first, again passing through the middle of the acetabulum. This creates four quadrants (Fig. 10.11).

Structures at risk

Posterior superior – **the safe zone**
- At risk – sciatic nerve and superior gluteal neurovascular bundle

Posterior inferior – safe if screws < 20 mm
- At risk – inferior gluteal and internal pudendal neurovascular bundles

Anterior superior – avoid screws
- At risk – external iliac vessels

Anterior inferior – avoid screws
- At risk – anterior inferior obturator neurovascular bundle

When all of the screws are properly seated, the liner can be inserted. The use of a 10° or 20° elevated rim can be selected if using a polyethylene liner. It should be remembered that this reduces the arc of motion and should not be an automatic action. Trials are available and should be used if there is any doubt. It is usual for the elevated lip to be situated posterosuperiorly or

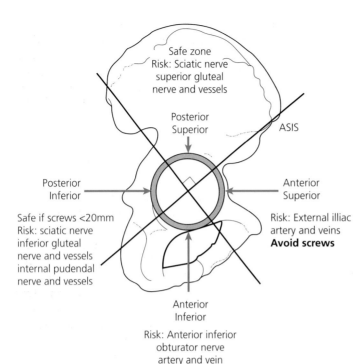

Safe zone
Risk: Sciatic nerve
superior gluteal
nerve and vessels

Posterior
Superior

ASIS

Posterior
Inferior

Anterior
Superior

Safe if screws <20mm
Risk: sciatic nerve
inferior gluteal
nerve and vessels
internal pudendal
nerve and vessels

Risk: External illiac
artery and veins
Avoid screws

Anterior
Inferior

Risk: Anterior inferior
obturator nerve
artery and vein
Avoid screws

Figure 10.11 *The quadrants of acetabular screw positioning. Redrawn with permission from Miller (2004)* Review of Orthopaedics. *Philadelphia: Saunders*

more posteriorly if a posterior approach has been used.

Technical points in cemented cup insertion

- Many acetabular components have a lip augment, which should be correctly orientated in the posterior to superior area. If the cup has a flange (which can help to prevent cement extrusion), this will need to be trimmed to the size of the reamed acetabulum.
- Drill holes into the ilium and ischium, but not the quadrilateral plate, and enhance the cement fixation. The bone surface is washed with pulsatile lavage and dried thoroughly. Many acetabular components have pegs on the medial surface; these are designed to ensure a uniform cement mantle of around 3 mm.
- The cement should be introduced from a cement gun with a short nozzle. It is first introduced to the keyholes in the ilium and ischium. This is done with the nozzle hard against the bone, to increase the pressure. It is then introduced to the rest of the acetabulum and pressurized with an impactor: most sets

have a polypropylene impactor to pressurize the cement into the acetabular bone.
- The surgeon should be aware of the properties of the cement that is being used to ensure that the cement and component are inserted at the appropriate time. It is vital that the component is held perfectly still while the cement is curing. Care should be taken to ensure that the introducer is able to be released without undue force, to reduce the stresses on the cement to component interface.
- Any excess cement should be removed.

Femoral preparation

In the posterior approach the assistant extends and internally rotates the hip while supporting the leg with the knee flexed. In the anterior approach, the leg is maximally adducted and the hip externally rotated; the knee is flexed to position the lower leg in the leg bag drape.

An entry point is created in the proximal femur, with a box chisel, to allow the insertion of reamers; it must be correctly situated to prevent varus malposition of the component. The starting

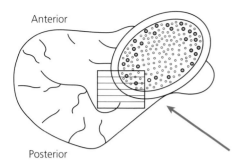

Anterior

Posterior

Figure 10.12 *The box chisel 'starting point' in femoral preparation*

point is further posterior than anterior, to allow for the anterior bow in the femur. It must also be lateral, so that it lies directly over the lateral margin of the medullary canal (Fig. 10.12). This allows instruments to run towards the medial femoral condyle, preventing varus malpositioning of the femoral component. This usually gives a starting point which enters the proximal portion of the greater trochanter.

The femur is initially prepared with a tapered reamer to remove a cone of medullary bone within which rasping is begun. The smallest reamer is inserted into the medullary canal. The reamer is allowed to run down the lateral cortex, thus following the medullary canal, but the tip of the reamer should be angled slightly medially, as if trying to come out through the medial femoral condyle. This is, again, to prevent eventual varus malposition of the femoral component. If the reamer will not follow the canal, further bone needs to be removed from the greater trochanter. The entry point position and angle should be checked and adjusted if necessary. The usual requirement is for removal of cancellous bone from the greater trochanter with a curette. Sequentially larger tapered reamers are then used to increase the diameter, until contact with cortical bone is felt. At this point, the reamer becomes more stable within the femur, such that the instrument and bone move as one.

The next step is shaping of the proximal femur to receive the implant, whether it is to be cemented or uncemented, with particular care paid to the anteversion of the rasp within the proximal femur. This is done with rasps. The rasps

are positioned to provide around 15° of anteversion. In the posterior approach, this is done by angling the medial side of the rasp downwards 15°; in the lateral approach it is angled 15° upwards. Rasps are used to the point where stability can be achieved with the definitive component.

Technical points in uncemented stem insertion

- The rasps used are specific to each stem design.
- The version must be precisely controlled throughout rasping.
- A small rasp is used to begin with and the size increased until stability is achieved. Impaction is with controlled hammer blows, watching the progress of the impactor. When the rasp stops progressing, it should not be impacted further as this may lead to proximal femoral fracture. When stable, the rasp is a tight fit within the canal and rotation of the component rotates the femur with no 'toggle' between the two.
- The templated size should be borne in mind.
- Excessive anteversion will tend to give a poor fit. Selection of a prosthesis several sizes smaller than that achieved on templating may indicate this to be the case.
- The depth of the rasp is noted. This should be such that the cutting teeth are at or just below the level of the neck cut.
- Trial reduction is carried out, with a variety of offset options available on most uncemented systems (see below for details).
- The rasp is removed and the definitive prosthesis can be inserted, following the version of the rasps. The canal is not washed out, as the bone swarf aids in union across the implant to bone interface.

Technical points in cemented stem insertion

- The rasps allow for a 2–3 mm cement mantle to be created between the component and bone. The technique is similar to that in uncemented stems, with increasing size of rasp used until stability is achieved.
- If using a collared stem, the final broach is sunk to the required depth and the 'calcar cutter' is used. This attaches over the final rasp and

provides a smooth, stable neck cut at the level upon which the collar will be supported.

- The height of the final rasp can be gauged in respect to both the greater trochanter and the medial extent of the femoral neck cut. It is vital to be able to reproduce these relationships with the definitive stem, when it is cemented *in situ*.
- Trial reduction is carried out (see below for details).
- A cement restrictor is used to occlude the medullary canal distally. The depth of insertion is obtained by measurement against the final rasp used, aiming for 1–2 cm of clearance to allow for distal cementing. The canal must now be thoroughly washed with pulse lavage, using a long nozzle to clean debris and fat from the entire length of the prepared bone. Suction is used to remove the saline cleaning solution. The canal is then dried and packed with swabs or a preformed absorbent sponge.
- Cementation is performed with a double mix of polymethylmethacrylate cement, using a cement gun with a long nozzle. The cement is introduced when it is of sufficient viscosity (when the cement does not stick to the surgeon's glove, the required viscosity has been reached – typically after around 2–3 minutes).
- The nozzle is introduced up to the cement restrictor then cement is pumped firmly to introduce it into the canal. The cement gun is not withdrawn, rather it is allowed to be pushed out by the cement as it fills the canal. Use of suction removes the fluid extruded from the canal.
- When the cement reaches the proximal femur, the nozzle is withdrawn and cut. A proximal cement pressurizer is placed over the remaining nozzle and reintroduced into the femoral canal, occluding the proximal femur. Further cement is introduced under pressure, as the restrictor occludes the femoral cavity, for around 30 seconds.
- The definitive stem should be checked and correctly assembled on its introducer. The correct time for introduction of the stem is determined by the type of cement and ambient temperature conditions. It is usually at around 4–6 minutes.

- The cement gun and pressurizer are removed and the femoral component is introduced in the correct version and manually inserted to the correct depth. The version must remain constant and the movement is a smooth, even application of force. If the stem will not reach the desired depth with manual pressure, a mallet can be used on the introducing handle to seat the implant at the correct depth. The end result should be a reproduction of the depth of the trial at time of rasping.
- The implant must be held perfectly still within the femur until the cement has cured, typically after 10–12 minutes.

Trialling and reduction

Trial reduction is a vital step in total hip replacement (THR). The assessment is essentially of stability, range of motion and leg length.

Reduction is carried out with appropriate trial components, usually consisting of the last rasp left *in situ* and a trial head. Reduction is via the surgical assistant applying in-line traction followed by rotation of the head into the acetabulum. The traction is assisted by the surgeon pushing on the femoral head with a conical pusher. If reduction cannot be achieved, a shorter femoral head and/or a neck with less offset is selected and the manoeuvre repeated.

Once the THR trial is reduced, assessment is made of the stability. The position of the head with respect to the greater trochanter is noted and compared with that on preoperative templating.

The hip is passed through a functional range of motion and must not dislocate in any position. The hip can then be forced into non-physiological positions to assess the point at which dislocation can occur. In the lateral approach, the hip should remain in joint even when the leg is replaced in adduction and external rotation, back into the sterile 'leg bag'. In the posterior approach, the hip is tested in slight adduction and forced internal rotation; the degree of internal rotation to dislocation should be noted and should be no less than 40°.

The tissue tension is assessed by the 'shuck test' – the femur is pulled sharply downwards and the degree of telescoping of the femoral head away from the acetabular socket is noted. Any more than a few millimetres of movement suggests that instability may be present. In this case, further trial with a longer trial femoral head is recommended.

The lateral tissue tension can be assessed with the 'lateral shuck test'. A dislocation hook is passed around the femoral neck and the component sharply pulled laterally. Again, excessive movement indicates instability and the need for a higher offset neck to be used.

The operated leg is placed against the opposite leg in order to compare leg length. Gross differences suggest incorrect head selection. Note that stability and range of motion are of higher importance than subtle differences in leg length, but lengthening of the operated leg to greater than 1 cm longer than the other leg is associated with significant patient dissatisfaction.

If a stable hip is not achievable in a functional range of motion, consideration must be given to the following factors:

- Component position – are the stem and socket in the right degree of version? Is the cup sufficiently medialized? Is the stem at the correct height? If they are not, they may need to be repositioned.
- Use of a lip augment on the acetabulum. In uncemented acetabula, exchange of the liner is relatively simple. The use of a 10° or 20° lip augment can prevent dislocation.
- Use of a larger femoral head will increase the stability of the hip.
- The use of a constrained prosthesis is a last resort and not usually appropriate in primary hip surgery.

Closure of posterior approach

If the capsule has been preserved, it is sometimes possible to repair this directly, using a heavy absorbable suture. Proper repair of the short external rotators to the shaft of the femur is vitally important. The rotators should be intact and easily identified by the sutures passed through their tendons prior to their division. If these sutures are left long at the time of their insertion, they can be used to reattach the muscles. If not, four sutures are secured to the cut ends of the short external rotators.

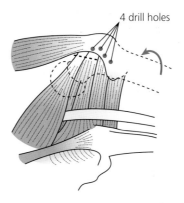

Figure 10.13 *Position of drill holes for reattachment of the short external rotators*

A small (e.g. 2.5 mm) drill is passed through the greater trochanter, from anterior to posterior, in the line of attachment of the small external rotators (Fig. 10.13). A suture passer is then passed through the drill hole, opened and used to pull one of the sutures through – both ends of the same suture are pulled through the one hole. Three further drill holes are created and the three remaining sutures pulled through.

Both ends of the upper two sutures are then tied to each other, then the same procedure carried out with the lower two sutures. This is done with the leg in around 10° of abduction and only a few degrees of external rotation, which allows approximation of the tendon to the greater trochanter without causing a fixed rotation deformity. The split fibres of the gluteus maximus are loosely approximated with absorbable sutures.

If a surgical drain is to be used, it is inserted now. Closure of the fascia lata is performed with the hip in slight abduction. Superficial closure utilizes absorbable sutures to approximate the subcutaneous fat, then cutaneous sutures or surgical staples. An occlusive dressing is applied.

Closure of lateral approach

If the capsule is repairable, this is performed first. The gluteus medius anterior and posterior flaps are approximated. These are then tightly sutured together with the leg in around 10° of abduction.

Superficial closure uses the same technique as that for the posterior approach.

POSTOPERATIVE CARE AND INSTRUCTIONS

The patient is returned to the supine position and an abduction pillow inserted between the legs. Any straps present on these pillows should not be used, due to the risk of peroneal nerve damage. Precautions against thromboembolism should be used. Common options include aspirin, low molecular weight heparin, graduated compression stockings and foot or calf intermittent compression pumps. Early mobilization should be encouraged in all patients. Two further doses of the same antibiotic given upon induction are given intravenously. Haemoglobin levels should be monitored and transfusion considered as necessary.

Weightbearing is begun immediately in those patients with a cemented stem, regardless of the cup used. Six weeks of avoidance of weightbearing is recommended in many uncemented stem arthroplasties, though some are permitted early partial or even full weightbearing. The patient is allowed to walk but asked to avoid crossing of the legs or excessive flexion of the hips. To this end, they are provided with a raised toilet seat and instructed to avoid low seats. **Particular care is recommended when putting on socks and shoes –** a common cause of early dislocation. Return to work is allowed after around 6 weeks for sedentary jobs, but may be delayed to 3 months or more in active work. Follow-up is recommended at 6 weeks, 6 months and 1 year after surgery. Continuation of follow-up is typically at 5 years, 10 years, 15 years and then at yearly intervals. The patient should be cautioned to return to clinic if there is pain or functional deterioration.

RECOMMENDED REFERENCES

Barrack RL, Mulroy RD Jr, Harris WH. Improved cementing techniques and femoral component loosening in young patients with hip arthroplasty. *J Bone Joint Surg Br* 1992;**74**:385–9.
Charnley J. Arthroplasty of the hip: a new operation. *Lancet* 1961;**1**:1129–32.
Hardinge K. The direct lateral approach. *J Bone Joint Surg Br* 1982;**64**:17–9.
Lidwell OM, Lowbury EJ, Whyte W, *et al.* Effect of ultraclean air in operating rooms on deep sepsis in the joint after total hip or knee replacement. *BMJ* 1982;**285**:10–4.
Murray DW, Carr AJ, Bulstrode CJ. Which primary total hip replacement? *J Bone Joint Surg Br* 1995;**77**:520–7.
Pellicci PM, Bostrom M, Poss R. Posterior approach to total hip replacement using enhanced posterior soft tissue repair. *Clin Orthop Relat Res* 1998;(355):224–8.
The Swedish Hip Arthroplasty Register. Online. Available at: www.jru.orthop.gu.se.

REVISION TOTAL HIP ARTHROPLASTY

This section refers extensively to sections in the primary hip arthroplasty section and is not intended as a standalone text to enable all surgeons to revise all hips. It aims to provide some useful directions as to appropriate techniques that can be applied to solve some problems, but cannot cover all potential problems.

PREOPERATIVE PLANNING

Indications

Revision hip replacement is indicated for painful failure of a primary arthroplasty. The most common causes are:
- Aseptic loosening of the socket and/or stem
- Deep infection (see later section)
- Instability, resulting in recurrent dislocation
- Fracture of either the implant or the proximal femur.

Contraindications

- Continuation of preoperative pain after hip arthroplasty (this suggests that the original diagnosis may have been wrong and warrants further investigation).
- Pain-free loosening is a relative contraindication, except in cases associated with significant and progressive osteolysis.

Consent and risks

- Nerve injury: 3–7 per cent.

- Infection: quoted up to 30 per cent, 5 per cent is a more commonly accepted figure
- Thromboembolism: 3 per cent
- Dislocation: 7 per cent
- Aseptic loosening: 10–30 per cent at 10 years
- Fracture
- Limb length discrepancy

Operative planning

Revision arthroplasty is more challenging than primary surgery so requires even more precise planning. Recent radiographs are essential. 'Judet views' can be very helpful in assessing acetabular bone loss. If there is significant bone loss, a fine cut computed tomography (CT) scan is used to assess and quantify it. The patient should have been seen in outpatients recently so that the functional status has been noted. This is as vital as the osseous imaging in decision making.

The soft tissue status must be assessed and any signs of infection need investigation and treatment. It is not always necessary to revise all components in aseptic failures; consideration should be given to keeping any well fixed and functional prosthetic component. If the prosthesis is infected, a two-stage procedure is preferred (see below).

Templating should be carried out with great care. It is necessary to be prepared for unexpected findings at the time of surgery and a wide range of implants should be available to the surgeon.

There are a number of extra instruments which can be useful in revision procedures. The surgeon should consider ordering any, or all of the following, in particular:
- Image intensifier
- Extraction instruments for the existing implant
- Bone allograft, for morcellized or block grafting
- Cement removing osteotomes and ultrasonic cement removal systems
- Supplementary metalwork, including cabling systems, trochanteric fixation devices, acetabular reconstruction rings and plates, cages, mesh and even computer-aided design/computer-aided manufacturing (CAD CAM) implants
- Thin, curved osteotomes for removing cementless hips.

Anaesthesia and positioning

This is the same as in primary arthroplasty, except that the initial antibiotic dose is usually delayed until after microbiological samples have been taken.

SURGICAL TECHNIQUE

Approach

Either the posterior or lateral approach can be used. Some surgeons argue that the posterior approach is best for posterior acetabular defects.

A trochanteric osteotomy can be required, particularly in highly complex revisions or in removal of a well-fixed cementless stem. The greater trochanter is removed with gluteus medius and minimus attached, allowing it to be mobilized well out of the way. The length of the osteotomy required is dependent on the implant that you are trying to get out and may be as long as the implant itself, which can be judged with image intensifier or from preoperative planning (Fig. 10.14).

Identification of the sciatic nerve is important, particularly in the posterior approach. The nerve can be isolated by carefully passing a vascular sloop around it, thus ensuring that its location is known at all times.

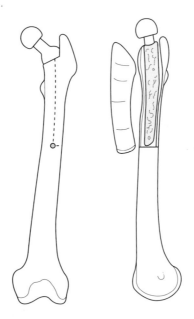

Figure 10.14 An 'extended' trochanteric osteotomy

Procedure

Following dislocation, the femoral head of a modular component is removed with a head and neck separator. Many implants have a specific extraction device and, if available, these should be used.

Removal of a cemented stem

It is sometimes possible to simply pull the implant out of the cement mantle. If this is not the case, some of the proximal cement mantle will need to be removed from the lateral margin of the implant. This is almost always necessary if removing a curved femoral stem. This is usually relatively easily achieved with cement osteotomes.

The rest of the cement can be left *in situ* at this time as it tamponades bleeding from the femoral canal. When cement is to be removed, it is done with cement osteotomes and an ultrasonic cement remover. The cement restrictor must also be removed.

Removal of a cementless stem

This can be very difficult in well-fixed stems, particularly if extensively coated.

The use of specialized, flexible osteotomes or high-speed burs is recommended. Care must be taken to avoid unnecessary breach of the proximal femoral cortex. Following removal, the femoral canal is packed with swabs to tamponade bleeding.

Assessing femoral bone loss

The two most commonly used grading systems are the Paprosky and the American Academy of Orthopedic Surgeons (AAOS) systems. Table 10.1 shows the Paprosky system together with possible solutions.

Table 10.1 Paprosky classification of femoral defects at revision hip surgery

Paprosky grade	Diagram	Treatment options
Type I – *has an intact metaphysis and isthmus*		*Typically treated with a primary implant*
Type II – *has metaphyseal damage but an intact isthmus*		*Long stem cemented implant; distally fixed uncemented stem*

Type IIIA – *distal fixation can be achieved at the isthmus, despite damage to the isthmus and the metaphysis*

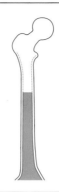

Long stem cemented implanted with impaction allograft; long stem distally fixed uncemented stem

Type IIIB – *damage to the metaphysis and isthmus prevent distal fixation from being achieved*

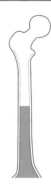

Long stem cemented implant with morcellized and corticocancellous strut graft; long stem distally fixed uncemented stem with corticocancellous strut graft; massive tumour prosthesis proximal femoral replacement

Type IV –*extensive metaphyseal damage and an eroded isthmus*

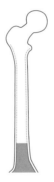

Proximal femoral replacement

Removal of a cemented socket

If the acetabular component is loose, it will often come free with minimal effort, typically along with the majority of its cement attached.

In a well-fixed socket, a curved osteotome is used to develop a plane between the cup and the cement. Alternatively, a pilot hole can be drilled into the centre of the component and a slap-hammer screwed into it. Once loose, the socket is removed and the cement is then removed piecemeal with small osteotomes. This method gives the least bone loss and minimizes the likelihood of acetabular fracture.

If the above method also fails, the acetabular socket is cut into quarters with a power saw and can then be removed. It is important that all cement is also removed.

Removal of an uncemented socket

If the cup is well-fixed, it should be remembered that it may not need to be removed. In this case, the liner can be removed but this must be done carefully to avoid damage to the liner to socket locking mechanism. If the locking mechanism is still functioning, a simple liner exchange can be performed, remembering that the replacement liner need not be of the same internal diameter or have the same augment or 'lip' size'. A controversial measure, in a well-fixed socket with a destroyed or obsolete locking mechanism, is cementation of a smaller liner within the shell.

If there is significant osteolysis behind the screw hole in the socket, it is possible to apply morcellized bone graft through the screw holes to aid in reducing this. If the socket is to be removed, any screws are removed first. The well-fixed socket is carefully removed by developing a plane between the bone and the implant with curved osteotomes. Care must be taken to avoid excess bone loss.

The use of a suitable removal system, such as Explant (Zimmer, Warsaw, IN, USA), can minimize the bone destruction.

Assessing acetabular bone loss

The most commonly used grading system is the AAOS system. Table 10.2 shows the AAOS system together with possible solutions.

Table 10.2 American Academy of Orthopedic Surgeons (AAOS) classification of acetabular bone loss at revision hip surgery

AAOS grade	Diagram	Treatment options
Segmental		Small defects, allowing for 70 per cent implant to bone contact, require no additional treatment; larger defects can require the use of structural allograft or asymmetric acetabular shells, e.g. the S-ROM oblong (DePuy, Warsaw, IN, USA); Loss of the medial wall can be managed with a malleable mesh and morcellized allograft as long as there is peripheral support
Cavitatory		If small, these are usually reamed to provide contact in 70 per cent or more of the bone surface. An uncemented cup with screw augmentation is a typical prosthesis used; larger defects require grafting – this can be with morcellized graft obtained from fresh frozen femoral head allograft. It can need structural graft, again usually obtained from femoral head or distal femoral allograft, fixed with screws or a buttress plate
Combined		The segmental defect is first reconstructed to provide a stable rim; persisting cavitatory loss is grafted with morcellized allograft
Pelvic discontinuity		This is a difficult problem, requiring reconstruction with plates and screws or even an entire acetabular allograft; CAD CAM sockets can be very useful to provide fixation to the ilium, ischium and pubis

CAD CAM, computer-aided design/computer-aided manufacturing.

Revision of infected implants

If the revision is for infection, this is usually carried out in two stages. The initial stage is removal of all implants and cement. It is vital that multiple samples from around all implants are sent for microbiological assessment. The whole surgical field should be thoroughly debrided and then washed out with a minimum of 6 L of saline pulsatile lavage.

A polymethylmethacrylate cement spacer is then inserted. This can be preformed or can be made with moulds of varying sizes. The cement should contain heat-stable antibiotics, such as gentamicin or tobramycin. Closure is performed and the patient may mobilize, although usually only partially weightbearing.

The patient should be followed up clinically and have regular checks of inflammatory markers. Postoperative antibiotics can be given once the microbiological sensitivities have been received. These cases often require combination antibiotic therapy. Once the inflammatory markers are normal, the second stage can be undertaken, with reconstruction depending on the extent of femoral and acetabular bone loss. Particular care must be taken with the soft tissues as multiple procedures will often have taken their toll on the surrounding musculature. Many surgeons prefer the use of a cemented stem in this situation as extra antibiotics can be added to decrease the chance of recurrence.

CLOSURE AND POSTOPERATIVE CARE

These are broadly in line with the guidelines for primary hip arthroplasty. It may be necessary to consider additional precautions, particularly in limitation of range of motion and weightbearing. It is usual to continue antibiotics until microbiological results are available.

RECOMMENDED REFERENCES

Gruen TA, McNeice GM, Amstutz AC. 'Modes of failure' of cemented stem-type components: a radiographic analysis. *Clin Orthop Relat Res* 1979;(141):17–27.
Jasty M, Harris WH. Total hip reconstruction using frozen femoral head allografts in patients with acetabular bone loss. *Orthop Clin North Am* 1987;18:291–9.
Valle CJ, Paprosky WG. Classification and an algorithmic approach to the reconstruction of femoral deficiency. *J Bone Joint Surg Am* 2003;85(Suppl 4):1–6.

HIP RESURFACING

Hip resurfacing can be more challenging than THR but shares many similar principles. Details of the approach can be found in the section on THR above.

PREOPERATIVE PLANNING

Indications and contraindications

The indications and contraindications for surface replacement of the hip are the same as those for THR. In addition, there are further contraindications that reflect the need to maintain the femoral neck:

- Femoral head cysts >1 cm diameter
- Osteoporosis – recommended to investigate with dual energy X-ray absorptiometry (DEXA or DXA) in perimenopausal women/high-risk groups
- Neck length of <2 cm
- Significant lateral head–neck remodelling
- Head:neck ratio <1.2.

Consent and risks

- The risks and consent are equivalent to THR
- In addition the risks of femoral neck fracture or intraoperative conversion to THR (e.g. due to notching or size mismatch) must be mentioned

Operative planning

Recent radiographs and templating are essential. The surgeon should have a guide available to check the compatibility of the femoral and acetabular components.

Anaesthesia and positioning

This is performed as for THR.

SURGICAL TECHNIQUE

Surface replacement is possible through any of the common approaches to the hip. The posterior approach is commonly used and the following description is based on it.

The dissection is exactly as described in the THR section. In order to gain visibility around the whole of the femoral neck, some further steps are applied:

- The quadratus femoris should be released prior to dislocation.
- The gluteus maximus tendon can be released off its insertion into the linea aspera, allowing more rotation and visualization.
- The capsular incision is much more significant. This is essential in order to allow 360° visualization of the neck to check that notching is not going to occur.
- The capsulotomy is carried out from superior to inferior around the femoral neck, carrying on down the inferior neck as far as can be visualized.
- This incision is then carefully continued with heavy 'capsulotomy' scissors, releasing the capsule inferiorly and medially. Great care is taken to stay close to the bone of the femoral neck.
- The hip is dislocated and the capsulotomy continued until the capsule is released right around the femoral neck, such that the head and proximal femur can be viewed all the way around (Fig. 10.15).

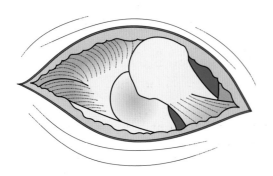

Figure 10.15 *Extensive release of the hip capsule to allow full delivery of the femoral head into the wound*

Femoral head displacement

In order to gain sight of the acetabulum, the femoral head must be displaced. If there are any particularly large osteophytes, these should be removed at this stage. A pocket is created for the femoral head, lying under the gluteus medius and upon the iliac wing above the acetabulum. This can be created by sweeping a blunt periosteal elevator or bone spike under the gluteus medius. Once a sufficient pocket is created, the leg is lowered sufficiently to place a sharp retractor over the anterior lip of the acetabulum. This is used to lever the femur anteriorly as the leg is dropped down onto the table and the head is guided into the pocket created for it.

If the head is very large, it can be debulked further by the initial stages of femoral head preparation (described later) prior to displacing it into the pocket created.

Acetabular preparation

This is very similar to the technique described in the section on THR for uncemented cup insertion and the position is the same. Care should be taken not to over-ream the acetabulum as the implants are press-fit and cannot be augmented with screws. In addition, selection of the femoral head size is guided by the size of the acetabular component as they must fit together.

Femoral preparation

Femoral shaping is done to create a cut surface which will fit with the femoral component. A variety of jigs are available depending upon the implant manufacturer and reference to the individual technical guides is recommended. They all aim to place a guidewire in the centre of the neck, in both the anteroposterior and mediolateral planes. This entry point will be some way above the fovea, which does not correspond to the midpoint of the neck. This critical step can be helped by drawing a line up the centre of the posterior and lateral margins of the neck and carrying this up onto the head as a guide. The position to aim for is equal to the native anteversion and 0–10° of valgus compared with the patient's femoral neck.

Once the guidewire is passed, a jig is placed over it and swept around the entire neck to ensure that there is clearance around the whole diameter, i.e. it will not be notched. If the entry point or angle is incorrect, the guidewire is removed and replaced.

Once the guidewire is correctly positioned a post drill is used to create a central hole for the post to be inserted into the femoral head. This is then the guide for further cuts. Again, equipment varies but all have specific cutters and reamers for shaping of the proximal femur. Care should be taken that the size chosen fits with the acetabular component and that notching is prevented. If a significant notch is created, the surgeon must change to a total hip replacement. While cutting and shaping, drapes should be placed over the surrounding soft tissues to prevent bone swarf from entering tissue planes.

A profile reamer is then used to shape the head and a step drill to create around six holes in the bevelled edge, to act as cement keys. The intended final resting place of the component is marked on the femoral head–neck junction.

The head is thoroughly washed with pulsed normal saline and the appropriate head is cemented *in situ*, typically with low viscosity cement. It is impacted up to the previously created mark to ensure that it is in place. The hip is reduced and assessed for stability.

At closure, the gluteus maximus tendon and quadratus femoris are closed, then closure is as in THR. Postoperative care and complications are also equivalent to total hip replacement.

HIP ARTHRODESIS

PREOPERATIVE PLANNING

Below is a description of one common technique although there are many described in the literature.

Indications

Hip arthrodesis is rapidly becoming a procedure of historical interest only as improvements in THR allow implantation in younger patients. It has limited indications now but was used in young adults in order to allow return to manual labour. Continuing indications are:
- Failed arthroplasty
- Sequelae of infection, particularly tuberculosis
- Sickle cell anaemic arthropathy.

Contraindications

- Contralateral hip disease
- Ipsilateral knee disease
- Pre-existing lower back pain
- Inflammatory arthropathy – relative.

Consent and risks

- Lower back pain: 60 per cent
- Leg length discrepancy: 100 per cent (typically up to 5 cm)
- Knee pain: 45 per cent
- Failure of fusion: 2 per cent clinically but up to 30 per cent radiographically
- Malpositioning (it has been shown that the rates of back pain are higher in malpositioned hips)

The patient must understand that walking will be abnormal and running impossible. There is a significant reduction in walking speed and increase in energy expenditure.

Operative planning

Planning of the position of fusion is vital. The position is:
- Flexion of 20–25°
- Rotation neutral to 10° of external rotation
- Adduction of 0–5°.

A variety of techniques can be used, with intra-articular or extra-articular fusion achieved.

Anaesthesia and positioning

This is performed as for THR.

SURGICAL TECHNIQUE

Approach

The lateral approach is used, as described in the primary arthroplasty section. The patient is positioned supine, rather than in the lateral position; a sandbag is placed under the ipsilateral buttock. This position allows for more accurate assessment of leg length and, upon removal of the sandbag, the surgeon can perform a Thomas' test at the end of the fusion in order to assess the position of arthrodesis.

Procedure

The gluteus medius and minimus complex is left attached to the greater trochanter and their anterior and posterior borders defined carefully. An oscillating saw is used to create an osteotomy, separating the greater trochanter from the proximal femur. The abductors remain attached to the greater trochanter. The greater trochanter and abductor complex are reflected upwards; this may require some dissection of the undersurface of the abductors away from the superior capsule.

The acetabulum is dissected of soft tissues, carefully defining from the sciatic notch at the back, around the superior border and round to the anterior border. A blunt Hohmann retractor is inserted into the sciatic notch (this protects the sciatic nerve and the superior gluteal vessels) and another is hooked around the iliopectineal eminence anteriorly. A horizontal osteotomy is carefully created between the two retractors, running just above the superior surface of the acetabulum. This can be begun with an oscillating saw but should be completed with an osteotome to reduce the danger of sciatic nerve injury.

A corresponding horizontal surface is created on the top of the femoral head by removing a small portion of the head with an oscillating saw. Curettes are used to remove any areas of persistent cartilage on the femoral head and the acetabulum. A retractor is inserted into the pelvic osteotomy and used to lever the osteotomy and displace the distal portion approximately 1 cm medially with respect to the proximal ilium. By removing the sandbag from under the buttock, the position for arthrodesis can be accurately assessed.

The cobra plate is attached over the osteotomy site; this only requires one screw into the pelvis and one into the femur at this stage. Careful palpation of the pelvis, patella and malleoli is carried out to confirm the correct position of the leg before the arthrodesis. The author

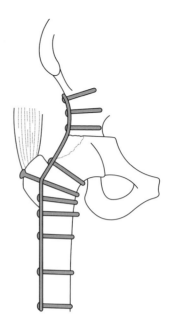

Figure 10.16 *A hip arthrodesis with cobra plate*

recommends the use of an image intensifier at this stage to further confirm positioning.

The flexion position of 20–25° is confirmed by performing the Thomas test. The greater trochanter is then repositioned at the anatomical site. This can now be attached back onto the femur with a screw through the greater trochanter and the cobra plate (Fig. 10.16). The remaining screw holes are drilled and further cortical screws inserted to strengthen the arthrodesis.

Closure

Closure is similar to the lateral approach for total hip replacement: a layered closure followed by the surgeon's choice of skin closure.

POSTOPERATIVE CARE AND INSTRUCTIONS

Thromboembolism should be prevented by early mobilization and the addition of chemical or mechanical measures in patients at increased risk. Two further doses of the antibiotic given at induction should be given at 8 hours and 16 hours after surgery.

Early mobilization is non-weightbearing, with the aid of crutches. Radiographic signs of union are sought before a return to weightbearing is allowed. This often takes around 3 months. If the patient has significant shortening, i.e. greater than 15 mm, a shoe raise insert can be provided and used as the patient deems necessary.

RECOMMENDED REFERENCES

Murrell GA, Fitch RD. Hip fusion in young adults. Using a medial displacement osteotomy and cobra plate. *Clin Orthop Relat Res* 1994;(300):147–54.
Sponseller PD, McBeath AA, Perpich M. Hip arthrodesis in young patients: a long term follow up study. *J Bone Joint Surg Am* 1984;**66**:853–9.

EXCISION HIP ARTHROPLASTY (GIRDLESTONE PROCEDURE)

PREOPERATIVE PLANNING

Indications

- It is a last resort operation and used as a salvage procedure, generally in patients with resistant infections or comorbidities which necessitate a quick operation.
- Sepsis of either THR or the native hip
- Aseptic loosening of THR
- Painful hip conditions in a patient otherwise immobile, particularly in degenerative neuro-muscular conditions.

Consent and risks

- Nerve injury
- Limb length discrepancy: it is usually 3–12 cm, depending on resection
- Recurrence of infection (if a septic indication): 10 per cent
- Nearly all will be reliant on walking aids after surgery; many have poor function but most have good pain relief

Anaesthesia and positioning

This is performed as for THR.

SURGICAL TECHNIQUE

One of the approaches for THR is selected. If the hip is septic, a thorough washout and debridement of infected tissue is essential.

The excision is carried out as in THR femoral head resection. All non-viable bone should be resected but results are best if as much proximal femur as possible is maintained, so it is advisable not to be overly aggressive in the excision.

POSTOPERATIVE CARE AND INSTRUCTIONS

This is similar to THR in many respects. Traction is often used for the first 2 weeks after surgery. Almost all patients will require walking aids and shoe raises.

FEMOROACETABULAR IMPINGEMENT SURGERY

PREOPERATIVE PLANNING

Indications

- Pain and/or restricted range of motion associated with a recognized anatomical deformity.

This can be of two types: cam or pincer; these can also coexist (Fig. 10.17). The cam deformity of the femur is also referred to as a 'pistol grip' deformity. The most typical presentation is groin pain worse on prolonged flexion e.g. sitting. The impingement test of the hip is usually positive. (The hip is held in 90° flexion and passively internally rotated and adducted.)

Contraindications

- Active infection
- Moderate or severe existing arthritis on radiographs.

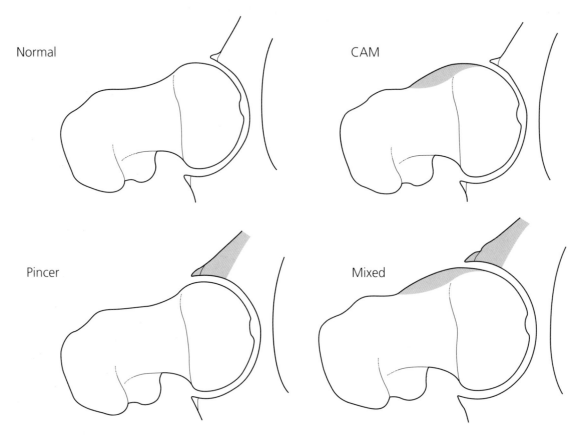

Normal

CAM

Pincer

Mixed

Figure 10.17 *The common variants of femoroacetabular impingement*

Consent and risks (as applicable to open femoroacetabular impingement surgery)

- DVT: <1 per cent
- Infection: <1 per cent
- Femoral neck fracture: incidence related to amount of femoral 'bump' removed
- Avascular necrosis of the femoral head: unknown incidence (many studies of open surgery show 0 per cent)
- Heterotopic ossification: 3 per cent
- Progression to frank osteoarthritis: up to 100 per cent

Operative planning

Recent radiographs must be available – antero-posterior views of the hip and a shoot-through lateral with the leg in maximal internal rotation best demonstrate the anatomy. Magnetic resonance imaging (MRI), MR arthrography or arthroscopy are often used to examine for labral pathology. Conventional arthrography and local anaesthetic injection are frequently used to provide evidence that the pain is originating in the hip.

The surgeon must decide the approach to be taken. There are three common options:
- The arthroscopic approach (see 'Hip arthroscopy', next section).
- The lateral open approach, using a trochanteric flip osteotomy, as popularized by Ganz. The hip is then dislocated to reveal the impingement.
- A more recent approach has been a 'mini-open' modified Smith–Peterson approach. This has the advantage of visualization without dislocation of the hip. This approach is described below, as an example.

Anaesthesia and positioning

Anaesthesia is general with supine positioning. The use of an intraoperative image intensifier is optional.

SURGICAL TECHNIQUE

Landmarks

The anterior superior iliac spine is palpated. Slight external rotation of the hip aids location of the interval between the tensor fascia lata and sartorius.

Incision

A 7–10 cm incision is created, running from just below the anterior superior iliac spine, running in the border between the tensor fascia lata and sartorius. This should not stray medially into the area overlying sartorius and it is preferable to create the incision a few millimetres lateral to the border of sartorius to ensure that this does not occur. The direction of incision is towards the lateral border of the patella.

Superficial dissection

Structure at risk

- Lateral femoral cutaneous nerve

Dissection is continued through fat and superficial fascia. The lateral femoral cutaneous nerve is identified, running over the fascia between the tensor fascia lata and sartorius. The nerve is retracted medially and the fascia incised between the two muscle bellies. This provides an interval with the muscle belly of the tensor fascia lata laterally and that of the sartorius medially.

The dissection is continued down between the tensor fascia lata and sartorius, until the direct and reflected heads of the rectus femoris are identified.

Deep dissection

Structures at risk

- Femoral nerve and artery – these lie medial to the sartorius, anterior to the pectineus muscle. They will not be damaged if dissection is lateral and deep to the sartorius
- Medial femoral circumflex artery – 1 cm proximal to the lesser trochanter, underlying the iliopsoas tendon. If not identified and accidentally damaged, profuse bleeding can be expected

The reflected head of the rectus femoris is identified and dissected off its origin on the superior acetabular margin. Its fibres also blend with the anterior hip capsule and these fibres are dissected free from the capsule. The direct head is retracted medially to reveal the iliopsoas tendon. This also requires dissection free from the capsule as it is attached by the iliocapsularis tendon. Subsequently, this too can be retracted medially.

The underlying capsule is exposed and can be incised in line with the femoral head–neck junction. This is most easily identified at the anteromedial portion of the femoral head as the impingement bump in a cam-impinging hip will prevent palpation of the head–neck junction laterally. Thus, it is advisable to begin the incision medially and proceed laterally.

PROCEDURE

The osteoplasty of the head–neck junction is carried out with a small (10–15 mm) osteotome. An assistant internally and externally rotates the hip to allow complete excision of the bump. The resection is directed distally to produce a bevelled resection, restoring the offset between the femoral head and neck. This creates a 'V'-shaped valley over the anterior head–neck junction. The depth of the valley can be assessed by bringing the hip back into the position of the impingement test. The aim is a gain in both internal rotation and flexion of the hip by over 10°. If the valley is not deep enough, it can be further deepened in a similar manner. The aim is complete excision of the protuberant bump, until the remaining femoral head is spherical and no longer impinging on the anterior acetabular rim. Similarly, if there is evidence of pincer impingement, the acetabular osteophytes or calcified labral tissue can be removed with an osteotome and excised.

Bleeding from exposed bone can be reduced by application of bone wax. The wound is thoroughly irrigated and any loose bone and cartilage carefully removed.

Closure

- The capsulotomy is closed with absorbable suture.
- The reflected head of rectus femoris is reapproximated with absorbable suture.
- The tensor fascia lata–sartorius interval is closed with absorbable suture.
- Skin closure.

POSTOPERATIVE CARE AND INSTRUCTIONS

The patient may begin mobilization as soon as comfortable – this should be touch-weightbearing, with crutches, for 6 weeks. Active flexion is avoided for 6 weeks to allow healing of the reflected head of rectus femoris. Active abduction is begun straight away. Mobilization without crutches is slowly begun after 6 weeks. High-impact sports, including running, are not permitted for 6 months.

HIP ARTHROSCOPY

PREOPERATIVE PLANNING

Indications

Hip arthroscopy is indicated in a variety of painful conditions of the hip. The most frequent are:
- Undiagnosed hip pain in the young
- Osteoarthritis
- Labral pathology
- Osteochondral defect
- Removal of loose bodies
- Synovectomy or synovial biopsy.

Contraindications

- Infection of overlying skin
- Lack of proper instrumentation. The instruments are specific to hip arthroscopy and surgery should not be attempted without fluoroscopy, appropriate portal instruments, a long arthroscope (30° or 70°) and distraction equipment
- Gross osteoarthritis is a relative contra-indication.

Consent and risks

- Nerve injury: <1 per cent. The lateral femoral cutaneous nerve (anterolateral portal) or the femoral nerve (anterior portal) are at risk
- Vascular injury: <1 per cent
- Infection: <1 per cent. As risk is very low, prophylactic antibiotics are not recommended
- Trochanteric bursitis: 1 per cent
- Iatrogenic injury/failure: 2 per cent Injury to articular cartilage or labrum is possible. A small number of patients cannot be sufficiently distracted for arthroscopy to be performed

Operative planning

Recent radiographs and, where taken, MR images and MR arthrograms, should be available. The equipment must be available; this should be checked by the surgeon.

Anaesthesia and positioning

Anaesthesia is general, and the supine position is used. A peroneal post is well padded and then inserted to provide counter-traction. The hip and knee are extended and the hip slightly externally rotated. The foot is placed in a foot holder on a traction table. This should have a simple mechanism for internal or external rotation as it is useful for an assistant to be able to move the hip during arthroscopy.

Under fluoroscopic control the hip joint is distracted, aiming for 10 mm of opening. The surgical field is prepared with a germicidal solution and draped.

SURGICAL TECHNIQUE

Landmarks

The greater trochanter is palpated and outlined with a cutaneous marker. Lines should be marked to indicate the anterior, middle and posterior thirds of the greater trochanter. The anterior superior iliac spine is also palpated and marked.

Approach

A variety of portals have been described. The details of most are beyond the scope of this book.

The 'workhorse' portals are two lateral portals (described below), although anterior portals can be added in specific situations. The anterior portal is created at the intersection of a line descending vertically from the anterior superior iliac spine and a line passing horizontally from the pubic symphysis.

The lateral portals are created just above the superior surface of the greater trochanter hence they are sometimes known as superolateral portals. Using a long, 14 G spinal needle, an approach is made lying just above the anterior third of the greater trochanter (Fig. 10.18). Fluoroscopy can be used at this stage to confirm entry into the joint.

The approach must be relatively flat (i.e. parallel to the floor) to avoid the superior acetabular labrum. Normal saline is injected through the needle, both to confirm entry and to further distend the joint. Another 14 G spinal needle is passed over the superior edge of the greater trochanter, this time in line with the posterior third. It should be passed at the same angle. A guidewire is placed through each spinal needle and the needles removed. Dilators are then used to enlarge the portal in a controlled manner e.g. a 5 mm, 7 mm then 10 mm dilator.

The final dilator is removed and the arthroscopic cannula is inserted into the anterior portal. A similar process is completed with the more posterior portal. The two portals are generally referred to as the anterolateral and the lateral portals, to avoid confusion with true anterior portals and the rarely used and more dangerous posterior portals. Initially, the anterolateral portal will be used for introduction of instrumentation and the lateral portal will contain the arthroscope.

Either a 30° or 70° arthroscope can be used. Some authors advocate a 70° scope as it can overcome some of the limitations in the viewing field with hip arthroscopy. The water flow should be controlled with an inflow pump on the posterior portal and an outflow integrated within the anterior cannula.

Procedure

A systematic approach is essential if pathology is not to be missed. The author recommends beginning posteriorly, following the posterior labrum and acetabulum. The arthroscope is then drawn superiorly, again specifically viewing the acetabulum and its labrum, then anteriorly.

Throughout the process the femoral head can also be viewed centrally, as the acetabular labrum is seen in the periphery of the view. A hooked probe is introduced and used to assess the soft tissues, particularly the labrum and the articular cartilage.

Specific instruments can be used for removal of loose bodies or debridement of labral tissues (Fig. 10.19).

Closure

Non-absorbable suture is used to close the skin defects.

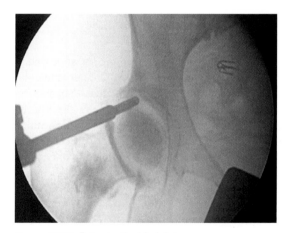

Figure 10.18 *Entry to the hip joint*

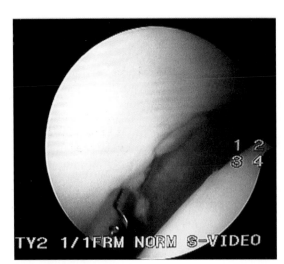

Figure 10.19 *Arthroscopic debridement*

POSTOPERATIVE CARE AND INSTRUCTIONS

The patient is fully weightbearing as tolerated. Specific precautions are rarely required.

RECOMMENDED REFERENCES

Mason JB, McCarthy JC, O'Donnell J, *et al.* Hip arthroscopy: surgical approach, positioning, and distraction. *Clin Orthop Relat Res* 2003;(406):29–37.

McCarthy JC, Lee JA. Hip arthroscopy: indications, outcomes, and complications. *J Bone Joint Surg Am* 2005;87:1137–45.

McCarthy JC, Lee JA. Hip arthroscopy: indications, outcomes, and complications. *Instr Course Lect* 2006;**55**:301–8.

HIP ARTHROGRAPHY

PREOPERATIVE PLANNING

Indications

- Osteoarthritis/rheumatoid arthritis – to assess the degree of cartilage loss
- Sequelae of paediatric disorders, particularly developmental dysplasia of the hip and Perthes disease
- Impingement syndrome
- Assessment of loose total hip implants, including aspiration in suspected sepsis.

Contraindications

- Contrast allergy
- Uncontrolled bleeding dyscrasias.

Operative planning

Preoperative anteroposterior and lateral views of the pelvis and hip should be available. A fluoroscope and contrast need to be available.

Anaesthesia and positioning

Hip arthrography is uncomfortable. It is recommended that it is performed under at least sedation but a short general anaesthetic is preferred. The supine position is used. The hip is placed in the position of maximum joint volume to aid injection:
- 10° abduction
- 10° flexion
- 10° internal rotation.

The fluoroscope is positioned over the hip.

SURGICAL TECHNIQUE

Landmarks

Three centimetres below the mid-inguinal point.

Procedure

Using a long, 22G spinal needle an approach is made through the above landmark, perpendicular to the skin. A 'pop' is felt as the needle penetrates the capsule. The correct position is checked by injecting a small amount of contrast and checking that it is intra-articular with fluoroscopy. Once the position is confirmed, several millilitres of contrast are injected and the needle is removed. The hip is manipulated to distribute the contrast throughout the joint.

Imaging is performed; a typical series includes:
- Anteroposterior hip

- Anteroposterior in internal and external rotation in flexion and extension
- Shoot-through lateral.

If impingement is suspected, an image in flexion and internal rotation is taken.

If the arthrogram is taken for planning an osteotomy, live screening can be used to locate a position of best fit of the femoral head in the acetabulum. This is particularly useful in cases of Perthes disease.

If imaging a total hip implant, digital subtraction can be used by taking a plain view prior to injection of contrast and overlaying it on the contrast anteroposterior view. This will show areas of contrast intrusion around the implant while removing the image of the implant and cement.

POSTOPERATIVE CARE AND INSTRUCTIONS

The patient may fully weightbear immediately. Risks are very low, with infection and contrast reaction both significantly <1 per cent.

RECOMMENDED REFERENCE

O'Neill DA, Harris WH. Failed total hip replacement: assessment by plain radiographs, arthrograms, and aspiration of the hip joint. *J Bone Joint Surg Am* 1984;**66**:540–6.

Viva questions

1. How does revision surgery differ when infection is suspected?

2. What are the indications, benefits and drawbacks for hip arthrodesis?

3. What are the surgical options for a 50-year-old man with symptomatic osteoarthritis of the hips?

4. Describe the anatomy of the sciatic nerve around the hip.

5. How do you classify bone loss around a femoral/acetabular component of a hip replacement?

6. What complications do you warn the patient about prior to hip replacement? What are their incidences?

7. What are the indications for Girdlestone's procedure?

8. When would allograft be used in hip replacement? What types of allograft are used and why?

9. Which approach do you use for total hip replacement and why?

10. What factors influence your choice of hip implant for total hip replacement?

11. What are the contraindications to total hip replacement?

12. What factors affect the quality of the cement mantle in cemented hip replacement?

13. Which nerves can be injured in hip surgery?

14. What factors contribute to dislocation in total hip replacement?

15. Describe the portals used in hip arthroscopy.

16. How do you perform a hip arthrogram?

17. What are the potential advantages of hip resurfacing over total hip replacement?

18. What imaging would you consider before revising a total hip replacement?

19. What are the options for reconstruction of cavitary bone loss in acetabular revision surgery?

20. How can femoroacetabular impingement be treated surgically?

11

Surgery of the knee

Lee David and Timothy W R Briggs

	Range of motion	Position of arthrodesis
Flexion	*150°*	*10–15°*
Extension	*0–(–5)°*	
Int/Ext Rotation	*10°*	*10°*

PRIMARY TOTAL KNEE REPLACEMENT

PREOPERATIVE PLANNING

Indications

Total knee replacement is indicated in the treatment of pain and deformity from the following conditions, when non-operative management has failed or is futile:
- Degenerative osteoarthritis
- Post-traumatic osteoarthritis
- Rheumatoid arthritis
- Other degenerative and inflammatory arthropathies.

Contraindications

- Active or recent local or generalized infection
- Critical arterial ischaemia
- Non-functioning extensor mechanism
- Severe neurological disorders (relative)
- Age (relative). Very young or very old patients should be carefully selected depending on severity of arthritis, level of symptoms and quality of life.

Severe deformity or instability may be a contra-indication to the use of an unconstrained, condylar implant and may require the use of a semi-constrained and stabilized or a constrained, hinged prosthesis.

Consent and risks

- Infection: 1–2 per cent
- Bleeding: approximately 1.5 L on average; it has local or general effects. Haematoma formation increases the risk of wound problems, arthrofibrosis and infection. Hypovolaemia and anaemia may cause cardiovascular, cerebral or renal complications
- Venous thromboembolism – below knee deep vein thrombosis (DVT) occurs in approximately two-thirds of patients following total knee arthroplasty. The risk of fatal pulmonary embolism (PE) is approximately 0.1 per cent. The prevention of DVT and PE remains a controversial topic but it is almost universally accepted that mechanical thromboprophylaxis should be used and that chemical thromboprophylaxis should be used in high-risk groups
- Neurovascular injury can be caused by direct laceration, traction or pressure. Discrete arterial damage is rare (approximately 0.05 per cent) but must be recognized and dealt with immediately. Distal arterial thromboembolism must be promptly recognized, pressure dressings released and a vascular surgical opinion sought. Common

peroneal nerve injury has an incidence of approximately 0.5 per cent and should initially be managed by release of pressure dressings with exploration indicated if caused by haematoma. If caused by traction, equinus deformity should be prevented and nerve conduction studies may be performed at a later date

- Fractures: the risk of fracture is increased in osteoporosis and rheumatoid arthritis. Significant notching of the anterior distal femoral cortex increases the risk of postoperative periprosthetic fracture. Excessive patella resection during resurfacing increases the risk of patella fracture. Intraoperative fractures usually require immediate fixation and the use of stemmed implants
- Extensor mechanism injury – avulsion of the patella tendon is a disastrous complication and must be avoided as it severely compromises the outcome following total knee replacement. In the event of this occurring, the tendon must be reattached to the tibial tuberosity and protected, although the result is usually poor
- Stiffness may be caused by true arthrofibrosis but other causes, including infection and mechanical problems, e.g. 'overstuffing' the knee, patellofemoral maltracking or inadequate bone resection must be ruled out. Treatment depends on the underlying problem
- Instability may be caused by unequal flexion/extension gaps, soft tissue imbalance, ligamentous insufficiency, insufficient insert thickness, polyethylene wear or patellofemoral maltracking. Treatment depends on cause
- Wear
- Loosening
- Pain

OPERATIVE PLANNING

Clinical examination should pay careful attention to alignment, deformity, instability, range of movement and extensor mechanism function. Scars should be carefully noted and a distal neurovascular assessment must be performed.

Recent weightbearing anteroposterior, lateral and skyline patella radiographs must be available and long-leg alignment views may be helpful to establish the mechanical axis of the leg (Fig. 11.1). It is imperative that the patient's symptoms should correlate with the radiographic findings. Templating of preoperative radiographs should be performed if possible, and it is the responsibility of the surgeon to ensure that the required implants are available.

There are many implants available for total knee replacement, and it is the surgeon's responsibility to ensure that he or she is familiar with the implants used, that all necessary equipment is available and that the appropriate range of sizes are readily to hand.

Anaesthesia and positioning

Anaesthesia is usually general, regional or combined, depending on the preferences of the

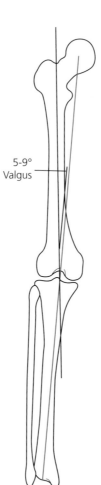

5-9°
Valgus

Figure 11.1 *The mechanical and tibiofemoral axes of the lower limb*

anaesthetist and surgeon and the patient's co-morbidities.

The patient is positioned supine on the operating table with a lateral thigh support and foot bolster, allowing free flexion and extension of the knee. Pressure areas should be protected with gel pads. Provided that there are no contra-indications (e.g. arterial calcification) a padded pneumatic tourniquet is applied around the thigh as proximally as possible and secured. A dose of an appropriate antibiotic is administered intra-venously prior to the inflation of the tourniquet. The skin in the area of the incision should be shaved immediately prior to surgery. The limb is exsanguinated and the tourniquet inflated to the desired pressure, with the tourniquet time clearly documented.

The surgical field is prepared with an antiseptic solution. The foot should either be thoroughly prepared or wrapped with an impervious 'shut off' drape. Appropriate waterproof drapes should be carefully applied. An antibacterial, transparent adhesive drape is applied to the surgical field. Ideally, the incision should be marked with a sterile pen.

SURGICAL TECHNIQUE

By far the most common approach to the knee joint in total knee arthroplasty is the medial parapatellar approach, which is discussed below. The subvastus, midvastus and direct lateral approaches are used much less frequently. Other extensile approaches are discussed in the section 'Revision total knee replacement'.

Landmarks and incision

The position of the patella, patella tendon, and tibial tubercle should all be noted. An anterior midline longitudinal incision is made, usually with the knee in flexion. The incision needs to be long enough to allow adequate exposure and avoid excessive skin stretching: this runs proximally, from the level of the tibial tubercle for approximately 20 cm, although the length is heavily dependent on the patient's build.

DISSECTION

Structures at risk

The medial collateral ligament (MCL) may be damaged during medial release. The risk of this can be minimized by careful subperiosteal release either using a periosteal elevator or coagulating diathermy.

The patella tendon may be damaged during excision of the fat pad, which can be prevented by always cutting away from the tendon itself. The patella tendon may be avulsed at its insertion to the tibial tubercle during eversion of the patella and flexion of the knee. This is a disastrous complication and can be prevented by extending the deep dissection proximally, dividing any lateral plicae and by performing a lateral parapatellar release to allow eversion of the patella. External rotation of the tibia also relaxes the extensor mechanism.

Dissection continues in the midline, until the quadriceps tendon is identified. The medial and lateral skin, subcutaneous fat and deep fascia should be reflected in matching thick flaps to allow exposure of the quadriceps tendon, medial patella retinaculum and patella tendon.

The medial parapatellar incision is extended from the quadriceps tendon proximally, through the medial parapatellar retinaculum and along the

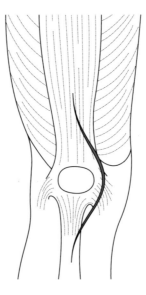

Figure 11.2 *The medial parapatellar approach to the knee*

medial border of the patella tendon distally (Fig. 11.2). There should be at least a 3 mm cuff of quadriceps tendon left attached to vastus medialis and a cuff of medial retinaculum attached to the patella to allow adequate closure.

The medial capsule is released subperiosteally off the proximal tibia to gain exposure to the medial compartment. In a varus knee, this dissection should include the deep medial collateral ligament and extend to the posteromedial corner. In a valgus knee this medial release should be minimized to the anteromedial corner in order to gain adequate exposure.

With the knee in extension, the patella is everted and the knee flexed. The retropatellar fat pad may be partially or fully excised if necessary. The visible remnants of the medial and lateral menisci may be resected at this stage and the anterior cruciate ligament (ACL) must be divided and resected. If a posterior cruciate substituting implant is to be used the posterior cruciate ligament (PCL) can be resected now by dissecting it from its femoral attachment with diathermy. Osteophytes may be debrided at this stage.

PROCEDURE

The primary goals of surgery are pain relief, restoration of function and longevity of the prosthesis. The immediate technical aims of the operation are: anatomical alignment, good range of motion, good stability and ligamentous balancing throughout the range and good patella tracking. Achievement of all these goals can only be accomplished by accurate bone cuts, equal flexion/extension gaps, correct soft tissue balancing, adequate fixation of implants and by addressing any patellofemoral problems, while minimizing the risk of any adverse intraoperative events. The surgeon must appreciate that a total knee replacement is as much a soft tissue operation as a bony procedure.

Bone cuts

Structures at risk

- The MCL must be carefully protected during bone cuts
- Patella tendon

- The common peroneal nerve is in danger from injudicious lateral retractor positioning
- Popliteus tendon can be divided during posterior femoral condylar or tibial bone cuts
- The popliteal vessels and tibial nerve can be at risk during posterior osteophyte removal, posterior capsular release, PCL resection and when cutting the posterior tibial cortex with the saw, if not protected. The anatomy of the popliteal artery in relation to the knee joint is extremely variable

In the vast majority of cases, the bony cuts can be made in the conventional manner with the use of standard instrumentation. Whether the femoral or tibial cut is made first depends on the surgeon's preference and type of prosthesis used.

Femoral cuts

The femur should be prepared with the use of an intramedullary alignment jig if at all possible. The tibial cut can be made by using intra- or extramedullary alignment jigs, depending on the surgeon's preferred method and the degree of extra-articular deformity of the tibia. There is evidence to show that intramedullary referencing of the tibial cuts is more accurate but it has also been shown to increase the risk of fat embolism.

Femoral preparation is undertaken with the knee flexed and the patella everted. A large drill-bit is used to create entry point in the distal femoral canal at a point approximately 1 cm anterior to the insertion of the PCL within the trochlear notch. The entry point can be slightly widened with a rotational movement of the drill. The intramedullary rod should be inserted into the canal with care, especially if a previous total hip replacement has been performed. The distal femoral cutting jig is positioned over the rod and adjusted so that **the distal cut is set at a 5–9° valgus angle** to the appropriate side of the knee to be replaced (Fig. 11.3). Ideally, this should be chosen to match the anatomical axis of the contralateral limb, if normal.

The distal cutting jig is secured with two or three pins which should be fully inserted to ensure that the saw is not hampered and to allow the saw blade to make ample excursion to complete the cut. The amount of distal femoral

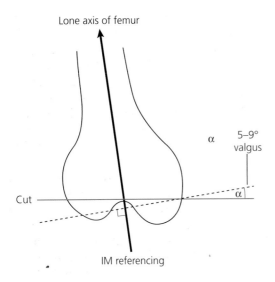

Lone axis of femur

α   5–9°
valgus

Cut

α

IM referencing

Figure 11.3 *Distal femoral resection*

resection performed depends upon the thickness of the implant and any fixed flexion deformity present (see later) but is usually at least 9 mm. Most jigs are slotted to allow for accurate saw blade advancement and have multiple slots and holes at different levels to allow adjustment of the amount of distal femoral resection desired. It is imperative that the medial and lateral soft tissues are retracted and protected with either Hohmann or Trethowan retractors. The cut bone surface needs to be of sufficient surface area and quality to allow adequate fixation with either a cemented or uncemented femoral component and must expose trabecular bone. If the distal femur is particularly sclerotic in parts, a 'second pass' with the saw blade may be required to achieve a flat surface, but one must bear in mind that repeated passes with a power saw generates heat, necrosis and metal debris from the jig.

The distal femur must then be sized to enable placement of the appropriate cutting block. Sizing jigs generally work on an anterior or posterior referencing system, using either the anterior distal femoral cortex or the posterior femoral condyles as the baseline, measuring the amount of anteroposterior resection required accordingly. The typical sizing jig has an anterior stylus that must be seated down onto the anterior cortex, and it may be necessary to remove the overlying synovium in order to ensure that the component

is not oversized. When the desired size is estimated, marker holes are made on the distal femur through the appropriate holes on the jig, to enable positioning of the distal femoral cutting block. The distal femoral cutting block should be positioned in slight external rotation and some implants have the marker holes set at 3° of external rotation on the distal femoral sizing jig. This can be checked by correlation with the transepicondylar axis or Whiteside's line. The reasons for this are explained below.

The cutting block of the estimated size is placed onto the cut surface of the distal femur, with pegs sitting into the previously drilled marker holes. In order to avoid notching of the distal femur during cutting, a cutting guide, commonly referred to as an 'angel wing', can be placed through the chosen cutting slot to estimate the exit point of the anterior cut (Fig. 11.4). The cutting block is firmly impacted until seated flat onto the cut surface of the distal femur and secured with obliquely placed pins. Again, the soft tissues must be carefully retracted during the placement of instrumentation. If there is any difficulty in seating either the sizing jig or cutting block, the surgeon must check that all osteophytes are removed, that there is adequate meniscal resection, that the bone cuts are complete and that the soft tissues are retracted sufficiently. The anterior cut should be made first, followed by the posterior condyles, anterior chamfer and finally posterior chamfer cuts. If it is apparent that there will be significant notching of the distal femur the cutting block should be removed and the sizing reassessed (Fig. 11.4). If there is a possibility of

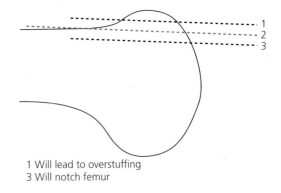

1
2
3

1 Will lead to overstuffing
3 Will notch femur

Figure 11.4 *The anterior femoral cut*

minor notching occurring, this should be controlled and any sharp edge of anterior cortex should be smoothed off with the saw or a bone file. The cut bone fragments can then be removed with knife and forceps and the posterior condylar cuts can be removed with a broad osteotome. The distal femur is then examined to ensure that the cuts are complete. Large posterior osteophytes apparent on the preoperative lateral radiograph or evident after bone cuts can be removed by lifting up the femur and carefully using a broad osteotome or saw under direct vision.

Tibial cut

The tibial cut should be made perpendicular to the axis of the tibia in the coronal plane with an anteroposterior slope of approximately 3° in the sagittal plane (Fig. 11.5). If intramedullary referencing is used, the entry point should be made with a drill at the centre point of the tibia. The intramedullary rod should be inserted comfortably into the tibial canal and the cutting block adjusted in a varus knee to allow resection of approximately 10 mm from the more normal lateral compartment and approximately 2 mm

from the more abnormal medial compartment. In a valgus knee the amount of tibial resection can be more difficult to estimate, but should generally extend to the level of the tip of the fibula head on the lateral side. When at the correct height, as confirmed with a stylus passed through the slot on the tibial cutting block and onto the tibial plateau, the cutting block can then be fixed with pins, advanced closer to the tibial surface, locked in place and the intramedullary rod removed.

The angle of the tibial cut can then be checked with an extramedullary alignment rod. If extramedullary referencing alone is used, the rod should be in line with the anterior tibial spine and the distal tip of the rod should lie just medial to the centre of the ankle joint (as this is where the mechanical axis of the limb passes). Using anatomical landmarks in the foot, such as the second metatarsal, is less reliable as rotation can occur within the hindfoot and midfoot. With extramedullary referencing, the anteroposterior slope of the tibial cut can be introduced either by use of an angled cutting block or by adjustment of the extramedullary jig itself. If the femoral cuts have already been made, the tibia can be externally rotated and subluxed anteriorly to allow exposure of the entire articular surface of the tibia. If the PCL must be preserved, a small portion of bone adjacent to the PCL attachment can be protected with a broad retractor and preserved during the tibial cut.

After the tibial resection is complete, the remaining meniscal remnants can be excised and the tibial component is sized and, following a trial of the components, the tibia can be prepared to accept the stem or keel of the prosthesis. The tibial component should lie in slight internal rotation on the tibia, with the midpoint of the tibial baseplate being in line with the medial third of the patella tendon to optimize patellofemoral tracking.

Flexion/extension gaps

The femoral and tibial cuts should be made such that the rectangular spaces created are the same in both full extension and 90° of flexion (Fig. 11.6). The fact that the mediolateral tibial slope in the coronal plane is 3° to the perpendicular means that the posterior femoral bone cut in flexion

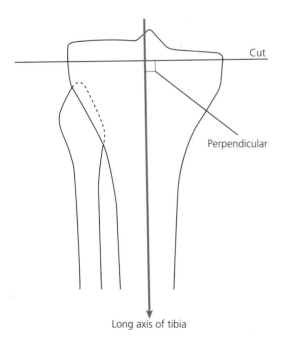

Figure 11.5 *The tibial cut*

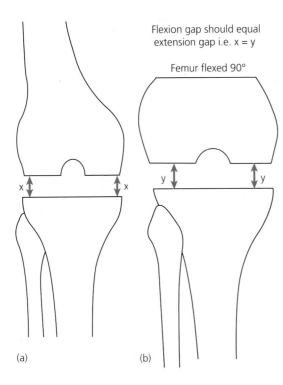

Flexion gap should equal extension gap i.e. x = y

Femur flexed 90°

(a)   (b)

Figure 11.6 *Flexion and extension gaps*

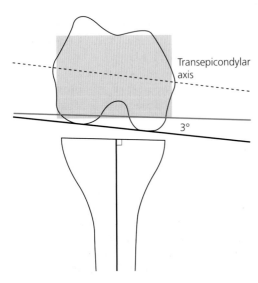

Transepicondylar axis

3°

Figure 11.7 *The effect of external rotation of the femoral cutting block*

should be in 3° of external rotation in order to obtain two parallel surfaces in flexion (Fig. 11.7). Some prostheses use the principle of a tensiometer in flexion and extension to establish the correct bone cuts in order to obtain equal flexion and extension gaps whereas others use spacer blocks or trial inserts.

The most common problems are:
- Tight in extension, flexion satisfactory
  - Solution: increase distal femoral resection. Release posterior capsule off femur. Recess or resect the PCL. Beware of raising the joint line with excessive distal femoral resection.
- Tight in flexion, extension satisfactory
  - Solution: downsize the femoral component by re-cutting the distal femur (beware of notching the femur when downsizing implants). Increase the anteroposterior tibial slope.
- Tight in flexion and extension
  - Solution: increase tibial resection. Beware of losing too much tibial surface area.
- Loose in flexion and extension
  - Solution: increase thickness of insert. Beware gross ligamentous instability.

Soft tissue balancing

Clearly, achieving anatomical alignment and equal flexion/extension gaps is a combination of accurate bone cuts and correct soft tissue balancing. Correcting malalignment and fixed flexion deformity improves the biomechanics of the knee, minimizes wear and therefore loosening, and subsequently improves the long-term outcome and longevity of the prosthesis.

Soft tissue balancing is essentially required in three scenarios; varus deformity, valgus deformity, fixed flexion deformity. Fixed flexion deformity can be present in a varus or valgus knee. The releases involved can be performed at different stages of the operation; initial releases to gain exposure, further releases to establish flexion/extension gaps and final release after trialling of implants.

Varus deformity

This is by far the most common deformity in the osteoarthritic knee. Bone loss is usually from the medial tibial plateau. An important part of the medial release involves excision of the medial osteophytes from the distal femur and proximal tibia with either an osteotome or bone nibbler. As described above, the preliminary soft tissue release is performed during the initial exposure and involves the medial capsule and deep MCL, released subperiosteally off the proximal medial tibia from anterior to posterior using either a periosteal elevator or diathermy. The next stage should be extension of the medial release distally to release the superficial MCL and pes anserinus. If further releasing is required, one should consider releasing the PCL as this can often be a deforming force.

Valgus deformity

> ### Structure at risk
>
> The common peroneal nerve is at risk following correction of a fixed valgus and fixed flexion deformity.

This is the most common deformity in rheumatoid arthritis and can occur in osteoarthritis. Bone loss is usually from the lateral femoral condyle. A lateral parapatellar approach is rarely required. It is commonly necessary to use a PCL sacrificing implant or, if the MCL is non-functional it may even be necessary to use a constrained prosthesis. There should be minimal medial releasing only to allow exposure, due to attenuation of the medial stabilizing structures. Osteophytes should be removed from the distal femur and proximal tibia. The distal femoral cut can be set at 5° to 'overcorrect' the deformity. The lateral patellofemoral ligament may need to be released to allow eversion of the patella. The lateral border of the tibia should be demarcated with a knife or diathermy to release the lateral capsule. If the knee is tight laterally in extension, which is common, the iliotibial band should be released off Gerdy's tubercle. If the knee is tight laterally in flexion, which is less common, the popliteus tendon should be released. The PCL can be a deforming force and at this stage if alignment cannot be corrected the PCL should be released. If there is attenuation of the MCL and a thick insert is needed to achieve stability, the PCL may need to be recessed or resected to allow full extension. Occasionally, the lateral collateral ligament needs to be released off the femur and if there is severe fixed deformity with associated fixed flexion, the posterolateral capsule and lateral head of the gastrocnemius must be released off the femur.

Fixed flexion deformity

Fixed flexion deformity is caused by contracture of the posterior structures of the knee and posterior distal femoral osteophytes. If fixed flexion is present the amount of distal femoral resection needs to be increased by approximately 1 mm for every 2–3° of fixed flexion present to increase the extension gap. This is limited by the fact that increasing distal femoral resection elevates the joint line. If there is severe fixed flexion deformity, it is usually necessary to resect the PCL. The posterior capsule can be released subperiosteally with a curved osteotome following bone cuts. Posterior condylar osteophytes can be excised with an osteotome and removed carefully with Kocher forceps (Table 11.1).

Table 11.1 The stages of soft tissue releases in deformity correction

Varus deformity	*Osteophytes, deep medial collateral ligament, superficial medial collateral ligament, pes anserinus, posterior cruciate ligament, posteromedial capsule, semimembranosus*
Valgus deformity	*Osteophytes, lateral capsule, iliotibial band, popliteus, lateral collateral ligament, posterior cruciate ligament, intermuscular septum, biceps tendon, lateral head of gastrocnemius*
Fixed flexion deformity	*Distal femoral resection, posterior osteophytes, posterior capsule, posterior cruciate ligament*

Patella

Whether the patella should be resurfaced is still a controversial issue. Some surgeons always resurface, some never resurface and some do if there are patellofemoral symptoms or if the retropatellar surface is severely affected.

The vast majority of patella buttons used are polyethylene. There are two types of patella button – onlay and inlay. As the respective names suggest, these designs utilize a prosthesis that is implanted either *onto* or *into* the resected retropatella surface. To resurface the patella, the knee should be extended and the patella fully everted. Peripheral osteophytes can be removed with a bone nibbler to demarcate the actual articular surface. The thickness of the patella should be measured and the amount of bone/cartilage removed should approximately correspond to the thickness of the implant, although if there is severe damage it may be less. Resecting too little bone runs the risk of overstuffing the knee and if a sclerotic surface is left behind, fixation is compromised, whereas resecting too much increases the risk of fracture. Many implants now have calibrated clamps and jigs that help indicate the correct resection level.

To avoid an increase in the 'Q'-angle and therefore reduce the likelihood of maltracking, the patella button should be slightly medialized and both the femoral and tibial components should be lateralized and slightly externally rotated. When trialing the implants and checking the patellofemoral tracking the 'rule of no thumbs' should be employed, i.e. the knee should be put through a range of movement and the patella should not sublux laterally even before the medial parapatellar reticulum is closed and without the use of a guiding thumb to 'aid' tracking. If the patella maltracks laterally, a lateral parapatellar retinacular release is usually required. This should be performed with a diathermy (as it may lead to significant bleeding and bruising postoperatively), and should be carried out from distal to proximal and from deep to superficial. There are often palpable fibrous bands and release of these is sometimes enough. To enable the release to be performed, the patella is lifted anterolaterally with the knee in extension. If possible, the superior lateral geniculate artery should be preserved to avoid devascularization of the patella. Superficial releasing with a resultant subcutaneous flap and undermining of the lateral skin should be avoided.

Where total knee arthroplasty is performed following a previous patellectomy, a PCL substituting implant should be used in order to avoid excessive anterior subluxation of the femur on the tibia due to an already relatively attenuated extensor mechanism.

Implantation of prosthesis

Condylar knee replacement systems can be cemented, uncemented or a hybrid design that usually has a cemented tibial component and an uncemented femur. Uncemented implants now often have a hydroxyapatite coating. The polyethylene insert can either be modular or monoblock (all polyethylene or metal backed), and can be of fixed or mobile bearing design.

In cemented knee arthroplasty, two mixes of antibiotic-impregnated polymethylmethacrylate (PMMA) bone cement should be used. **The surgeon should be familiar with the biomechanical properties of the cement and its mixing technique.** Following satisfactory trials, the selected components are checked by the surgeon and opened. The knee is flexed and the patella everted allowing the tibia to be subluxed anteriorly, with a Hohmann retractor or similar, and the prepared surface of the tibia exposed medially and lateral with spiked retractors. The knee is washed out thoroughly with normal saline pulsed lavage in order to expose the bone trabeculae and maximize the mechanical fixation of the cement. If sclerotic bone surfaces are present, a small drill can be used to make multiple small 'key holes'. When intramedullary referencing has been used, many surgeons insert a bone block into the medullary canal to reduce blood loss. The knee should be thoroughly dried with suction and swabs. The cement can then be mixed and the whole surgical team should change the outer layer of gloves. In most situations, cementing of both components can be performed simultaneously, but on occasions it may be desirable to perform cementing of the components separately with different mixes of cement.

To ensure a satisfactory and efficient cementation process, everything should be prepared and ordered in a logical fashion. The tibial component is usually implanted first. Cement can be applied onto the tibial surface either via a gun with short nozzle or with a spatula. The tibial component is positioned in the correct orientation and firmly seated with a soft impactor and hammer. Excess cement is removed. A trial insert is then applied to the tibial baseplate and the femur lifted up. Cement can be applied to both the exposed distal femur and implant, but as it is difficult to remove cement from the posterior aspect of the knee following implantation, in this region it is preferable to place the cement onto the prosthesis rather than onto bone. The femoral component must be positioned carefully in relation to the distal femur; in particular flexion of the femoral component should be avoided. The femoral component must be firmly impacted and any excess cement should be removed. The knee is then fully extended and axial compression applied (note: hyperextension leads to uneven cement pressurization and may cause posterior 'lift-off' of the tibial baseplate). If the patella is resurfaced the orientation should be checked and once positioned, the patella is compressed and held with a clamp. The knee can then be flexed again and any further cement extruded can be removed quickly. The knee is then extended and further axial compression applied. The trial insert is removed and the baseplate inspected to ensure that there is no cement or soft tissue present which may impede the insert. The definitive insert can then be positioned correctly and impacted fully using the appropriate instrumentation.

In uncemented knee arthroplasty, there must be good bone stock and accurate bone cuts in order to allow good primary press fit and secondary osseointegration of the implant.

Closure

Once the cement has set, the knee can be washed out again with pulsed lavage. Some surgeons prefer to deflate the tourniquet and gain haemostasis prior to closure. However, most surgeons favour closure of the knee over a reinfusion drain and application of a pressure bandage prior to deflating the tourniquet. If a drain is used, placing the drain in the lateral gutter reduces the chance of stitching the drain in when closing the medial parapatellar retinaculum.

The actual closure technique varies with surgical preference but it is important that the repair is watertight and that range of motion is maintained with no patella maltracking. Closure of the knee in flexion ensures that the correct tension is achieved. The deep layer is closed with a heavy suture (e.g. no. 1 Vicryl), by means of a continuous repair of the quadriceps tendon, interrupted repair of the parapatellar retinaculum and continuous repair of the medial capsule to patella tendon. The deep fascia can be closed as a separate layer if desired or the subcutaneous fat can be opposed with deep interrupted sutures. The deep dermal layer is closed with a continuous absorbable suture to allow tension-free closure of the skin with surgical staples or a continuous absorbable subcuticular suture. A sterile occlusive dressing and a padded compression bandage is applied and the drain secured with adhesive tape.

POSTOPERATIVE CARE AND INSTRUCTIONS

Regular neurovascular, cardiovascular and respiratory observations are mandatory. Urine output, temperature and drainage should also be monitored. Adequate analgesia should be administered. Mechanical and, if indicated, chemical thromboprophylactic measures are taken. Two further doses of prophylactic antibiotics are administered at 8 hours and 16 hours after surgery. The use of a reinfusion drain allows for autologous blood transfusion. Haemoglobin levels should be checked 24–48 hours after the procedure. Any drains, urinary catheters, epidural lines and intravenous cannulae should be removed as soon as appropriate to avoid unnecessary portals of infection. Pressure dressings should be reduced and ice applied. Full weightbearing and active range of motion exercises should be commenced as soon as possible. The wound should be inspected and check radiographs performed prior to discharge. The patient must be declared safe for discharge and for routine cases should be able to straight leg raise and flex the knee from 0° to 90°.

Skin clips should be removed 10–14 days after surgery and an outpatient appointment should be arranged approximately 6 weeks post operatively. Ideally, patients undergoing total knee arthroplasty should be followed up for life with serial radiographs, but in reality this is rarely possible.

RECOMMENDED REFERENCES

Anonymous *Knee Replacement: A Guide to Good Practice.* British Orthopaedic Association and British Association for Surgery of the Knee: London, 2002.

Bargren JH, Blaha JD, Freeman MAR. Alignment in total knee arthroplasty. *Clin Orthop Relat Res* 1983;**173**:178.

Dorr LD, Boiardo RA. Technical considerations in total knee arthroplasty. *Clin Orthop Relat Res* 1986;**205**:5.

Scuderi GR, Insall JN. Total knee arthroplasty. *Clin Orthop Relat Res* 1992;**276**:26.

Scuderi GR, Insall JN, Windsor RE, *et al.* Survivorship of cemented knee replacement. *J Bone Joint Surg Br* 1989;**71**:798.

REVISION TOTAL KNEE REPLACEMENT

This section is not intended as a comprehensive guide to revision of all knee replacements but covers the principles of revision knee arthroplasty and refers extensively to the section 'Primary total knee replacement' (p. 172).

PREOPERATIVE PLANNING

Indications

Revision total knee replacement is indicated in the treatment of pain, stiffness or instability from a failed total knee arthroplasty. The cause of failure must be diagnosed prior to embarking on revision surgery. There may be several causal factors present in combination. The common causes of failure and indications for revision are:
- Aseptic loosening
- Polyethylene wear
- Osteolysis
- Ligamentous instability
- Patellofemoral dysfunction
- Mechanical stiffness

- Periprosthetic fracture
- Infection.

Contraindications

- Medically unfit for surgery or anaesthetic
- Active or recent local or generalized infection
- Critical arterial ischaemia
- Non-functioning extensor mechanism
- Unexplained pain
- Insufficient skin coverage (relative)
- Severe neurological disorders (relative)
- Age (relative) – very elderly patients should be carefully selected depending on severity of symptoms, quality of life and options available.

Consent and risks

All of the risks and complications of primary total knee replacement occur at increased rates following revision knee arthroplasty. The overall complication rate for revision knee replacement is approximately 25 per cent, while the outcome is significantly inferior to the results of primary total knee replacement. In revision for infection, the best results for eradication rate are in the region of approximately 95 per cent.
- Infection (or failure to eradicate)
- Bleeding
- Venous thromboembolism
- Wound problems
- Neurovascular injury
- Fractures
- Extensor mechanism injury
- Stiffness
- Instability
- Wear
- Loosening
- Pain

OPERATIVE PLANNING

A thorough history and examination is essential to rule out pain referred to the knee from elsewhere and to assess the level of pain and functional disability. Special consideration should be given to potential risk factors and realistic goals identified.

The examination should pay careful attention to ligamentous instability, range of movement and extensor mechanism function. Infection must be excluded. Scars should be carefully noted and a distal neurovascular assessment must be performed. If the skin over the knee is of poor quality it may be necessary to consult a plastic surgeon.

Recent weightbearing anteroposterior, lateral and skyline patella radiographs must be available and long-leg alignment views are helpful in guiding alignment. Computed tomography may occasionally help. It is absolutely essential that a cause for the failure is found. Templating of preoperative radiographs should be performed if possible and it is the responsibility of the surgeon to ensure that the required implants are available.

The choice of implant is extremely important and is essentially governed by the degree of bone loss and ligamentous instability present. In most cases, due to osteolysis in the metaphyseal region and suboptimal surfaces for fixation, stemmed implants are used, which can either be cemented or uncemented and press-fit with flutes for rotational stability. Small, contained defects can be filled with cement or bone graft but uncontained defects need to be restored with augments or wedges. Massive bone loss may require a distal femoral or proximal tibial endoprosthetic replacement. The use of a PCL substituting design is usually recommended. If there is some degree of ligamentous laxity a semi-constrained implant with a high post should be used to give valgus/varus stability but in the case of MCL deficiency a rotating hinged prosthesis should be used. Infected total knee replacements should ideally be revised as a two-stage procedure.

Anaesthesia and positioning

See 'Primary total knee replacement' (p. 173). The operation is likely to last longer than a primary knee replacement, leading to more physiological disturbance. It can be helpful to exsanguinate the leg after preparation and draping to save tourniquet time.

SURGICAL TECHNIQUE

Although many revision procedures can be performed via the medial parapatellar approach, as described in primary total knee arthroplasty,

other extensile approaches may be required to gain adequate exposure.

Landmarks and incision

All scars should be marked with a sterile pen. If possible, a generous midline incision is used. If there are multiple longitudinal incisions in front of the knee the most lateral scar should be used to avoid necrosis of the intervening strip of skin due to the fact that the blood supply passes from medial to lateral. The incision needs to be long enough to allow adequate exposure and avoid excessive skin stretching. It may be desirable to excise the old scar.

Superficial dissection

Skin flaps should be kept as thick as possible and should not be undermined. The quadriceps and patella tendons should be defined. It may be necessary to extend the incision until 'virgin' tissue is found, in order to find the correct tissue plane.

Deep dissection

Structures at risk

- The medial collateral ligament is at risk from aggressive synovectomy and medial release
- The patella tendon is usually thickened, tight and at risk of avulsion. The patella tendon and quadriceps tendon should be thinned down by excision of any thickened fibrous tissue and the articulating surface of the patella should be exposed. If the patella does not evert or sublux easily, one or more of the measures below needs to be performed
- All other important structures around the knee are at greater risk of injury during revision surgery than in the primary procedure due to scar tissue, difficulty in exposure and stiffness or laxity

The standard medial parapatellar approach is usually performed initially but an alternative is the Insall approach, which extends longitudinally over the patella at the junction of the medial one-third and lateral two-thirds. The medial retinaculum is dissected subperiosteally off the patella to allow a cuff for repair. It is usually necessary to perform an extensive synovectomy in order to improve exposure and to recreate the suprapatellar pouch and medial and lateral gutters. The fat pad is excised. Medial release should be performed to allow exposure to the tibia. There is usually a plane visible between the pseudocapsule and normal tissue and this can be developed with knife or diathermy and the pseudocapsule carefully pulled away under tension. As the PCL is usually sacrificed, this can be performed following implant removal.

Lateral parapatellar release

It is almost always necessary to perform a lateral parapatellar release to allow eversion of the patella. It is usually beneficial to perform the lateral parapatellar release early on. The release should be performed from deep to superficial and from distal to proximal, alongside the lateral border of the patella tendon and lateral parapatellar retinaculum. To reduce subsequent blood loss, it can be performed using diathermy. Full thickness lateral release should be avoided if possible, but if this is necessary to gain exposure the superior lateral geniculate artery should be left intact and the lateral parapatellar retinaculum should be closed later.

Quadriceps snip

This involves a lateral incision into the quadriceps tendon from the proximal extent of the standard medial parapatellar approach (Fig.11.8a). A quadriceps snip can be performed in combination with a more distal lateral release, provided that the superior lateral geniculate artery is preserved.

Quadriceps turndown

This consists of an incision passing distally and laterally from the proximal extent of the standard medial parapatellar approach (Fig. 11.8b). The superior lateral geniculate artery should be preserved. The inverted V thus formed can be

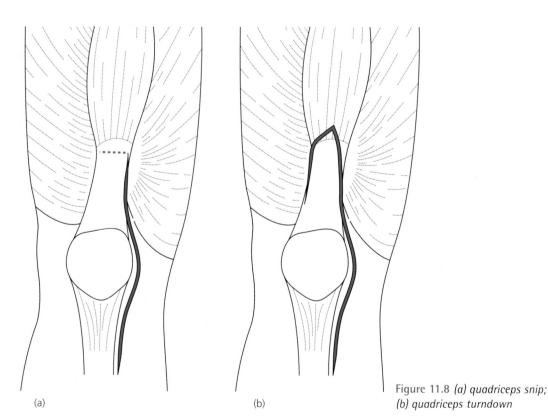

(a)

(b)

Figure 11.8 (a) quadriceps snip; (b) quadriceps turndown

closed as a Y, thereby advancing the quadriceps tendon and patella distally.

Tibial tubercle osteotomy

This requires an osteotomy of approximately 6 cm of the tibial tuberosity, hinging on the lateral soft tissues in order to maintain vascularity (Fig. 11.9). The osteotomy can be elevated in a case of patella baja. The osteotomy may be performed with a saw or sharp osteotome from the medial side and should be wide enough to include the patella tendon insertion, tapering distally along with the anatomy of the tibial tubercle. It needs to be fixed with screws or wires at the end of the procedure.

Procedure

The ultimate goals of revision knee replacement are pain relief, functional stability and eradication of infection, if present. In order to achieve these goals, the important factors are: preservation of bone stock, reconstruction of defects, adequate fixation of implants, ligamentous balancing and restoration of the joint line. The choice of prosthesis is of crucial importance and essentially

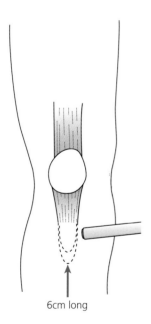

6cm long

Figure 11.9 *Tibial tubercle osteotomy (leaving the lateral soft tissues undisturbed)*

depends on the amount of bone loss and ligamentous instability present.

Implant removal

Safe and careful implant and cement removal should involve preservation of as much bone stock as possible. It is necessary to use fine, sharp osteotomes and it may be helpful to have cement-splitting osteotomes, a thin saw blade, Gigli saw and burr available. If a modular polyethylene insert is present it can be removed prior to the cemented components. It is usually preferable to remove the femoral component first as this facilitates easier extraction of the tibial component. With adequate retraction, the bone–cement interface should be carefully disrupted with osteotomes of appropriate width. If the implant is well fixed it may be safer to disrupt the implant–cement interface and remove the cement separately. Only when fully loosened, should the implant be removed with the appropriate extraction device using a longitudinal distraction force. The tibial component can be removed in a similar manner. The tibial component should never be 'levered' out of bone. It is usually necessary to remove the cement from around the tibial keel and stem with cement-splitting osteotomes or gauges. If a polyethylene patella button has been used it should be removed if significantly worn, in cases of infection, or if there is a patellofemoral problem. Metal-backed patella components can be very difficult to remove and are often best left if possible.

Reconstruction

Following successful removal of implants and cement, any fibrous membrane on the distal femur and proximal tibia is carefully removed with a small, sharp curette and bone nibblers. Ideally, the remaining bone surfaces should consist of trabecular bone to allow optimum cementation. Any small, contained, cavitatory defects can be filled with morsellized bone graft or cement but larger, uncontained, segmental defects need to be reconstructed with augments or wedges (Fig. 11.10). Where there is massive bone loss extending into the metaphyseal region a modular endoprosthetic implant may need to be used with distal femoral or proximal tibial replacement and

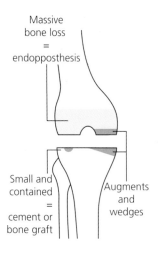

Massive
bone loss
=
endopposthesis

Small and
contained
=
cement or
bone graft

Augments
and
wedges

Figure 11.10
*Reconstructive
options for bone loss
in revision knee
surgery*

this necessitates the use of a constrained, rotating-hinged device.

The tibia should be prepared first with the knee flexed, the proximal tibia exposed and subluxed anteriorly and the patella everted if possible. The canal is opened with a drill. Sequential reamers are used to the desired stem length until there is good endosteal engagement of the reamer. Using stable intramedullary referencing, which may be in the form of an intramedullary rod and sleeve, the proximal tibia is then resected to the correct level. If a tibial cutting jig is used with an inherent anteroposterior slope, the rotation should be referenced from the medial third of the tibial tubercle. Tibial resection should usually be conservative, but depends on the previous resection level and bone stock. If a flat, level cut cannot be achieved a wedge may be used.

Attention is then turned to the femur. The canal is prepared as above. Distal femoral cuts are made with intramedullary referencing and a cutting jig. If the condyles are resected at different levels, the additional resection must be compensated for by an augment of that size. The femoral anterior, posterior and chamfer cuts are then performed with the cutting block positioned in the correct rotational orientation. This can be estimated from the transepicondylar axis or by referencing from a spacer block placed onto the flat proximal tibial surface. This is essential to ensuring a symmetrical flexion gap. Again, augments can be used to make up differences in resection levels of the posterior condyles.

Thought must constantly be given to achieving equal flexion and extension gaps (see 'Primary total knee replacement', p. 175) and to restoration of the joint line. If the knee is looser in flexion than extension, the femoral component is upsized with posterior augmentation. If the knee is loose in extension compared with flexion, the distal femur is augmented. This is preferred to using a thicker insert and elevating the joint line. The level of the joint line should be approximately one fingerbreadth below the inferior pole of the patella or at the level of the meniscal scar.

Some revision knee systems incorporate anteroposterior offset options for the femoral component and mediolateral offset options for the tibial component. Final trials should be performed with all trial stems, augments and wedges in place and the thickness of insert can be determined and final ligamentous releases performed. If the patella is to be revised, care must be taken with further resection. It is commonplace to cement the tibial component first and use a separate batch of cement for the femur.

Two-stage revision for infection

Revising a total knee replacement for infection is even more challenging. Two-stage revision maximizes the chance of eradicating infection, although some units report good eradication rates with one-stage revision and better functional outcome.

At the first stage, all implants and cement are removed. Aggressive debridement is performed with excision of all infected looking tissue and multiple fluid and tissue samples are sent to microbiology and histopathology. The knee is thoroughly washed out. It may be helpful to perform preliminary bone cuts at this stage. A premoulded antibiotic-impregnated cement spacer is inserted and lightly cemented in place to avoid displacement. Appropriate antibiotics are continued and inflammatory markers checked on a regular basis. The knee should be mobilized to preserve range of motion if possible. When confident that infection has been eradicated, the second stage revision can be performed with implantation of the definitive prosthesis. Occasionally, if not settling, the first stage may need to be repeated.

Closure

Routine cases can be closed in a similar fashion to primary knee replacements. Occasionally, especially after repeated revision cases or following infection, closure can be difficult and it may even be necessary to consider gastrocnemius muscle flap coverage and skin grafting, where the assistance of a plastic surgeon may be required.

POSTOPERATIVE CARE AND INSTRUCTIONS

If a standard approach has been used, in aseptic cases, the postoperative regimen is similar to that following primary knee replacement. The results of microbiology samples must be obtained.

If a quadriceps turndown or tibial tubercle osteotomy has been performed, flexion should be limited for approximately 6 weeks to allow the tendon or osteotomy to heal and active quadriceps extension should be avoided.

RECOMMENDED REFERENCES

Back DL, David L, Hilton A, *et al.* The SMILES prosthesis in salvage revision knee surgery. *Knee* 2008;**15**:40–4.

Hanssen AD. Managing the infected knee: as good as it gets. *J Arthroplasty* 2002;**17**(Suppl 1):98–101.

Rand JA. Revision total knee arthroplasty using the total condylar III prosthesis. *J Arthroplasty* 1991;**6**:279–84.

Saleh KJ, Rand JA, Ries MD, *et al.* Revision total knee arthroplasty. *J Bone Joint Surg Am* 2003;**85**(Suppl 1).

Younger AS, Duncan CP, Masri BA. Surgical exposures in revision total knee arthroplasty. *J Am Acad Orthop Surg* 1998;**6**:55–64.

PATELLOFEMORAL KNEE REPLACEMENT

PREOPERATIVE PLANNING

Indications

Patellofemoral replacement is indicated in the treatment of pain from isolated patellofemoral osteoarthritis when non-operative or more conservative operative management has failed.

The lateral facet of the patella and trochlea are most commonly involved and there is commonly some degree of dysplasia, malalignment or laxity present as a predisposing factor.

Contraindications

General contraindications to knee arthroplasty (see 'Primary total knee replacement', p. 172).
• Tibiofemoral osteoarthritis
• Inflammatory arthritis.

Consent and risks

• See 'Primary total knee replacement' (p. 172)
• Progression of arthritis may require revision to total knee arthroplasty (5 per cent incidence at 5 years)
• Specific problems with the patellofemoral articulation include: patella fracture; lateral subluxation; impingement; anterior knee pain

Operative planning

Recent weightbearing anteroposterior, lateral and skyline patella radiographs must be available and Schuss views may be helpful. Schuss views are anteroposterior weightbearing X-rays taken with the knee in 30° of flexion and may be more sensitive in picking up tibiofemoral osteoarthritis. It is essential that the symptoms and signs should be consistent with patellofemoral osteoarthritis. It is sometimes necessary to perform magnetic resonance imaging or arthroscopy to assess the rest of the joint surfaces, although in most cases the decision can be made from the history, examination and plain radiographs. Occasionally, however, the final decision is made at the time of operation.

Anaesthesia and positioning

Anaesthesia, positioning, preparation and draping are similar to that for primary total knee replacement.

SURGICAL TECHNIQUE

Patellofemoral replacement should be performed via a medial parapatellar approach.

Landmarks and incision

The position of the patella, patella tendon, and tibial tubercle should all be noted. An anterior midline longitudinal incision is made with the knee in flexion. It is not usually necessary to extend the excision as far distally as in total knee arthroplasty, but it needs to be long enough to allow eversion of the patella and adequate exposure of the distal femur.

Superficial dissection

The medial and lateral skin, subcutaneous fat and deep fascia should be reflected in a thick flap to allow exposure of the quadriceps tendon, medial patella retinaculum and patella tendon and to allow mobilization of the patella.

Deep dissection

Structures at risk

- The anterior horns of the medial and lateral menisci should be carefully preserved, unlike with total knee replacement where they are sacrificed. The incision at the level of the joint line must be done with great care not to extend into meniscal tissue
- The medial femoral condyle can be damaged during the medial parapatellar approach
- If the patella tendon is contracted, there may be a risk of patella tendon avulsion from the tibial tubercle during eversion of the patella. This can be prevented by extending the deep dissection proximally, dividing any lateral plicae and by performing a lateral parapatellar release to allow eversion of the patella

The medial parapatellar incision is extended from the quadriceps tendon proximally, through the medial parapatellar retinaculum and along the medial border of the patella tendon distally. There

should be an adequate cuff to ensure a good soft tissue repair. The retropatellar fat pad can be incised or partially excised to facilitate eversion of the patella and it may be necessary to perform a lateral parapatellar release. Osteophytes may be debrided at this stage.

Procedure

The aims of the operation are pain relief, good patella tracking and patellofemoral stability. This is achieved by accurate bone resection, correct alignment of implants and parapatellar soft tissue balancing.

Patella

To resurface the patella, the knee should be extended with the patella fully everted and held with a clamp. Peripheral osteophytes can be removed with a bone nibbler to demarcate the articular surface. It is often difficult to accurately assess the amount of patella to be resected, as the articular cartilage wear is usually not uniform. If the median ridge is of normal height, the thickness of the patella should be measured and the amount of bone and cartilage removed should correspond to the thickness of the implant. If there is severe damage, a measured resection technique is unreliable. In this situation, the insertions of the quadriceps tendon and the lateral border of the patella tendon can be exposed carefully with a diathermy and used as reliable landmarks. Resection 2 mm above this plane results in 66 per cent of the original patella thickness being left behind. Resecting too little bone runs the risk of overstuffing the knee and if a sclerotic surface is left behind, fixation is compromised, whereas resecting too much increases the risk of fracture. A clamp is then applied and used as a cutting guide. The amount of resection should be carefully inspected and adjusted if necessary. There will usually be more bone resected from the medial than lateral facet and the remaining cut surface may be sclerotic. This can be roughened with a saw or burr and small drill holes made to improve cement fixation. The patella is then subluxed or everted and the knee flexed to allow the distal femur to be prepared. Care must be taken to avoid fracture of the patella during flexion if the remaining patella is thin.

Femur

To expose the distal femur, two Hohmann retractors are placed medially and laterally. The anterior surface of the distal femur is exposed by excising the overlying synovium with coagulating diathermy. The femoral component should sit flush with the anterior distal femur without notching, with the correct degree of rotation to ensure restoration of the lateral ridge and good tracking. The implant should not be situated too far distal within the notch, as this can cause impingement and catching of the patella in full flexion. The femoral bone cuts can be based on either intramedullary or extramedullary referencing. Individual implants rely on different anatomical landmarks for rotational alignment, e.g. long axis of tibia, transepicondylar axis of distal femur, and specific instruction manuals should be referred to. Most bone cuts are made using sizing jigs and cutting guides.

Trials are then performed and tracking assessed. Final adjustments and preparations can then be made including lateral parapatellar release if necessary. Components are cemented in place.

Closure

If a lateral parapatellar release has been performed a drain should be inserted. The knee should be closed in flexion in a similar manner to a primary total knee replacement.

POSTOPERATIVE CARE AND INSTRUCTIONS

As for primary total knee replacement.

RECOMMENDED REFERENCES

Ackroyd CE, Newman JH, Evans R, *et al.* The Avon patellofemoral arthroplasty: five-year survivorship and functional results. *J Bone Joint Surg Br* 2007;**89**:310–15.

Cartier P, Sanouiller JL, Khefacha A. Long-term results with the first patellofemoral prosthesis. *Clin Orthop Relat Res* 2005;(436):47–54.

UNICOMPARTMENTAL KNEE REPLACEMENT

PREOPERATIVE PLANNING

Indications

Unicompartmental knee replacement is indicated in the treatment of painful osteoarthritis when non-operative management has failed. The following criteria must be met:

- Osteoarthritis mainly confined to one compartment
- Varus or valgus deformity must be correctable to normal
- Fixed flexion deformity less than 10°
- Minimum flexion of 105°
- Intact knee ligaments.

Contraindications

- General contraindications to knee arthroplasty (see 'Primary total knee replacement', p. 172)
- Inflammatory arthritis
- Failure to meet criteria above
- Patellofemoral osteoarthritis – relative. This is a controversial and debatable issue, with some evidence showing no detrimental effect of the presence of patellofemoral osteoarthritis on results.

Consent and risks

- Most risks and complications of primary total knee replacement can occur in unicompartmental knee replacement
- The rate of conversion to total knee replacement is around 3 per cent at 3 years
- Medial knee pain is common and usually resolves with time. Persistent anteromedial knee pain may be associated with a degree of MCL damage intraoperatively
- Dislocation of the insert can occur with mobile bearings, especially if ACL laxity is present
- Progression of arthritis may require revision to total knee replacement. Although this can be relatively straightforward, there is often

significant bone loss, especially around the tibial baseplate and it may be necessary to use a stem and wedge

OPERATIVE PLANNING

Recent weightbearing anteroposterior, lateral and skyline patella radiographs must be available and stress views may be helpful. It is essential that the site of pain should correlate with radiographic findings. It is sometimes necessary to perform magnetic resonance imaging or arthroscopy to assess the integrity of the ACL and the rest of the knee, although in most cases the decision can be made by the history, examination and plain radiographs. However, the final decision is made at the time of operation.

Anaesthesia and positioning

This is essentially similar to that described for total knee replacement. However, as unicompartmental knee replacement is usually performed via a less invasive approach, the use of regional anaesthesia can be avoided, if desired, by the administration of local anaesthetic into the wound and deep tissues. Some surgeons prefer to use a leg holder with the knee flexed, the hip abducted and the leg over the side of the operating table or the foot of the table removed. This allows the knee to be stressed and can improve exposure.

SURGICAL TECHNIQUE

Medial unicompartmental knee replacement

Landmarks and incision

With the knee flexed, a longitudinal incision is made along the medial border of the patella tendon from patella to tibial tubercle and can be extended proximally or distally as required.

Dissection

The incision is deepened along the same line and the medial border of the patella and tendon identified. It is continued along the medial border of the patella tendon and proximally up to the medial parapatellar retinaculum. The medial capsule is dissected subperiosteally off the proximal tibia to gain exposure to the medial compartment. The dissection should not extend beyond the anteromedial corner and should not involve any release of the MCL. The medial portion of the fat pad can be excised. The anterior two-thirds of the medial meniscus can be excised at this point, with the posterior horn removed later following bone cuts. This should give adequate exposure of the medial compartment and it should be possible to inspect the ACL, patellofemoral joint and lateral compartment.

This operation can usually be performed through a relatively minimally invasive approach, with the skin incision being used as a 'mobile window' to gain access to the femur or tibia with varying degrees of knee flexion. However, if exposure is difficult, the skin incision and deep dissection should be extended to allow the patella to be subluxed laterally, although it should not usually be necessary to involve the quadriceps tendon or vastus medialis.

Procedure

Structures at risk

- The MCL must be protected throughout
- The ACL is at risk during the sagittal tibial cut with the reciprocating saw and should be retracted
- The patella tendon can be damaged during reaming of the femoral condyle

Osteophytes on the medial tibial plateau and femoral condyle are excised. The exact nature and sequence of bone preparation is dependent on the implant used and manufacturer's recommendations but the aims are the same as in any knee arthroplasty; anatomical alignment, equal flexion/extension gaps, optimum range of motion and good fixation of implants.

The tibial cut is usually made first, with extramedullary referencing and a tibial cutting guide. The vertical cut is performed, with a reciprocating saw, just medial to the ACL insertion. The horizontal cut utilizes an oscillating saw, perpendicular to the long axis of the tibia. The wedge of tibia can then be removed with a Kocher forcep.

The femoral preparation uses femoral intramedullary alignment and the tibial cut as a combined reference (Fig. 11.11). The flexion gap is set by making the posterior condylar cut first. The initial reaming of the distal femur is then carried out in order to position the trials in place and the flexion and extension gaps are equalized by taking more bone off the distal femur.

Final trials and preparations can then be made and the definitive implants inserted. If there is impingement of the bearing anteriorly on the femoral condyle in full extension, the condyle can be fashioned to allow clearance. The majority of unicompartmental knee replacements are cemented and medial unicompartmental knee replacements are usually mobile bearing.

Closure

Closure is done in layers, with continuous absorbable sutures and a continuous subcuticular suture or staples to the skin. It is not usually necessary to use a drain.

Lateral unicompartmental knee replacement

This is much less commonly performed than medial unicompartmental knee replacement. It can either be performed via a midline approach with the patella everted, or a direct lateral parapatellar approach. The procedure itself is analogous to that of medial unicompartmental surgery. Due to the increased excursion of the lateral compartment during knee movement, the use of a fixed bearing is required.

POSTOPERATIVE CARE AND INSTRUCTIONS

Patients should be encouraged to mobilize the knee and weightbear as quickly as possible. As there is minimal soft tissue disruption, the patient should recover function relatively quickly.

RECOMMENDED REFERENCES

Koskinen E, Eskelinen A, Paavolainen P, *et al.* Comparison of survival and cost-effectiveness between unicondylar arthroplasty and total knee arthroplasty in patients with primary osteoarthritis: a follow-up study of 50,493 knee replacements from the Finnish Arthroplasty Register. *Acta Orthop* 2008;**79**:499–507.

Murray DW, Goodfellow JW, O'Connor JJ. The Oxford medial unicompartmental arthroplasty: a ten-year survival study. *J Bone Joint Surg Br* 1998;**80**:983–9.

Steele RG, Hutabarat S, Evans RL, *et al.* Survivorship of the St Georg Sled medial unicompartmental knee replacement beyond ten years. *J Bone Joint Surg Br* 2006;**88**:1164–8.

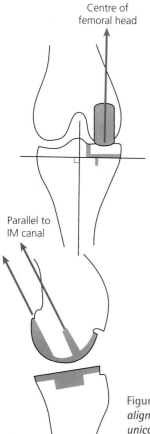

Centre of femoral head

Parallel to IM canal

Figure 11.11 *Component alignment in unicompartmental knee replacement*

DISTAL FEMORAL OSTEOTOMY

PREOPERATIVE PLANNING

Distal femoral osteotomy is used to correct valgus deformity of the knee and consists of a varus osteotomy which may either be a medial closing wedge or a lateral opening wedge. The authors' preference is the lateral opening wedge varus osteotomy and this is described below.

Indications

Distal femoral osteotomy is indicated in the treatment of pain and deformity caused by valgus osteoarthritis in relatively young patients when non-operative management has failed.

It can also be used to correct malunion following supracondylar fractures of the femur.

Contraindications

- Distal lower limb ischaemia
- Significant medial or patellofemoral osteoarthritis
- Flexion limited to less than 90°
- Fixed flexion deformity greater than 15°
- Inflammatory arthritis
- Osteoporosis
- Inability to comply with the rehabilitation protocol.

Consent and risks

- Delayed/non-union
- Inadequate/loss of correction
- Failure of fixation
- Stiffness
- Iliotibial band irritation
- Progression of arthritis may require revision to total knee replacement. Although this can be relatively straightforward, it may be advisable to remove the metalwork at a separate operation prior to performing total knee replacement
- There may be difficulty in achieving the desired valgus intramedullary alignment of the distal femoral bone cut following distal femoral osteotomy

- Infection
- Bleeding
- Venous thromboembolism
- Neurovascular injury

Operative planning

Recent weightbearing anteroposterior, lateral and skyline patella radiographs must be available. Long-leg alignment films must be performed and stress views may be helpful. It is essential that the symptoms and signs should correlate with radiographic findings. It is sometimes necessary to perform magnetic resonance imaging or arthroscopy to assess the integrity of the ligaments and the state of the joint surfaces. Although instability has historically been thought of as a contraindication to osteotomy, it may be performed as a precursor to or in association with ligament reconstruction, as correcting any bony malalignment is an important part in stabilizing the knee. Templating of the alignment films is important to have an idea of the correction required. Each millimetre of opening corresponds to 1° of correction.

Anaesthesia and positioning

General anaesthesia is used. Regional anaesthesia can be avoided, if desired, by the administration of local anaesthetic into the wound and deep tissues. The patient is positioned supine on the operating table. Provided that there are no contraindications, a tourniquet is applied as proximally as possible. An image intensifier is needed throughout the operation.

Prior to preparation and draping, in order to reference the mechanical axis of the limb, the centre of the femoral head can be screened with the image intensifier and a radio-opaque electrocardiogram (ECG) sticker is placed on the skin directly overlying the centre of the femoral head. If a tri-cortical wedge of iliac crest bone graft is to be used the iliac crest must be prepared, draped and exposed to allow bone graft harvesting.

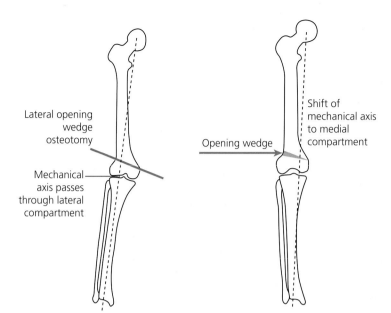

Lateral opening
wedge
osteotomy

Mechanical
axis passes
through lateral
compartment

Opening wedge

Shift of
mechanical axis
to medial
compartment

Figure 11.12 *Lateral opening
wedge distal femoral osteotomy
in a valgus knee*

SURGICAL TECHNIQUE

The aim of a varus osteotomy is to correct valgus malalignment, shift the mechanical axis to the medial compartment and offload the diseased lateral compartment (Fig. 11.12). The goal is to overcorrect to a tibiofemoral angle of 0°. A distal femoral osteotomy should be used rather than a proximal tibial osteotomy as this achieves a horizontal joint line.

Landmarks and incision

An opening wedge osteotomy is performed via a lateral approach to the distal femur. A longitudinal incision is made over the lateral aspect of the thigh in the supracondylar region. Correct placement of the incision site is ensured by screening with the image intensifier.

Dissection

The incision is deepened along the same line until the fascia lata is exposed. The fascia lata is split and the vastus lateralis can either be divided or incised and lifted off the femur at its posterior border. Any blood vessels encountered should be coagulated and subperiosteal dissection is

continued anteriorly and posteriorly around the femur. Insertion of the appropriate retractors anteriorly and posteriorly gives good exposure of the distal femur.

Procedure

Structures at risk

- The popliteal artery must be protected by the subperiosteal retractor throughout the procedure. The risk of major arterial injury may be reduced by performing the osteotomy with the knee in flexion as the artery moves away from the posterior femur
- The medial distal femoral cortex should be left intact. If breached, a staple can be inserted to maintain stability

The ECG sticker placed over the femoral head is palpated through the drapes and an alignment rod can be placed to lie between this point and the centre of the articular surface of the ankle joint. When the osteotomy is opened by the correct amount, the mechanical axis is shifted to the desired point, i.e. the centre of the medial tibial plateau. This improves the efficiency of the use of fluoroscopy, minimizes X-ray exposure and helps to minimize operation time.

A first guide wire is inserted with the power driver from the lateral cortex in a medial and slightly caudal direction. The wire should emerge in the metaphyseal region of the distal femur at the junction of the medial femoral condyle and the supracondylar ridge. A second wire is then introduced to lie exactly superimposed on the first on a true anteroposterior fluoroscopic image, indicating that the wires are exactly parallel to the joint surface. This second wire can be introduced through a parallel guide.

The osteotomy can then be performed with an oscillating saw, using either the guide wires or cutting jig to help control the saw. The saw is placed on the proximal side of the wires and advanced approximately two-thirds of the distance across the femur under fluoroscopic control. Care must be taken not to penetrate the medial cortex. The osteotome is then used to complete the osteotomy through the anterior and posterior cortices, but should stop approximately 1 cm short of the medial cortex. The blade of the osteotome can be marked at a level where penetration of the far cortex will not occur and this marking can be observed carefully as the osteotome advances.

The osteotomy is then opened with distraction osteotomes using a screwdriver under fluoroscopic control. When the osteotomy is opened, metal wedges can be gently inserted into the osteotomy to the desired level. The amount of correction can be checked with the image intensifier using the alignment rod as previously described. A locking plate with interposition wedge of the desired size is then inserted into the osteotomy in the correct position and screws inserted and checked with fluoroscopy. The opening wedge can be filled with bone graft or calcium triphosphate wedges.

Closure

Closure is performed in layers with continuous absorbable sutures and a continuous subcuticular suture or staples to the skin. It is not usually necessary to use a drain.

POSTOPERATIVE CARE AND INSTRUCTIONS

As for proximal tibial osteotomy.

RECOMMENDED REFERENCES

Backstein D, Morag G, Hanna S, *et al.* Long-term follow-up of distal femoral varus osteotomy of the knee. *J Arthroplasty* 2007;**22**(Suppl 1):2–6.

Brouwer RW, Raaij van TM, Bierma-Zeinstra SM, *et al.* Osteotomy for treating knee osteoarthritis. *Cochrane Database Syst Rev* 2007;**18**:CD004019.

Puddu G, Cipolla M, Cerullo G, *et al.* Osteotomies: the surgical treatment of the valgus knee. *Sports Med Arthrosc* 2007;**15**:15–22.

PROXIMAL TIBIAL OSTEOTOMY

PREOPERATIVE PLANNING

Proximal tibial osteotomy is used to correct varus deformity of the knee and consists of a valgus osteotomy which may either be a lateral closing wedge or a medial opening wedge. The authors' preference is the medial opening wedge valgus osteotomy and is described below.

Indications

Proximal tibial osteotomy is indicated in the treatment of pain and deformity caused by varus osteoarthritis in relatively young patients when non-operative management has failed.

Contraindications

- Distal lower limb ischaemia
- Significant lateral or patellofemoral osteoarthritis
- Significant bone loss from the medial tibial plateau
- Flexion limited to less than 90°
- Fixed flexion deformity greater than 15°
- Inflammatory arthritis
- Osteoporosis
- Inability to comply with rehabilitation protocol.

Consent and risks

Progression of arthritis may require revision to total knee replacement. Although this can be relatively straightforward, it may be advisable to remove the metalwork prior to performing total knee replacement.

There may be problems caused by patella baja. Other specific complications include:

- Infection
- Bleeding
- Venous thromboembolism
- Common peroneal nerve injury (usually associated with fibular osteotomy in closing wedge proximal tibial osteotomy).
- Major arterial injury
- Compartment syndrome
- Lateral tibial plateau fracture
- Delayed/non-union
- Inadequate/loss of correction
- Overcorrection
- Failure of fixation
- Stiffness

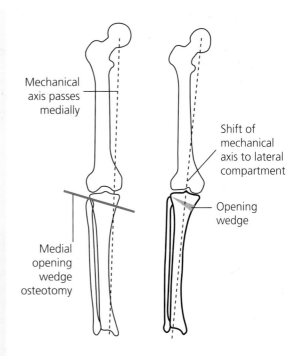

Figure 11.13 *Medial opening wedge proximal tibial osteotomy in a varus knee*

Operative planning

As for distal femoral osteotomy.

Anaesthesia and positioning

As for distal femoral osteotomy.

SURGICAL TECHNIQUE

The aim of a valgus osteotomy is to correct malalignment, shift the mechanical axis to the lateral compartment and offload the diseased medial compartment (Fig. 11.13). The goal is to correct to a tibiofemoral angle of 5–9°. The advantages of an opening wedge valgus osteotomy include the fact that there is no need for a fibular osteotomy, there is more control over the correction and that it may correct instability in anterior or posterior cruciate ligament deficiency by adjustment of the tibial slope. It has the disadvantage of creating a degree of patella baja.

Landmarks and incision

A medial opening wedge valgus osteotomy is performed via an anteromedial approach to the proximal tibia. A longitudinal or oblique incision is made over the anteromedial aspect of the proximal lower leg in the region of the insertion of the pes anserinus and 3 cm medial to the lower border of the tibial tubercle.

Dissection

The incision is deepened until the fascia overlying the pes is exposed. The fascia is incised and the pes anserinus is reflected posteriorly, with the superficial medial collateral ligament. Any blood vessels encountered should be coagulated and subperiosteal dissection is continued anteriorly and posteriorly around the tibia. Insertion of the appropriate retractors anteriorly and posteriorly gives good exposure of the proximal tibia and protects the patella tendon anteriorly with the popliteal artery and tibial nerve posteriorly.

Procedure

Structures at risk

- Popliteal artery: the risk of major arterial injury may be reduced by performing the osteotomy with the knee in flexion as the artery moves away from the posterior tibia
- Patella tendon
- Superficial MCL
- The lateral tibial cortex should be left intact. If breached, a staple should be inserted laterally to maintain stability
- The lateral tibial plateau can be fractured if the anterior cortex has not been fully osteotomized prior to distraction of the osteotomy. If this occurs, the osteotomy should be advanced and the fracture stabilized with one or more interfragmentary screws from the lateral side

The ECG sticker placed over the femoral head is palpated through the drapes and an alignment rod can be placed to lie between this point and the centre of the articular surface of the ankle joint. When the osteotomy is opened by the correct amount, the mechanical axis is shifted to the desired point, i.e. at the junction of the medial two-thirds and lateral third of the articular surface of the tibia. Using an alignment rod to show the mechanical axis improves the efficiency of the use of fluoroscopy, minimizes X-ray exposure and helps to minimize operation time. It is imperative that a 'true' anteroposterior radiograph of the knee is obtained in order to gauge the anteroposterior slope of the tibia.

A first guide wire is inserted, with the power driver, from the medial cortex in a lateral and slightly cephalad direction. The wire should emerge in the metaphyseal region of the proximal tibia at the level of the tip of the fibula head. A second wire is then introduced to lie exactly superimposed on the first on a true anteroposterior fluoroscopic image, indicating that the wires are exactly parallel to the joint surface. This second wire can be introduced through a parallel guide.

The osteotomy can then be performed with an oscillating saw, using either the guide wires or a cutting jig to help control the saw. The saw is placed on the distal side of the wires and advanced approximately two-thirds of the distance across the tibia under fluoroscopic control. Care must be taken not to penetrate the lateral cortex. The osteotome is then used to complete the osteotomy through the anterior and posterior cortices, but should stop approximately 1 cm short of the lateral cortex. The blade of the osteotome can be marked at a level where penetration of the far cortex will not occur and this marking can be observed carefully as the osteotome advances.

The osteotomy may pass above the insertion of the patella tendon, but if it crosses the anterior tibial cortex at the level of the tibial tuberosity it may be necessary to make a step cut beneath the tuberosity from the transverse osteotomy proximally to ensure that the tuberosity and patella tendon insertion remain intact (Fig. 11.14).

The osteotomy is then opened with distraction osteotomes using a screwdriver under fluoroscopic control. When the osteotomy is opened, metal wedges can be gently inserted into the osteotomy to the desired level. The amount of correction can be checked with the image intensifier using the alignment rod as previously described. A locking plate with interposition

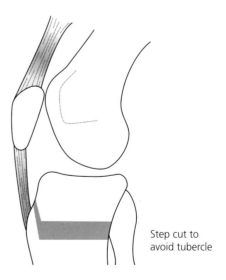

Figure 11.14 *A step cut to avoid tibial tuberosity*

Step cut to avoid tubercle

wedge of the desired size is then inserted into the osteotomy in the correct position and screws inserted and checked with fluoroscopy. The opening wedge can be filled with bone graft or calcium triphosphate wedges. Autograft is still advocated for larger corrections or revision procedures.

Closure

Closure is undertaken in layers with continuous absorbable sutures and a continuous subcuticular suture or staples to the skin. It is not usually necessary to use a drain.

POSTOPERATIVE CARE AND INSTRUCTIONS

Regular neurovascular observations should be performed and the patient carefully monitored for signs of compartment syndrome. Adequate analgesia is administered. Mechanical and chemical thromboprophylaxis is recommended. Two further doses of prophylactic antibiotics are administered at 8 hours and 16 hours postoperatively. The wound should be inspected and check radiographs performed prior to discharge. If the fixation is stable, range of motion exercises are encouraged from day 1 postoperatively. Patients should remain non-weightbearing in a hinged knee brace for 2 weeks. Repeat radiographs are taken and clips removed at this stage. Touch weightbearing only is commenced in a hinged knee brace for a further 4 weeks. If radiographs are satisfactory at 6 weeks, partial weightbearing can be commenced and if the osteotomy has united at 12 weeks the patient can build up to full weightbearing.

RECOMMENDED REFERENCES

Brinkman JM, Lobenhoffer P, Agneskirchner JD, *et al*. Osteotomies around the knee: patient selection, stability of fixation and bone healing in high tibial osteotomies. *J Bone Joint Surg Br* 2008;**90**:1548–57.
Coventry MB, Ilstrup DM, Wallrichs SL. Proximal tibial osteotomy. A critical long-term study of eighty-seven cases. *J Bone Joint Surg Am* 1993;**75**:196–201.
Fisher DE. Proximal tibial osteotomy 1970–1995. *Iowa Orthop J* 1998;**18**:54–63.

KNEE ARTHRODESIS

PREOPERATIVE PLANNING

Indications

The most common indication for knee arthrodesis is **as a salvage procedure** in failed revision knee arthroplasty either where infection has been resistant to eradication or when there is a non-functioning extensor mechanism.

In the past and currently still in some parts of the world, knee arthrodesis is more commonly performed in patients with post-infective arthritis, tuberculosis, poliomyelitis and severe trauma.

Contraindications

- Critical arterial ischaemia
- Extensive bone loss (relative)
- Ipsilateral hip arthrodesis (relative).

Consent and risks

- Infection (or failure to eradicate existing infection)
- Bleeding
- Venous thromboembolism
- Wound problems
- Neurovascular injury
- Fractures
- Delayed or non-union
- Pain
- Immobility
- Risk of subsequent amputation

Operative planning

The indication for arthrodesis, severity of bone loss and adequacy of soft tissue coverage all need to be taken into account prior to deciding on whether the arthrodesis should be a single or staged procedure, an intramedullary or extramedullary fixation and whether it is necessary to enlist the help of a plastic surgeon.

The patient should be thoroughly counselled before the operation.

Anaesthesia and positioning

See 'Revision total knee replacement' (p. 183).

SURGICAL TECHNIQUE

This depends on indication, type of fixation and need for bone grafting.

Landmarks and incision

A longitudinal, anterior midline incision is used, usually through a previous total knee replacement scar.

Dissection

The quadriceps tendon and patella tendon are split and a patellectomy performed. A synovectomy can be carried out and ligaments released or divided to gain exposure.

Procedure

The goals of arthrodesis are pain relief, eradication of infection and sound bony fusion in the correct alignment. In order to achieve these goals the important factors are: good apposition of healthy bone surfaces, preservation of bone stock and stable fixation with compression.

Implants are removed as described in the section 'Revision total knee replacement' (p. 185). It is important to preserve as much bone as possible. Bone surfaces must be viable. In the presence of infection, it is usually desirable to perform a two-stage procedure with the first stage involving thorough debridement, insertion of an antibiotic-impregnated cement spacer and temporary fixation. Second stage involves the definitive arthrodesis. This is commonly achieved in one of two ways.

External fixation

The tibia is cut perpendicular to the long axis. The femur is cut to enable apposition at approximately 15° of flexion, 7° valgus and 10° external rotation. Bone graft may be used if desired. Compression must be achieved with the external fixator. Any form of external fixator can be used, from simple monoaxial fixators to fine wire frames.

Intramedullary fixation

Bone cuts are made as above. The femoral and tibial intramedullary canals are reamed. The distal femur/proximal tibia can be reamed in a concave/convex fashion to increase contact surface area. Fixation can be achieved either with a long nail or with a two-part nail with a locking device between the femur and tibia which can also provide compression and correct alignment. The nail can be locked proximally and distally.

Closure

In some cases closure can be difficult. Occasionally, especially after repeated revision cases or following infection, closure can be such a challenge that it may even be necessary to consider gastrocnemius muscle flap coverage and skin grafting, where the assistance of a plastic surgeon may be required.

POSTOPERATIVE CARE AND INSTRUCTIONS

The amount of weightbearing allowed depends on the stability of fixation, but generally touch weightbearing should be commenced immediately, gradually built up to partial weightbearing over approximately 6 weeks and to full weightbearing over the next 6 weeks.

RECOMMENDED REFERENCES

Conway JD, Mont MA, Bezwada HP. Arthrodesis of the knee. *J Bone Joint Surg Am* 2004;**86**:835–48.
Wiedel JD. Salvage of infected total knee fusion: the last option. *Clin Orthop Relat Res* 2002;(404):139–42.

Viva questions

1. What are the risks and complications of total knee arthroplasty?

2. What are the contraindications to total knee replacement?

3. Which total knee replacement would you choose and why?

4. Discuss the advantages and disadvantages of posterior collateral ligament retaining and sacrificing total knee replacement.

5. Describe how you would address an imbalance in flexion/extension gaps.

6. What releases would you perform to correct alignment in a valgus knee?

7. How do you deal with a fixed flexion deformity during total knee replacement?

8. What measures do you take to ensure correct patella tracking in primary total knee replacement?

9. How would you manage a patient with a painful knee replacement?

10. Describe the modes of failure of total knee replacement.

11. What extensile approaches are available in revision knee arthroplasty?

12. What is your rationale for choosing an implant in revision knee arthroplasty?

13. What are the treatment options for a 50-year-old man with medial compartment osteoarthritis?

14. What criteria need to be met for a medial unicompartmental knee replacement?

15. How would you select the ideal patient for a patellofemoral replacement?

16. How would you ensure adequate realignment in proximal tibial osteotomy?

17. Why is a distal femoral osteotomy preferred to proximal tibial osteotomy in a valgus knee?

18. Discuss the pros and cons of opening versus closing wedge proximal tibial osteotomy.

19. What are the indications for knee arthrodesis?

20. Describe the general principles and fixation options in arthrodesis.

12

Soft tissue surgery of the knee

Jonathan Miles and Richard Carrington

	Range of motion	Position of arthrodesis
Flexion	*0°*	*0–20°*
Extension	*140°*	*(10° ext rot)*

KNEE ARTHROSCOPY

PREOPERATIVE PLANNING

Indications

Knee arthroscopy is used as a diagnostic and interventional tool in a wide variety of conditions. Because of advances in other imaging modalities, particularly magnetic resonance imaging (MRI), it is becoming less common for arthroscopy to be used for diagnosis alone. The frequent indications include:
- Meniscal tears
- Cruciate ligament injury
- Chondral defects
- Removal of loose bodies
- Washout of sepsis
- Synovectomy, including cases of pigmented villonodular synovitis
- Patella realignment procedures
- Intra-articular knee fracture assessment and reduction.

Contraindications

- Infection – particularly cellulitis over the potential portal sites

- Ankylosis of the knee
- Rupture of the joint capsule (allows extravasation of the irrigation fluid).

Consent and risks

- Venous thromboembolism: <1 per cent
- Septic arthritis: <1 per cent
- Superficial wound infection: <1 per cent
- Neuropraxia (secondary to tourniquet use): <1 per cent
- Effusion: virtually universal and can last for several months

Operative planning

Any preoperative imaging should be available. Appropriate instrumentation should be available and checked by the surgeon, including the arthroscope, camera, light lead, arthroscopic instruments, irrigation fluid pump and the 'stack', which must include a functioning light source and monitor. The arthroscope used for knee arthroscopy has a 4 mm diameter and 30° viewing angle.

Anaesthesia and positioning

Anaesthesia is usually general, though regional anaesthesia is acceptable. The position is supine. A side support can be used, at the level of the upper to mid thigh, to provide a lever when opening up the medial compartment.

An appropriately padded tourniquet is applied and inflated at the level of the upper thigh. If the patient is hirsute, the anterior knee is shaved. The surgical field is prepared with a germicidal solution. Waterproof drapes are used with adhesive edges to provide a seal to the skin. The foot and lower leg are covered with a stockinette. The arthroscope is connected to the camera and light source. With the arthroscope applied against a clean white swab, the white balance button is pushed to prevent colour casts (unwanted colour tints affecting the picture) during the arthroscopy.

SURGICAL TECHNIQUE

Examination under anaesthesia

The first stage of any arthroscopy is vital and occurs before any incision is made. The knee is assessed for its full range of movement (which includes any hyperextension) and stability of its ligaments. The patella height and tracking are noted.

Landmarks

The patella, patella tendon, medial and lateral joint lines are palpated carefully with the knee in around 70° of flexion.

Portals

All arthroscopy requires at least two portals with by far the most common two being the anterolateral and anteromedial portals (Fig. 12.1). The anterolateral portal is almost always created first and other portals can be created under direct vision.

The **anterolateral portal** is created 1 cm above the lateral joint line and 1 cm lateral to the lateral border of the patellar tendon. This corresponds to a level just below the inferior pole of the patella. It can be palpated by pushing a thumb against the angle between the lateral border of the patella and the anterolateral border of the upper tibia. If the thumb is left on the upper tibial border, the incision can be made just above the thumb to guide the surgeon to the correct position. It is best done with a pointed, rather than curved, blade,

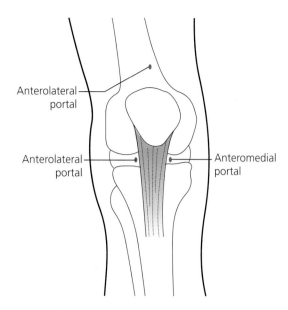

Fig. 12.1 *The three common knee arthroscopy portals*

with the blade facing away from the patella tendon. A vertical incision or horizontal incision is acceptable. If using a horizontal incision, once the skin is breached the blade is turned to face vertically upwards to perform the capsulotomy. This reduces the risk of damaging the lateral meniscus.

The **anteromedial portal** is created under direct vision with the arthroscope viewing the medial compartment. It lies 1 cm above the medial joint line and 1 cm medial to the medial border of the patellar tendon. A 16G needle is inserted at this point, facing slightly downwards towards the tibia. This can be visualized directly to ensure that it exits just above the medial meniscus. If it does not, it can be withdrawn and replaced correctly. Once the correct entry point has been identified, the needle is withdrawn and the scalpel used to enlarge the portal in the same fashion as the anterolateral portal.

The **superomedial portal** is 2 cm above the superior pole of the patella, in line with the medial border of the patella. It was historically used for an outflow cannula. These are rarely used now, as modern pumps obviate their use.

The **superolateral portal** is 2 cm above the superior pole of the patella, in line with the lateral border of the patella. It can be used in suprapatellar synovectomy or in surgery for patellar maltracking.

The **posteromedial portal** is 1 cm above the posteromedial joint line, in line with the lateral border of the medial femoral condyle. This represents the 'soft spot' between the tendon of semimembranosus, the medial head of gastrocnemius and the medial collateral ligament. The portal is created with the knee in 90° flexion, allowing the saphenous nerve to fall out of the surgical field. It can be used to visualize the posterior cruciate ligament (PCL) or posterior horn of the medial meniscus or in total synovectomy of the knee. It utilizes a longitudinal skin incision to avoid neurovascular damage. Following skin incision, an artery clip is used to dissect down to and through the capsule.

Structures at risk

- Sartorial branch of the saphenous nerve
- Long saphenous vein: can be transilluminated by the arthroscope to help its identification

These structures pass together, approximately 1 cm behind the portal incision.

The **posterolateral portal** is placed in a soft point between the lateral head of gastrocnemius, the lateral collateral ligament and the posterolateral tibial plateau. It is very infrequently used, but can be used to visualize the posterior horn of the lateral meniscus or retrieve a loose body from the posterior compartment of the knee. Again, a longitudinal incision is used.

Structures at risk

- Common peroneal nerve, running lateral to the lateral head of gastrocnemius, 15 mm below the portal
- Lateral superior and inferior geniculate arteries, passing just below and above the incision site, respectively

Insertion of the arthroscope

Structures at risk

- Articular cartilage
- Anterior horn of lateral meniscus

This is the only step of arthroscopy which must be carried out blind: it must be done with great care to prevent gouging of the articular surfaces. The anterolateral portal is created as described above. The trochar and sleeve are inserted at 70° of knee flexion. Firm, gradual pressure is applied until there is a reduction in resistance, indicating that the trochar has passed through the joint capsule. At this point the knee is extended to around 20° of flexion and the trochar advanced, passing through the patellofemoral joint. Its intra-articular position can be confirmed by sweeping the arthroscope gently from side to side – it can be felt to be beneath the patella. If it is outside the knee joint, it will not sweep from side to side. The position of the arthroscope should be confirmed before removing the trochar, introducing the camera and turning on the saline inflow.

Arthroscopic inspection of the knee

It is good practice to follow the same 'route' around the knee as this helps to prevent any omissions. It is the authors' practice to address any pathology as it is located, rather than to proceed with a full inspection before beginning intervention. Table 12.1 gives a suggested route, which many surgeons find the most effective one.

Closure

The portals are closed with either single nylon sutures or adhesive paper stitches. Adhesive dressings then wool and crepe are applied before the tourniquet is deflated.

POSTOPERATIVE CARE

Weightbearing mobilisation is begun early, together with range of motion exercises. Anti-thromboembolism stockings are recommended

Table 12.1 Arthroscopic inspection of the knee

Step	Area of inspection	Position of knee	Position of arthroscope	Structures to inspect	Technical notes
1	Suprapatellar pouch	20° flexion	Upright/upside down	Synovium; loose bodies	Turning the arthroscope through all angles allows visualization of the synovium throughout the whole cavity
2	Lateral gutter	20° flexion	Upright	Loose bodies	Best inspected at this stage so that it is not forgotten after tibiofemoral joint inspection
3	Patellofemoral joint	20° flexion	Upright/upside down	Medial + lateral patella facets; synovial plica; trochlea; patella tracking	The arthroscope is turned upside down to inspect the patellar cartilage and kept upright to view the trochlea. It must be withdrawn to just inferior to the patella to view tracking
4	Medial gutter	20° flexion	Upright	Loose bodies	
5	Medial compartment	90° flexion initially 30° flexion to view the posterior horn	Normal/viewing laterally to improve visualization of the posterior horn	Medial femoral condyle; medial tibial plateau; medial meniscus; loose bodies; creation of medial portal	Viewing the posterior horn is easier with the knee straighter and with the arthroscope swung to look laterally
6	Intercondylar notch	90° flexion	Upright	Anterior cruciate ligament (ACL); posterior cruciate ligament; loose bodies; both posterior horns	In ACL surgery, the portals are created a little closer to the patella tendon to improve access to the notch
7	Lateral compartment	Figure-four position	Upright/viewing medially	Lateral femoral condyle; lateral tibial plateau; lateral meniscus; loose bodies; popliteus tendon	Move the knee into the figure-four position with the arthroscope in the notch (Fig. 12.2). Drive into the lateral compartment as it opens and comes into view.

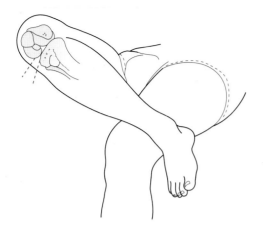

Fig. 12.2 *The figure-four position for lateral compartment viewing*

for 6 weeks. The wool and crepe are removed 24 hours after surgery, to increase mobility. Sutures are removed at 10–14 days after surgery.

RECOMMENDED REFERENCES

Jaureguito JW, Greenwald AE, Wilcox JF, *et al.* The incidence of deep venous thrombosis after arthroscopic knee surgery. *Am J Sports Med* 1999;**27**:707–10.

Kim SJ, Kim HJ. High portal: practical philosophy for positioning portals in knee arthroscopy. *Arthroscopy* 2001;**17**:333–7.

Kramer DE, Bahk MS, Cascio BM, *et al.* Posterior knee arthroscopy: anatomy, technique, application. *J Bone Joint Surg Am* 2006;**88**:110–21.

Moseley JB, O'Malley K, Petersen NJ, *et al.* A controlled trial of arthroscopic surgery for osteo-arthritis of the knee. *N Engl J Med* 2002;**347**: 81–8.

ARTHROSCOPIC MENISCAL KNEE SURGERY

PREOPERATIVE PLANNING

See 'Knee arthroscopy' (p. 200) for further details of consent and operative planning, as well as postoperative care.

Indications

- Acute tears of the meniscus – radial, longitudinal, complex and bucket-handle forms (Fig. 12.3)
- Degenerative tears of the meniscus (commonly posterior horn of medial meniscus)
- Meniscal repair – in non-degenerative, longitudinal tears within 3 mm of the periphery (i.e. within the vascular zone of the meniscus).

SURGICAL TECHNIQUE

Partial meniscectomy

Partial meniscectomy is the most common procedure performed by trainees throughout the developed world and is considered a required skill by trainers and programme directors. It must be part of a full diagnostic arthroscopy, as described in the previous section.

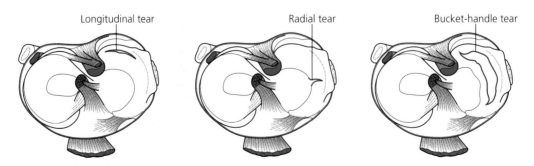

Fig. 12.3 *The common forms of acute meniscal tear*

Initial inspection of the meniscus can often reveal the presence, though not extent of a tear. The smooth outline of the meniscus will be lost. The first stage is to probe the meniscus with an arthroscopic probe. The probe is inserted under the meniscus and the hook turned to point upwards, into the meniscus; the probe is withdrawn and will catch any inferior tear that was not previously visible.

Large posterior horn tears and even displaced bucket-handle tears can flip into the intercondylar notch and will not be seen unless specifically looked for in the posterior part of the notch. Using the probe, the surgeon can determine the extent of the tear and decide on the boundary between unstable, torn meniscal remnants and well-fixed, stable, meniscal rim (Fig. 12.4).

The meniscus can be resected using a number of instruments. The author prefers to use simple punches for the majority of the resection and use an arthroscopic shaver to smooth over the final remnant. An 'upbiter' is very useful during resection of very posterior tears, particularly of the medial meniscus (Fig. 12.5).

The resection should be careful and methodical, leaving all stable meniscus behind. After resection, the meniscus must be probed again to ascertain that all remaining meniscus is stable.

Bucket-handle tear surgery

A bucket-handle tear is a large, longitudinal tear in which the internal portion is mobile and can flip over and become stuck in the intercondylar notch. It is three times as common in the medial as the lateral meniscus. The following discussion uses the medial meniscus as an example, though the principles are transferrable to the lateral meniscus.

Entry of the arthroscope into the medial compartment can be difficult. Careful creation of an anteromedial portal, as described, is recommended, followed by use of a probe through this portal to gently push the displaced fragment medially. This will usually afford a good view. Assessment can be made as to whether the tear is repairable (see the following section).

A probe is used to define the attachments of the tear, both posteriorly and anteriorly (Fig. 12.6). A punch is used to detach 90 per cent of the tear at

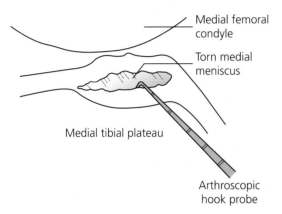

Fig. 12.4 *Use of an arthroscopic probe to show a horizontal tear*

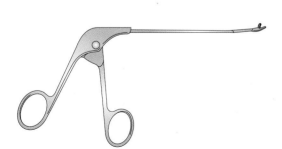

Fig. 12.5 *An 'upbiter' is useful in posterior horn resection*

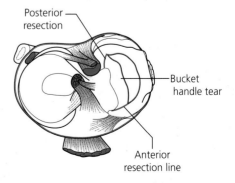

Fig. 12.6 *Resection points of a bucket-handle medial meniscal tear.*

its posterior origin. It is easiest to do this with an upbiter curved to the left for a left medial meniscus and to the right for a right medial meniscus. A straight punch or side-biter is used to resect completely through the anterior attachment. A strong, locking arthroscopic grasper is introduced through the medial portal and locked onto the middle of the torn remnant. The remnant is removed with a 'crocodile roll' – the graspers are rolled over several times while carefully watching with the arthroscope.

Once the meniscal remnant has been freed, it is removed through the medial portal. In large tears, this portal often requires enlargement. Careful inspection of the meniscal remnant is carried out, with debridement of any further unstable tissue.

Meniscal repair

Repair is possible if the tear is within 5 mm of the periphery, but more commonly undertaken if the tear is within 3 mm of the periphery, i.e. within the vascular zone. In order to be worthy of repair, the tear should be between 8 mm and 30 mm long.

The results of meniscal repair are better in patients with a concurrent anterior cruciate ligament (ACL) reconstruction than in repair alone. Repair should not be undertaken in a knee with ligament injury that has not been repaired. A variety of methods are described including outside-in, inside-out and all-inside suturing (Fig. 12.7). In addition, meniscal darts can be used. The details of this surgery are beyond the scope of this book. Sutures are placed, usually vertically, about 3–4 mm apart from each other.

Most surgeons recommended avoidance of weightbearing for around 4 weeks after surgery, particularly avoiding weightbearing in flexion.

Discoid meniscus surgery

Discoid malformation more frequently affects the lateral meniscus and is bilateral in one-fifth of cases. The majority are stable, i.e. have peripheral attachments to the rim. These are treated by partial menisectomy, if symptomatic, to create a more normal meniscus.

If a discoid meniscus becomes suddenly painful, it is likely that it is torn and should be examined and treated as such. The rarer unstable, or Wrisberg variant, discoid meniscus is hypermobile due to absent peripheral attachments. These are usually treated by complete excision as there is no stable rim to leave *in situ*.

POSTOPERATIVE CARE

See 'Knee arthroscopy' (p. 200).

Meniscal repair has a more controversial rehabilitation regimen. The author uses a brace, limited to 0–60° range for 1 month then full range of motion within the brace for a further 2 months. Return to sports is gradual following the initial 3 months in the knee brace.

RECOMMENDED REFERENCES

Fabricant PD, Jokl P. Surgical outcomes after arthroscopic partial meniscectomy. *J Am Acad Orthop Surg* 2007;**15**:647–53.

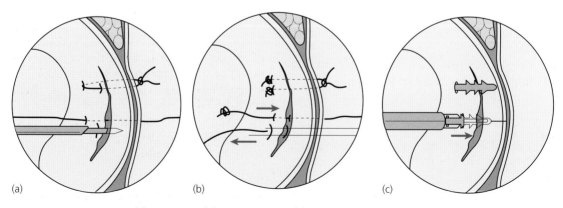

(a)   (b)   (c)

Fig. 12.7 *Meniscal repair: (a) outside-in; (b) inside-out; and (c) all-inside technique*

Min S, Kim J, Kim LM, *et al.* Correlation between type of discoid lateral menisci and tear pattern. *Knee Surg Sports Traumatol Arthrosc* 2004;**10**:218–22.

Rankin CC, Lintner DM, Noble PC, *et al.* A biomechanical analysis of meniscal repair techniques. *Am J Sports Med* 2002;**30**:492–7.

LATERAL PATELLAR RETINACULUM RELEASE

PREOPERATIVE PLANNING

Indications

Lateral release of the patella is indicated in patients with a tight lateral patellar retinaculum who meet the following criteria:
- Anterior knee pain
- Positive patella tilt test – less than 5°
- Failure of conservative measures, including physiotherapy specifically to strengthen the quadriceps and hamstrings.

Associated conditions that may worsen the symptoms include chondromalacia patellae, patella alta, abnormal Q angle and trochlear hypoplasia, but these alone are not sufficient to perform a lateral release. In cases of malalignment, it may need to be combined with more advanced procedures, including osteotomy or tibial tubercle transfer. It can also be performed in conjunction with medial patellofemoral ligament reconstruction and vastus medialis advancement.

Contraindications

Lateral release is not indicated in patients with generalized hypermobility or patellar hypermobility – it will worsen the symptoms.

Operative planning

Very careful history and examination is required to elucidate the features. Plain radiography, including patella views, is essential. If malalignment is suspected, reconstruction computed tomography is useful.

Anaesthesia and positioning

See 'Knee arthroscopy' (p. 200).

Consent and risks

- The complications are essentially those of any knee surgery: bleeding, infection, thrombosis and numbness, whether carried out open or arthroscopically
- Mention of haemarthrosis should be made in particular as it is very common and can be major
- Medial subluxation is a rare, late complication

SURGICAL TECHNIQUE

Open lateral release

Landmarks
- Lateral border of the patella
- Gerdy's tubercle (insertion of the iliotibial band on the lateral tibia).

Incision

A straight incision is created 1 cm from the lateral border of the patella, running from the level of the superior pole of the patella to 1 cm above Gerdy's tubercle. The incision is carried down to the lateral retinaculum.

Technique

The superficial lateral retinaculum is incised in line with the skin incision. The deeper fibres and synovium are not incised. The surgeon now assesses whether the release has been sufficient. If the patella is now able to be tilted 45° or more laterally it is sufficient.

If the release is insufficient, the superficial retinaculum is dissected off the deep retinaculum for 2 cm on the lateral side of the incision. The deep retinaculum can now be incised parallel to the superficial retinacular incision but 2 cm further lateral. If this is required, the lateral portion of the superficial retinaculum is sutured to the medial edge of the deep retinaculum – this helps to lessen haemarthrosis.

Closure

The subcutaneous fat is opposed with interrupted sutures and the skin closed with the surgeons chosen method. Occlusive dressing and heavy wool and crepe bandages are applied.

Arthroscopic lateral release

Technique

A complete arthroscopy is carried out first – the lateral release is done last as it causes bleeding. A tourniquet is not used as it interferes with patellar tracking and causes more bleeding postoperatively.

A horizontal line is drawn laterally from the superior pole of the patella and another line 1 cm away from the lateral border of the patella. A needle is inserted into the knee joint at the level where these lines cross.

Structures at risk

- The superior geniculate artery
The needle serves as a proximal limit of the release to prevent damage to the artery and subsequent bleeding that cannot be controlled arthroscopically.

Release is carried out, with cautery, running from the needle to the anterolateral portal; it is continued until subcutaneous fat is seen from within the knee.

Closure

The portals are closed with either single nylon sutures or adhesive paper stitches. Adhesive dressings then wool and crepe are applied.

POSTOPERATIVE CARE AND INSTRUCTIONS

Weightbearing is begun immediately. The wool and crepe are removed after 24–36 hours and range of motion exercises are begun early (to prevent lateral adhesions within the knee). The patient is referred to physiotherapy to reinstate medial quadriceps exercises.

RECOMMENDED REFERENCES

Kolowich PA, Paulos LE, Rosenberg TD, et al. Lateral release of the patella: indications and contraindications. Am J Sports Med 1990;18: 359–65.

Mulford JS, Wakeley CJ, Eldridge JD. Assessment and management of chronic patellofemoral instability. J Bone Joint Surg Br 2007;89:709–16.

CARTILAGE RECONSTRUCTION SURGERY

PREOPERATIVE PLANNING

Indications

- Articular cartilage injury (most common on the medial femoral condyle)
- Osteochondritis dessicans (most common on the lateral part of the medial femoral condyle)
- Atraumatic osteonecrosis of the knee.

Contraindications

- Degenerative knee changes – none of the techniques developed to date are successful on osteoarthritic lesions
- Age over 55 years – poor cartilage regeneration and may be more suitable for arthroplasty techniques
- Active infection.

Consent and risks

- As for 'Knee arthroscopy' (p. 200)
- Unpredictable outcome (worse if longstanding injury or high body mass index)
- Donor site morbidity (mosaicplasty and autologous chondrocytes transplants [autologous chondrocyte implantation; ACI])
- Need for second procedure (ACI)

Operative planning

Details of previous imaging and surgery should be available. Suitable equipment for the chosen technique of chondroplasty consists of:
- Microfracture picks / K-wire (microfracture)
- Plug harvest and implant equipment (mosaicplasty)
- Chondrocytes (ACI).

Anaesthesia and positioning

See 'Knee arthroscopy' (p. 200).

SURGICAL TECHNIQUE

Debridement

- Simple removal of loose chondral material and smoothing of the damaged edges.
- 'Roughening' of the underlying, subchondral bone may allow clot formation and encourage fibrocartilage formation.
- May be suitable for small lesions.

Microfracture

Following debridement, an awl is inserted into the ipsilateral arthroscope portal and used to create microfractures in the subchondral bone at the defect (Fig. 12.8). The microfractures are 5 mm apart and approximately 5 mm deep. This allows penetration of the tidemark and the release of pluripotential cells from the cancellous bone. This produces a more pronounced and longer-lasting healing response than abrasion alone and increases the prospect of fibrocartilage formation at the defect.

Mosaicplasty

Small plug grafts are taken from a non-weightbearing area of the knee, typically the

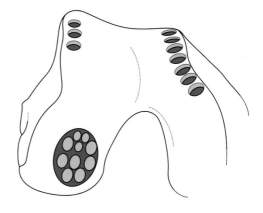

Fig. 12.9 *Femoral condylar defect treated with mosaicplasty*

peripheral areas of the superior trochlea, and grafted into the defect until it is filled. Grafts are taken with a core drill and are 4–8 mm in diameter and 20 mm deep. Matching cores are removed from the defect and the graft plugs impacted in a mosaic pattern (Fig. 12.9).

Care must be taken to leave the graft plugs flush with the surrounding cartilage. The defects between the plugs fills in with fibrocartilage. Results are variable and highly dependent on the skill of the surgeon. There are questions over its use in defects over 4 cm^2.

Autologous chondrocyte implantation

Autologous chondrocyte implantation is performed as a two-stage procedure. The first stage is arthroscopic and includes a diagnostic arthroscopy and debridement of any chondral flaps around the area of chondral damage. This should be done to provide a rim of stable or healthy cartilage all around the lesion and is essential for attachment of the graft. At the end of the first stage arthroscopy, small segments of healthy cartilage are harvested from the outer border of the anterosuperior femur, usually on the medial side of the trochlea. This is performed with a small gouge to loosen the segment and rongeurs to retrieve it. A venous blood sample is taken to screen for infectious diseases.

The chondrocytes can be prepared in a number of ways and can be provided suspended in

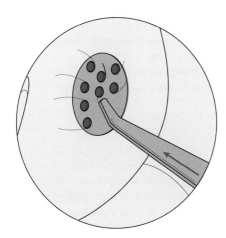

Fig. 12.8 *Microfracture of a chondral injury of the medial femoral condyle*

solution or can be implanted onto a membranous matrix. This usually takes 3–6 weeks. The steps of preparation are similar in each technique: collagenases dissolve the matrix to leave the chondrocytes, then the cells are washed and put in a culture medium derived from the patient's serum. The cells adhere to a culture surface and proliferate to provide a large number of healthy chondrocytes.

The second procedure is carried out once the chondrocytes have been grown and returned. This is a larger procedure and is performed open. The incision is dependent on the site: for example a medial femoral condyle defect requires an 8 cm medial parapatellar incision. The defect is exposed and any further loose material is debrided. The defect is then covered with an appropriately shaped membrane which is stitched or glued in place. If the cells are embedded on the membrane, this is the final stage; if the cells are in suspension, the liquid is injected under the membrane. The wound is closed in layers.

POSTOPERATIVE CARE AND INSTRUCTIONS

Movement encourages chondrocyte growth, so after ACI or mosaicplasty, the patient is rested for up to 2 weeks, in either a bulky dressing or a cylinder plaster, then passive mobilization is begun. In all cases, the patient is allowed to toe-touch weightbear for 6–8 weeks, to reduce the force on the grafts. Running is not allowed for 6 months and contact sports for 12 months after ACI or mosaicplasty.

RECOMMENDED REFERENCES

Briggs TWR, Mahroof S, David LA, *et al.* Histological evaluation of chondral defects after autologous chondrocyte implantation of the knee. *J Bone Joint Surg Br* 2003;**85**:1077–83.

Hangody L, Kish G, Karpati Z, *et al.* Mosaicplasty for the treatment of articular cartilage defects: application in clinical practice. *Orthopaedics* 1998;**21**:751–6.

Steadman JR, Briggs KK, Rodrigo JJ, *et al.* Outcomes of microfracture for traumatic chondral defects of the knee: average 11 year follow-up. *Arthroscopy* 2003;**19**:477–84.

ANTERIOR CRUCIATE LIGAMENT RECONSTRUCTION

PREOPERATIVE PLANNING

Indications

Anterior cruciate ligament reconstruction is indicated in patients with **symptomatic** instability of the knee with a proven ACL rupture. Specific indications include:

- High-level athlete (consider early reconstruction, without rehabilitation phase)
- Inability to return to sports, particularly those which involve twisting on a planted foot (e.g. rugby, football, racquet sports).
- Ongoing instability, giving way and pain resistant to a dedicated ACL rehabilitation physiotherapy programme.

Consent and risks

- Knee stiffness (due to arthrofibrosis, inaccurate tunnel placement or insufficient notchplasty)
- Arthrofibrosis: more common if early reconstruction used, rather than delayed
- Knee pain
- Kneeling difficulty (higher risk if bone–patellar–tendon–bone (B-T-B) technique is used
- Ongoing instability (11–25 per cent symptomatic, 60–89 per cent asymptomatic)
- Failure to return to previous level of sport (up to 30 per cent)
- Graft failure: impingement or enlargement of the tunnel with time (typically 2 years)
- Degeneration: found in 75 per cent of patients beyond 10 years after surgery

Operative planning

Careful examination and judicious use of investigations are essential, both to confirm the presence of ACL rupture and to search for associated injuries, particularly associated ligament injury. In many cases, surgery will have been preceded by a diagnostic arthroscopy and treatment of any associated irreparable meniscal tear.

The operation notes from prior surgery should be available, along with results of previous MRIs or other imaging. If there is an associated meniscal tear, consideration should be given to concurrent repair, as the results are improved in conjunction with ACL reconstruction.

Anaesthesia and positioning

General or regional anaesthesia is used. The patient is positioned supine with a side support or leg holder to hold the knee in supported flexion.

SURGICAL TECHNIQUE

The two common methods of reconstruction are with a B-T-B graft or a hamstring tendon graft. The harvesting of both grafts is described, along with the method of reconstruction via an open technique with B-T-B and an arthroscopic technique with the hamstrings graft.

As always, careful examination under anaesthesia is essential. The technique and portals of the arthroscopy are in common with that described in the previous sections. It is wise to carefully inspect the PCL and popliteus tendon in case of associated PCL or posterolateral corner injury.

B-T-B graft, open technique

Landmarks

Midline – superior pole of the patella, tibial tuberosity.

Incision and dissection

A midline incision is created from the superior pole of the patella to just below the tibial tuberosity. Dissection is continued to reveal the paratenon, which is then incised to expose the whole of the patella tendon. The central portion (usually 10 mm unless it is a narrow tendon – in which case use one-third of its width) of the tendon is dissected free for its entire length between the patella and the tibial tuberosity.

This dissection is continued across the patella for 30 mm proximally and the tibial tuberosity 30 mm distally. These incisions mark the sites of bone cuts for harvesting of proximal and distal blocks (Fig. 12.10).

Procedure

Structures at risk

- Anterior horns of the medial and lateral menisci, just posterior to the fat pad
- PCL: the olive-tipped drill passes over the PCL in the notch and it requires protection

With a 2 mm drill, drill two holes around 10 mm deep, in the centre of each area of bone between the dissected margins – these will be used to pass sutures for control of the graft at insertion. Using a narrow oscillating saw and then an osteotome (8–10 mm wide), dissect a block from the patella of 25 mm length. The osteotomes are directed 45° towards the midline when performing the cuts, in order to create a trapezoidal graft shape. Care must be taken to avoid a graft which is too deep, risking subsequent patella fracture, or too thin, risking failure of fixation of the graft. The aim is creation of a block 25 mm long, 8 mm wide and 5–8 mm deep. The bone block is trimmed to a uniform size and two heavy sutures are passed through the previously drilled holes.

The same technique is used to create two holes in and harvest the tuberosity bone block, which

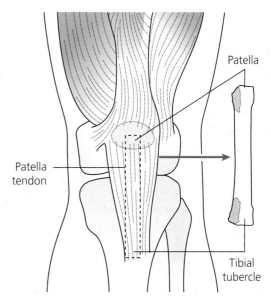

Fig. 12.10 *Bone–patellar-tendon–bone graft harvest*

should be of a similar size and shape. It is again trimmed and one heavy suture passed through one of the drilled holes (Fig. 12.11).

The graft is sized with a tunnel sizer, aiming for a snug but not too tight fit. If the grafts are of significantly different sizes, different tunnel widths can be used for the reconstruction; if this is done the tibial tunnel must be the larger one. The length of the entire graft and width of the two bone blocks should be written down and the graft wrapped in a saline-soaked gauze.

A self-retaining retractor is placed in the defect in the patella tendon, revealing the fat pad below it. The fat pad is then excised, revealing a good view of the notch and lateral wall of the notch (i.e. medial wall of the lateral femoral condyle) in particular. The ACL remnant, if present, is excised. It may be adherent to the PCL and care must be taken to avoid damage to the PCL when it is dissected free. The lateral wall is cleared of any further soft tissues and the back of the lateral wall indentified with a hook.

To prepare the proximal tibia for tunnel creation, the area of tibia medial to the patella tendon is exposed. Using subperiosteal dissection good bone exposure is obtained so that the tunnel jig will not slip. The ACL tibial tunnel jig is set at 50° and the aiming device placed at the posterior ACL stump, just anterior to the PCL. This is in line with the anterior attachment of the lateral meniscus (Fig. 12.12).

An ACL guidewire is drilled, through the jig, entering the knee just in front of the medial tibial spine; the jig will sit just anterior to the PCL. The guidewire is over-drilled with the tunnel drill of appropriate size for the graft – the reamings are saved to graft the patella defect from the graft harvest at the end of the procedure. A tunnel rasp is used to smooth any sharp bone edges present at

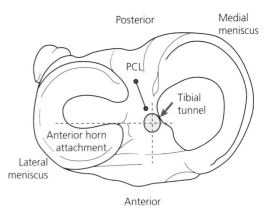

Fig. 12.12 *Site of the tibial tunnel for anterior cruciate ligament reconstruction. PCL, posterior cruciate ligament*

the joint surface. A probe is used to carefully identify the posterior wall of the lateral femoral condyle from within the notch. The guidewire is passed through the tibial tunnel with the knee flexed to 90° and drilled into the lateral wall of the notch at the isometric point of the ACL origin (Fig. 12.13). It is drilled through until it passes through the skin of the anterolateral thigh.

The position of the tunnel in the femur is absolutely critical. Its position is as posterior as possible without causing blowout of the posterior wall. This can be guided using an 'over the top guide'. These have an extension which passes around the posterior margin of the lateral condyle and provides a measure for insertion of the guidewire into the lateral wall. For example, if the tunnel is to be 8 mm, the over the top guide will create an offset of 5 mm from the posterior wall. This will leave 1 mm of posterior wall behind the 4 mm radius of the tunnel.

The position of the tunnel on the lateral wall is traditionally described by the position of the clock face. It is at 10.30 or 1.30 on the clock face depending on whether it is the left or right knee.

The femoral tunnel is drilled with the appropriate sized tunnel drill passing over the guidewire (Fig. 12.14). The length of the tunnel should be just over that of the length of the bone plug to be used in the tunnel – this is usually 35 mm. Again, any graft is saved and any rough edges smoothed with a tunnel rasp.

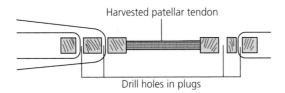

Fig. 12.11 *The harvested bone–patellar-tendon–bone graft*

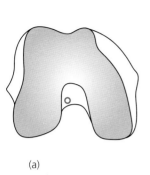
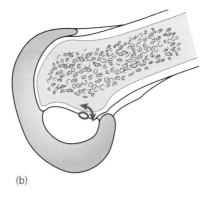

(a)   (b)

Fig. 12.13 *The isometric point for the femoral tunnel insertion: (a) anterior view; and (b) lateral view*

Returning to the graft, the junction of bone and tendon of the femoral block is marked with a surgical pen – the femoral block should be the smaller of the two. The two strong sutures in the femoral block are inserted into the eye of the guidewire and a Jacob chuck attached to the tip of the guidewire in front of the thigh. The guidewire is pulled through and the sutures recovered. A second suture is passed through the tibial bone block – this should be either a strong, braided non-absorbable suture or a steel wire.

The graft is firmly, but smoothly, pulled through into position, keeping the knee at 90° of flexion

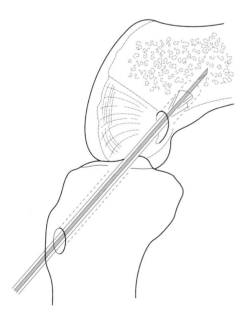

Fig. 12.14 *Drilling the femoral tunnel through the tibial tunnel*

and the cortical margin of the graft facing posteriorly in the tunnel. Inspection within the knee will reveal when the marking on the femoral plug has reached the margin of the femoral tunnel. An interference screw guidewire is passed anterior to the graft within the femoral tunnel to a depth of at least 25 mm. An interference screw of appropriate size is then passed over the guidewire to secure the graft within the femur. The position and security is checked by cycling the knee through flexion and extension several times.

The knee is held at 30–40° with the tibia in slight external rotation, to secure the graft in the tibia. While the graft is tensioned, a further interference screw is inserted. The abolition of the pivot shift phenomenon can be checked at this stage. The graft saved from the tunnels is packed into the defects in the patella.

Closure

The paratenon is closed with interrupted, absorbable sutures over the tendon. The tendon itself is not closed as this would shorten the patella tendon. A small drain is inserted and the skin is closed. Adhesive dressings then a wool and crepe dressing are applied.

HAMSTRING, ARTHROSCOPIC TECHNIQUE

Landmarks

- Tibial tuberosity
- Patellar tendon.

Incision and dissection

Structure at risk

The sensory branch of the saphenous nerve can often be seen traversing the wound at the site of graft harvesting – it should be preserved if possible.

A diagnostic arthroscopy is carried out to identify and treat associated injuries. The anteromedial portal is kept anterior, close to the patella tendon, in order to allow good visualization of the notch. The lateral wall is cleared with an arthroscopic shaver or a small curette. An arthroscopy hook is used to carefully identify the posterior wall.

A 50 mm incision, parallel with the patellar tendon, is created 20 mm medial to the tibial tuberosity. It should begin 60 mm below the joint line. Fat and deep fascia are dissected to reveal the tendons of the pes anserinus (Fig. 12.15).

An incision is created over the upper border of the tendons, taking care not to damage the tendons themselves. Dissecting scissors are used to develop the plane between the gracilis and semitendinosus tendons and the underlying medial collateral ligament.

Procedure

The tendons are then pulled forward with the scissors and a tendon hook passed over them in turn. It is recommended that a length of surgical tape is passed over semitendinosus, which is then released but freely rediscovered via pulling on the tape.

The tendons of gracilis and semitendinosus are dissected free of soft tissue attachments in turn. The tendons are harvested in turn with a tendon stripper. The gracilis tendon is held taught and the stripper carefully pushed over it, keeping the stripper parallel to the tendon. It is advanced until the tendon is released from its muscle belly, and then the same method is used to release the tendon of semitendinosus.

The tendons can then be dissected free of the pes medially, carefully preserving as much graft length as possible. This will give a graft of two tendons which are joined at one end and free at the other. Alternatively, the graft can be prepared *in situ*. Muscle tissue is scraped off the tendons. The two tendons are looped over a strong suture and folded in half. The four strands are sutured together, using a whip stitch, for 30 mm at either end (Fig. 12.16). The graft is then tensioned, in order to prevent stretching *in situ*. If a tensiometer is available, it is usually tensioned to 80 N (20 lb) for 10 minutes. Next, the graft is measured: most are 8–10 mm, with 7 mm being a minimum acceptable diameter.

The knee is positioned in 90° of flexion. The tibial jig is passed through the medial portal and positioned as for B-T-B reconstruction, with its aiming device passing through the previously

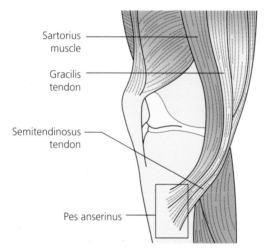

Sartorius muscle

Gracilis tendon

Semitendinosus tendon

Pes anserinus

Fig. 12.15 *Anatomy of the pes anserinus*

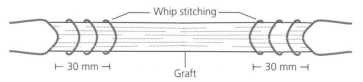

Whip stitching

⊢ 30 mm ⊣   Graft   ⊢ 30 mm ⊣

Fig. 12.16 *Prepared hamstring graft for anterior cruciate ligament reconstruction*

created graft harvest incision. With the arthroscope in the anterolateral portal, the tibial tunnel guidewire is inserted and its entry point into the knee confirmed to be within the posterior portion of the tibial stump on the tibial surface. The tibial tunnel is then drilled and any debris at its entrance into the knee cleared with an arthroscopic shaver. The guidewire is then drilled into the correct position in the lateral wall, as in the B-T-B technique.. This is again drilled to 30–35 mm depth, debris is removed and the posterior margin of the tunnel is checked.

The guidewire is threaded with the sutures from one end of the graft and pulled through the skin. The graft is pulled into place, until the 30 mm of whip stitch has entered the femoral tunnel, as viewed with the arthroscope. The graft can be fixed *in situ* with an interference screw, with a similar technique to that described in 'B-T-B graft, open technique' (p. 211).

Alternatively, a transfixion pin method can be used to introduce and fix the graft in the femoral tunnel. In this method a transfix guide is inserted 30 mm into the femoral tunnel and the cannulated guide is advanced to the lateral aspect of the thigh. The skin and iliotibial band are incised and the cannulated guide advanced to the lateral femur. A Beath pin is drilled through the guide, through the femur and out through the medial skin. The cannulated guide and sidearm are removed and the lateral cortex is drilled to accept the head of the

transfix screw. The Beath pin is left captured within the guide in the femoral tunnel. A thin wire is passed over the end of the Beath pin and then pulled through the femur and the guide, using a handle attached to the Beath pin medially. When the guide is pulled out of the femoral tunnel, the guidewire is pulled with it, through the tibial tunnel and out of the anterior tibial cortex (Fig. 12.17).

The graft can be looped over the wire and the two ends of the wire pulled apart to introduce the graft, through the tibial tunnel and into the femoral tunnel. When the wire passes freely from side to side, the graft has been fully advanced. A transfix pin passed over the wire, which is held tight, will now pass through the loop in the two graft strands, thus fixing it in the femoral tunnel (Fig. 12.18).

The position of the graft is checked arthroscopically and the graft fixed in the tibial tunnel as described in 'B-T-B graft, open technique' (p. 211).

Closure

Closure of wounds is with a combination of interrupted, absorbable deep sutures and the surgeon's chosen skin closure. The arthroscopy portals and exit wounds of guidewires can be closed with adhesive paper closure sutures alone. Adhesive dressings and a wool and crepe dressing are applied.

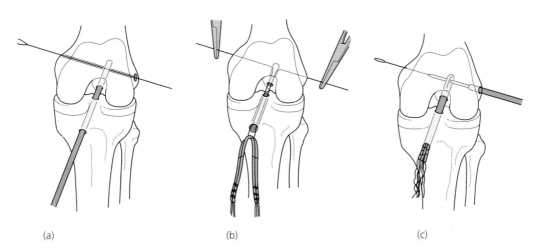

(a)   (b)   (c)

Fig. 12.17 *(a) Wire is advanced through femoral tunnel, (b) graft introduced into the femur and (c) transfix pin passed through the graft*

POSTOPERATIVE CARE AND INSTRUCTIONS

The patient is not put into a brace, rather early supervised range of motion exercises are begun. A drain, if used, is removed at 24 hours after surgery. At this time the bulky dressing is removed, leaving adhesive dressings over the wounds. With the aid of a physiotherapist, range of motion exercises are begun. The patient can be discharged once they have achieved a range from 0–90°. The wounds are inspected and sutures removed at 2 weeks after surgery.

The physiotherapist supervises gentle exercise, using closed chain exercises only for the first 6 weeks. After 6 weeks, the use of a rowing machine and exercise bike is permitted. The range of motion is increased up to full at around 12 weeks. After this period more aggressive exercise can begin. Running is not permitted for the first 3 months and contact sports not for the first 8 months after surgery. The use of proprioceptive exercises is encouraged and maintenance exercises

used to keep the thigh and calf musculature optimal.

RECOMMENDED REFERENCES

Frank CB, Jackson DW. Current concepts review – the science of reconstruction of the anterior cruciate ligament. *J Bone Joint Surg Am* 1997;**79**:1556–76.

Salmon LJ, Russell VJ, Refshauge K, *et al.* Long term outcome of endoscopic anterior cruciate ligament reconstruction with patellar tendon autograft. *Am J Sports Med* 2006;**34**:721–32.

Williams RJ, Hyman J, Petrigliano F, *et al.* Anterior cruciate ligament reconstruction with a four-strand hamstring tendon autograft. *J Bone Joint Surg Am* 2004;**86**:225–32.

Woo SL, Kanamori A, Zeminski J, *et al.* The effectiveness of reconstruction of the anterior cruciate ligament with hamstrings and patellar tendon: a cadaveric study comparing anterior tibial and rotational loads. *J Bone Joint Surg Am* 2002;**84**:907–14.

Viva questions

1. What equipment is required to perform a diagnostic arthroscopy?

2. Define the anatomy of the posterior knee arthroscopy portals.

3. Which structures are at risk in the posterior portals for knee arthroscopy?

4. What are the indications for meniscal repair?

5. Which techniques do you know for meniscal repair?

6. How are discoid lateral menisci classified?

7. What treatment do you use for a discoid lateral meniscus?

8. Which associated anatomical findings worsen a tight lateral retinaculum?

9. What are the advantages and disadvantages of arthroscopic over open lateral release?

10. What are the common indications for cartilage reconstruction surgery?

11. Describe the procedure of microplasty to the medial femoral condyle.

12. What are the advantages of autologous chondrocyte implantation over microplasty?

13. How are the cells provided for autologous chondrocyte implantation?

14. What risks do you describe to a patient consenting for anterior cruciate ligament reconstruction?

15. Describe the anatomy of the pes anserinus.

16. How are the hamstrings harvested for an anterior cruciate ligament graft?

17. What is the minimal acceptable graft thickness for anterior cruciate ligament reconstruction?

18. Where are the isometric points for the origin and insertion of an anterior cruciate ligament graft?

19. What position is the knee held in while an anterior cruciate ligament graft is tensioned and fixed?

20. Describe your postoperative regimen after anterior cruciate ligament reconstruction.

13

Surgery of the ankle

Laurence James and Dishan Singh

Movement	Range of motion
Dorsiflexion	*0–20°*
Plantarflexion	*0–45°*

Position of arthrodesis

- Neutral flexion
- 0–5° valgus
- 5–10° external rotation

ANKLE ARTHRODESIS

PREOPERATIVE PLANNING

Indications

- Arthropathy failing conservative management
- Failed arthroplasty
- Tumour reconstruction
- Sequelae of infection, particularly tuberculosis
- Avascular necrosis of talus
- Neuropathic joint
- Neurological conditions (resulting in instability).

Contraindications

- Infection
- Degeneration of subtalar and midfoot joints.

Consent and risks

- Failure of fusion: <2 per cent
- Malpositioning
- Metalwork prominence: may require further surgery
- Nerve injury is rare

The patient must understand that walking will not return to normal. There is a significant reduction in walking speed and increase in energy expenditure compared with normal.

Operative planning

Planning of the position of fusion is vital. The position is:
- 0° dorsiflexion
- 0–5° valgus hindfoot (varus positioning restricts midtarsal mobility)
- 5–10° external rotation (note: observe contralateral limb).

Posterior displacement of the talus allows for greater ease of 'rollover' at the end of the stance phase.

Anaesthesia and positioning

This is performed as for ankle replacement.

SURGICAL TECHNIQUE

Arthrodesis can be performed arthroscopically (see 'Ankle arthroscopy', p. 223), or via anterior (see 'Ankle arthroscopy', p. 221) and lateral transmalleolar open approaches. Internal fixation with screws, intramedullary nails and plates are used to give a good hold and adequate compression (Fig. 13.1). Thorough preparation of all joint surfaces is vital. This is achieved by removal of remaining articular cartilage and exposure of subchondral bleeding cancellous bone to aid biological union.

For surgical principles of joint surface preparation (see Chapter 14).

Lateral transmalleolar approach

Landmarks

- Tip, anterior and posterior border of fibula
- Base of fourth metatarsal
- Anterior to sural nerve.

Dissection

A longitudinal incision is made directly over lateral aspect of fibula, of sufficient length to avoid tension on the soft tissue flap. Distally the incision is angled toward the base of the fourth metatarsal to allow greater access to the ankle joint.

Procedure

Structures at risk

- Peroneal tendons
- Sural nerve

Subperiosteal dissection of the fibula is carried out, protecting the peroneal tendons posteriorly and distally at all times. **This also avoids damage to the sural nerve.** The joint line is identified, using an image intensifier, and is marked on the skin. The fibula is cut obliquely with a saw (superolateral to inferomedial ending at the level of the tibial plafond) and finished with an osteotome. The free distal end of the fibula is then reflected inferiorly and freed of soft tissues and ligamentous attachments. Care is taken not to divide the peroneal tendons at the tip of the distal fibula. Capsulotomy then allows access to joint surface. The bone of the distal fibula can then be used to harvest cancellous bone graft and the surgeon's choice of fixation is performed. For an isolated ankle fusion, with good quality bone, cannulated screws can be used. For poorer quality bone, or if the subtalar joint is to be included, a retrograde (pantalar) nail is a better choice (Fig. 13.2).

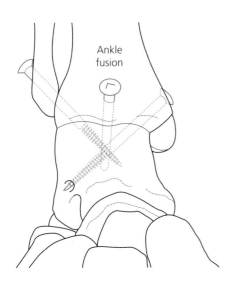

Figure 13.1 *Arthrodesis with screw fixation*

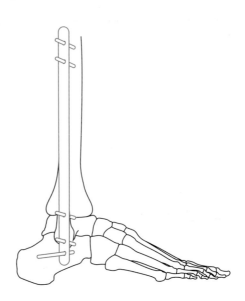

Figure 13.2 *Arthrodesis with nail fixation*

Closure

A layered closure is followed by the surgeon's choice of skin closure for open techniques. Nylon to skin is used to close arthroscopic fusion portals.

POSTOPERATIVE CARE AND INSTRUCTIONS

Thromboembolism should be prevented by early mobilization and the addition of chemical or mechanical measures in patients at increased risk. Two more doses of the antibiotic given at induction should be given at 8 hours and 16 hours after surgery.

Early mobilization is non-weightbearing, with the aid of crutches. Radiographic signs of union are sought before unprotected full weightbearing is allowed; this often takes around 3 months.

RECOMMENDED REFERENCES

Buck P, Morrey BF, Chao EY. The optimum position of arthrodesis of the ankle. *J Bone Joint Surg Am* 1987;**69**:1052–62.

Kitaoka HB, Patzer GL, Felix NA. Arthrodesis for the treatment of arthrosis of the ankle and osteonecrosis of the talus. *J Bone Joint Surg Am* 1998;**80**:370–9.

Mann RA. Arthrodesis of the foot and ankle. In RA Mann and MJ Coughlin (eds). *Surgery of the Foot and Ankle*. St Louis: Mosby Year Book, 1993.

Mann R, Rongstad AM. Arthrodesis of the ankle: a critical analysis. *Foot Ankle Int* 1998;**19**:3–9.

Scranton PE. An overview of ankle arthrodesis. *Clin Orthop Relat Res* 1991;**268**:268–96.

ANKLE ARTHROPLASTY

PREOPERATIVE PLANNING

Indications

Total ankle arthroplasty is indicated in painful conditions that have failed conservative management. The most frequent indications are:
• Osteoarthritis
• Inflammatory arthritis and other arthropathies.

Contraindications

• Ankle joint infection
• Avascular necrosis of a large part of the talar body
• Severe deformity that would not allow for good biomechanical function and lead to greater wear of the ultrahigh molecular weight polyethylene (UHMWPE) insert (greater the 15° varus/valgus deformity)
• Poor soft tissues
• Heavy manual occupation.

Consent and risks

• Loosening: revision surgery is required for loosening in up to 10 per cent at 10 years (approximately).
• Malpositioning
• Fracture: up to 10 per cent though they fare well with appropriate identification and management.
• Wound problems, pain and stiffness: 5 per cent
• Deep vein thrombosis (DVT)/pulmonary embolism/infection: 1 per cent

Operative planning

Assessment of the soft tissues, as well as vascular and neurological examination are mandatory on the day of surgery. Recent weightbearing radiographs must be available.

Availability of the implants and operative sets must be checked by the surgeon. Prophylactic antibiotics are administered on induction (the antibiotic of choice depends on local policy, but a common choice is cefuroxime).

Anaesthesia and positioning

Anaesthesia is usually general, regional or combined. A thigh tourniquet is used. The supine position is used with appropriate padding where necessary. Occasionally a sand bag under the ipsilateral buttock allows for greater ease of surgery. The knee should always be exposed and prepared (with a germicidal solution) to allow for intraoperative orientation of the implant.

The ankle should be sufficiently mobile for appropriate movement intraoperatively. Waterproof drapes are used with adhesive edges to provide a seal to the skin.

SURGICAL TECHNIQUE

Landmarks

These should be marked preoperatively:
- Tendons – tibialis anterior, extensor hallucis longus, extensor digitorum longus
- Dorsalis pedis – note: this is absent in 10 per cent of the population
- Cutaneous branches of the superficial peroneal nerve (variable course).

Incision

The anterior approach to the ankle is used. The skin is incised in the midpoint between the medial and lateral malleoli – from 3 cm above, extending 5 cm below the palpable ankle joint and avoiding cutaneous nerves where encountered.

Dissection

Structures at risk

- Dorsalis pedis artery
- Deep peroneal nerve

The extensor retinaculum is divided in the line of the incision. Large skin flaps are avoided to reduce the risk of necrosis. The approach is then developed either between the extensor hallucis longus (EHL) and the extensor digitorum longus (EDL) or (more commonly) between the tibialis anterior and the EHL. The key is protecting the dorsalis pedis artery and deep peroneal nerve – identification (and protection) of these structures more proximally, before they cross at the ankle joint itself may be required. A longitudinal capsulotomy is then performed.

Procedure

Several ankle prostheses are commercially available and the individual operative technique should be referred to. Although the designs vary, the principles of adequate bone preparation and implant positioning are the same. In general terms, an extramedullary guide is placed on the anterior surface of the tibia, in line with the crest and passing though the line of the second metatarsal ray distally – anatomical axis. This is strapped in place. The joint line is then identified and a fin is placed between the talus and tibia through the centre of the cutting block. Pins are used to fix the cutting guide to the tibia. This block ensures parallel cuts in the distal tibia and talar dome, without altering the joint line height – approximately 2–3 mm is resected from each surface. Guides then size the tibial and talar components, such that an appropriate sized window and accurate anterior and posterior chamfer cuts are made to the tibia and talus, respectively. Trial components and spacer (to assess stability and range of movement) are used prior to actual prosthesis placement.

Pitfalls to avoid include:
- **Varus/valgus positioning** of tibial and talar cutting guides, which can also lead to abnormal saggital plane tilting – early loosening.
- **Anterior/posterior placement of talar or tibial components** – early loosening.
- **Notching** of medial and lateral malleoli during tibial cuts – fracture.
- **Fracture of the anterior tibial cortex** when creating window to allow for tibial post during insertion of component.

Newer-generation systems are uncemented with three components (semi-constrained/mobile bearing), thus minimizing bone loss, stresses across components and early failure. Commonly used prostheses include: STAR (Scandinavian Total Ankle Replacement), Beuchal–Pappas, Ramses and Agility.

POSTOPERATIVE CARE AND INSTRUCTIONS

Patients are placed in a non-weightbearing, below knee plaster of Paris (changed at 2 weeks for wound inspection). Adequate pain relief and DVT prophylaxis are planned prior to departure from theatre.

Physiotherapy is commenced within 24–48 hours. Patients commence weightbearing after 4–6 weeks following clinical and X-ray review.

A return to work (and driving) would be expected after 3 months. Follow up is recommended at 6 weeks, 6 months and 1 year after surgery. Continuation of follow up is typically at 5 years, 10 years, 15 years then at yearly intervals. The patient should be cautioned to return to clinic if there is pain or functional deterioration.

RECOMMENDED REFERENCES

Carachiolo B. Design features of current total ankle replacements: implants and instruments. *J Am Acad Orthop Surg* 2008;**19**:530–40.

Hopgood P, Kumar R, Wood PL. Arthrodesis for failed ankle replacement. *J Bone Joint Surg Br* 2006;**88**:1032–8.

Spirt AA, Assal M, Hansen ST Jr. Complications and failure after total ankle arthroplasty. *J Bone Joint Surg Am* 2004;**86**:1172–8.

Wood PL, Deakin S. Total ankle replacement: the results in 200 ankles. *J Bone Joint Surg Br* 2003;**85**:334–41.

ANKLE ARTHROSCOPY

PREOPERATIVE PLANNING

Indications

- Undiagnosed ankle pain in the young
- Osteoarthritis
- Osteochondral defect
- Removal of loose bodies
- Synovectomy or synovial biopsy
- Impingement syndromes (bony and soft tissue)
- Arthrofibrosis (e.g. post traumatic)
- Fracture
- Meniscoid lesions
- Septic arthritis.

Contraindications

- Infection of overlying skin
- Lack of proper instrumentation
- Gross osteoarthritis is a relative contraindication
- Severe oedema.

Consent and risks

- Nerve injury: <1 per cent
- Vascular injury: <1 per cent
- Infection: <1 per cent. Risk is very low, so prophylactic antibiotics are not recommended

Operative planning

It is vital that the patient is examined before transfer to theatre. This allows for identification and marking of structures vulnerable to damage during portal insertion intraoperatively. These include:

- Tibialis anterior and EHL tendons
- Dorsalis pedis artery and associated deep peroneal nerve
- Traction on second and fourth toes usually demonstrates medial and lateral branches of the superficial peroneal nerve
- Saphenous vein and nerve
- Medial and lateral malleoli.

Recent radiographs and, where taken, magnetic resonance (MR) images, should be available.

The equipment must be available; this should be checked by the surgeon. Usually a 2.7 mm 30° arthroscope and 3.5 mm shavers are required. Water pressure is set at 50 mmHg.

Anaesthesia and positioning

Anaesthesia is usually general with intraoperative local anaesthetic infiltration into the joint at the end of the procedure. The supine position is used, with the hip flexed and a well-padded support under the thigh. The ankle distractor is applied with the knee at 90° of flexion and the ankle in a neutral position. Adequate padding avoids damage to skin and neurological structures. Too much traction (>15 kg) and excessive time can lead to irreversible nerve damage.

The surgical field is prepared with a germicidal solution. Waterproof drapes are used with adhesive edges to provide a seal to the skin.

SURGICAL TECHNIQUE

The ankle joint is filled with 20 mL of saline to aid access and avoid chondral surface damage. Small longitudinal skin incisions are made, then blunt dissection (with a clip) used to breech the ankle joint, thereby avoiding damage to the superficial nerves – unlike knee arthroscopy where a blade is passed directly into the joint.

Creation of portals

Structures at risk

- Nerves: deep peroneal, superficial peroneal branches, sural, tibial
- Arteries: dorsalis pedis, posterior tibial artery

A number of portal sites are described (Fig. 13.3). The central anterior portal is best avoided because of a high risk of neurovascular damage.

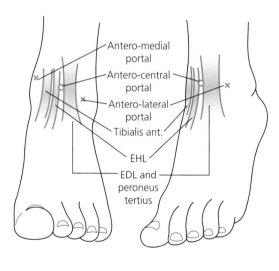

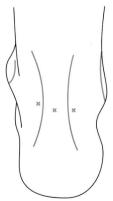

Figure 13.3 *Typical portal positioning (anterior above and posterior below)*

- **Anteromedial portal** – this lies medial to tibialis anterior. The joint line is initially identified by palpation and then a white needle is inserted into the joint to confirm the level. The needle is directed slightly superiorly to pass over the talar dome. The arthroscope and introducing trochar should be able to be swept across the joint from medial to lateral.
- **Anterolateral portal** – this lies lateral to extensor peroneus tertius and the neurovascular bundle (dorsalis pedis and deep peroneal nerve), avoiding the superficial nerves marked out preoperatively. The light source within the joint can be used as a guide, this will also help to **identify the dorsal lateral branch of the superficial peroneal nerve which is at risk**. A white needle is inserted as outlined above
- **Posterolateral portal** – this is located lateral to the Achilles tendon 1 cm above the tip of fibula. Insert prior to posteromedial portal – **risk of sural nerve damage**.
- **Posteromedial portal** – this is just medial to Achilles tendon at the level of the posterolateral portal. Flexor hallucis longus is used to sweep away the **tibial nerve and posterior tibial artery – the main structures at risk**.

Posterior portals are not as frequently used (because of the increased risk of neurovascular damage), but are helpful in visualizing the posterior ankle and subtalar joints.

Procedure

A systematic approach is essential if pathology is not to be missed. Initially the whole of the talar dome is inspected – ankle plantar flexion aids visualization of the posterior dome. The talar neck is then examined. Pathology on the corresponding articulating surface of the tibia is also documented, as well as the anatomy of the anterior aspect of tibia. The medial and lateral gutters are then inspected. Key features to identify include:

- Medial malleolus
- Deltoid ligament
- Lateral malleolus
- Anterior and posterior tibiofibular ligaments
- Anterior talofibular ligament
- Syndesmosis.

Closure

Non-absorbable suture is used to close the skin incisions.

POSTOPERATIVE CARE AND INSTRUCTIONS

The patient is fully weightbearing – as tolerated – unless the patient has a microfracture of an osteochondral defect, where range movement is encouraged in a non-loading manner so as to protect the developing fibrocartilage plug.

Specific precautions are rarely required.

RECOMMENDED REFERENCES

Ferkel RD, Karzel RP, Del Pizzo W, et al. Arthroscopic treatment of anterolateral impingement of the ankle. Am J Sports Med 1991;19:440–6.

Ferkel RD, Zanotti RM, Komenda GA, et al. Arthroscopic treatment of osteochondral lesions of the talus: Long-term results. Am J Sports Med 2008;36:1750–62.

Niek van Dijk C, van Bergen CJ. Advancements in ankle arthroscopy. J Am Acad Orthop Surg 2008;16:635–46.

Tryfonidis M, Whitfield CG, Charalambous CP, et al. Posterior ankle arthroscopy portal safety regarding proximity to the tibial and sural nerves. Acta Orthop Belgica 2008;74:370–3.

SURGERY FOR ACHILLES TENDINOPATHY

PREOPERATIVE PLANNING

There is an ever increasing incidence of tendon problems, most commonly seen in recreational runners (racket sports, track and field, volleyball and football) and competitive runners, who are 10 times more affected than age-matched controls.

Despite preventive measures, 7–8 per cent of top level athletes experience the problem at some stage in their career. The long-term prognosis is good with 84 per cent fully recovered at 8 years; 94 per cent remain asymptomatic.

Indications

Diagnosis is key. There are three common patterns of tendon pathology:
- **Overuse (non-insertional) tendinopathy** – this has a gradual onset classically with morning pain and stiffness that eases with activity and reoccurs at rest later. Associated with an increase in activity, change of surface or change of footwear/poor footwear.
- **Partial and complete ruptures** – there is a sudden onset of severe pain, marked disability and these ruptures are 10 times more common in males. With peak incidence in the 30s and 40s. Patients often describe hearing a 'pop' and feel an impact in the back of the leg or heel.
- **Insertional tendinopathy** (enthesopathy) – this can be mistaken for a number of pathologies including retrocalcaneal bursitis, Hagland disease (painful retrocalcaneal bursitis and a bony prominence), Achilles bursitis.

Be aware of the systemic enthesopathies/rheumatoid arthritis and spondyloarthropathies; it is an area where misdiagnosis is common and the differential diagnoses include:
- Posterior ankle impingement syndrome
- Accessory soleus
- Deep posterior compartment syndrome
- Sever's disease
- Stress fracture
- Inflammatory arthropathy
- Neurogenic referred pain.

Contraindications

Active infection.

Consent and risks

- 12 per cent complications (54 per cent wound related)

88 per cent return to function after a 6- to 12-month treatment programme.

Operative planning

Non-operative management

Once the diagnosis has been made, consideration

is given to whether operative treatment is the best option for the patient. These include:

- Older patients and those with low activity levels
- Those able to tolerate a rehabilitation regimen, which have an overall success rate of 75–85 per cent.
- Achilles rupture with a 10 mm gap when the ankle is in neutral and complete apposition of the ends with plantar flexion on ultrasound; treatment with 3 cm of hindfoot elevation for 8 weeks in a below knee cast and then a 1 cm elevation for an additional 3 months (75 per cent rate of return to normal function).

Poor outcomes occur in 17.5 per cent, these include:

- Ongoing pain
- Lengthening dysfunction
- A reduced calf size
- Re-rupture in 6.4 per cent.

For tendinopathies in the absence of rupture conservative management should include eccentric heel drops (Alfredson's painful eccentric heel-drop protocol):

- Three sets of 15 repetitions twice daily, 7/7, for 12 weeks
- Exercise until pain free then add load to create pain (up to 60 kg).

There is a 90 per cent cure rate.

Bursae are treated with non-steroidal anti-inflammatory drugs (NSAIDs), intrabursal cortisone injections and deep friction massage. Biomechanical treatment includes heel lifts. Other treatments include sclerosant injections, nitric oxide, corticosteroids and electrophysical agents.

Operative management

A rapid return to function and reduced long-term pain.

Anaesthesia and positioning

- General anaesthesia with local infiltration.
- Thigh tourniquet.
- Prone position with ankles resting of pillow.

SURGICAL TECHNIQUE

There is much debate about open versus percutaneous repair. The open technique is

described here, as an example. Ancillary procedures can be used to augment treatment; their details are beyond the scope of this book. The procedures include: calcaneoplasty, bursectomy, osteotomy and debridement of the tendon.

Landmarks

- Midpoint of the calcaneal tuberosity posteriorly where tendo-Achilles inserts
- Medial and lateral aspects of tendon traced proximally to bellies of gastrocnemius to identify aponeurosis.

Incision

Structure at risk

- Sural nerve

A 5–10 cm incision is created (at the level of the defect) along the medial border of the Achilles tendon. This avoids the sural nerve and allows access to plantaris.

Dissection

- Directly deepen to paratenon.
- Open paratenon and debride tendon.
- Thick flaps are vital for healing.

Procedure

It is necessary to address peritendinous adhesions and excise intratendinous lesions. A modified Kessler box suture is recommended. This consists of two standard Kessler sutures, at 90° to each other, ensuring the ends are tied inside not outside. It is best to use 1/0 PDS: this ensures good strength and slides easily. The repair is completed with a continuous epitendinous suture (3/0 Vicryl). A number of techniques are described for repair of tendon defects, including:

- Turn down flaps – this involves a centrally based fascial flap developed from the proximal segment and turned distally though 180° before suturing.

- V-Y advancement – a V-shaped incision is made in the aponeurosis. The limbs of the 'V' should be 1.5 cm longer than the gap to be filled. The intermediate segment is advanced distally and the proximal segment is closed as a 'Y' in the lengthened position (Fig. 13.4).

If the repair or augment is too compromised the flexor hallucis longus, peroneus brevis or an allograft made of polyglycol or carbon fibre can be used.

Closure

Closure is performed in thick layers with a non-absorbable suture for the tendon repair. Absorbable suture is used for the paratenon and skin closure.

POSTOPERATIVE CARE AND INSTRUCTIONS

Initially immobilize in equinus cast with strict elevation and neurovascular observation. This is followed by 6 weeks' non-weightbearing with serial casting to return the ankle to a plantigrade position. At 6 weeks, conversion to a removable boot allows the patient to fully weightbear and commence physiotherapy for another 6 weeks. The functional outcome is assessed in clinic at 3 months.

RECOMMENDED REFERENCES

Hufner TM, Brandes DB, Thermann H, *et al.* Long-term results after functional nonoperative treatment of Achilles tendon rupture. *Foot Ankle Int* 2006;**27**:167–71.

Manoli A, Graham B. The subtle cavus foot. *Foot Ankle Int* 2005;**26**:256–63.

Oyedele O, Maseko C, Mkasi N, *et al.* High incidence of Os peroneum in cadavers. *Clin Anat* 2005;**19**:605–10.

SURGERY FOR PERONEAL TENDINOPATHY

PREOPERATIVE PLANNING

The peroneus longus originates from the lateral tibial condyle and head of fibula to insert on the first metatarsal base and medial cuneiform. The peroneus brevis originates from the middle one-third of the fibula and tibia to insert on the base of the fifth metatarsal. Remember, at the ankle the peroneus brevis is sandwiched between bone and the peroneus longus – 'brevis to bone'.

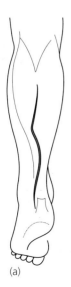
(a)

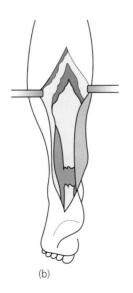
(b)

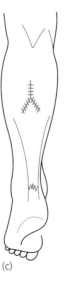
(c)

Figure 13.4 *V-Y advancement for repairs with defect*

Indications

A history of sprains is common. Other causes include: trauma, inflammatory arthritides, fibula anatomy (shallow fibular groove, sharp lateral ridge), hypertrophied peroneal tubercle, lateral ankle instability and peroneus quartus (overcrowding). Developmental varus hindfoot alignment is associated with increased incidence of peroneal disorders:

- Tenosynovitis (a static mass on examination)
- Tendinosis (a mass moving with the tendon, through sheath)
- Tears (present with pain and weakness)
- Subluxation (palpation along the length of the tendons noting any deviation of their course)
- Os peroneum syndrome: ossified in 20 per cent population. Articulates with inferior margin of cuboid. May be degenerative/osteochondritis or fractured, leading to pain in the plantar/lateral aspect of the foot.
- Eventually pain-related functional weakness will lead to deformity.

Contraindications

Varus deformity related to underlying peroneal weakness rather than tendinopathy.

Consent and risks

- Sural nerve injury during dissection and skin closure
- Painful scar
- Late re-rupture/subluxation
- Fracture to tip of fibula/disruption of retinaculum
- Tendinous adhesions

Operative planning

Radiographs are helpful, however MRI and ultrasound show: brevis flattening, thickening, nodules, tears, fluid in the peroneal sheath, dislocation, and the retrofibular groove anatomy in good detail (18 per cent have a shallow or convex surface). The presence of fluid around a normal tendon on imaging indicates tenosynovitis.

Depending on the quality of proximal and distal tendon, orthoses (lateral posting) and physiotherapy are usually successful. Conservative management of peroneal subluxation has <50 per cent success.

Anaesthesia and positioning

General with local infiltration, or spinal/epidural can be used. The patient is positioned prone with a thigh tourniquet and a sandbag under the ipsilateral buttock or, more usually, the lateral position with adequate supports and protection between leg pressure points.

SURGICAL TECHNIQUE

Landmarks

The tip of the fibula to the base of the fifth metatarsal.

Incision

A longitudinal incision parallel to the posterior border of the fibula. Distally, the incision is curved towards the base of the fifth metatarsal.

Dissection

Dissection is straight down, directly to the tendon sheath. Thick tissue flaps are reflected under minimal tension. The sheath is divided longitudinally and as posteriorly as possible, to aid repair and reduce scar tissue irritation when the tendons are mobilized under stress. Tendon hooks are used to isolate, deliver and clear individual tendons of adhesions.

Procedure

Surgical management for tendinopathy includes soft tissue procedures such as synovectomy, debridement or tubularization of tears. If greater than 50 per cent of the tendon is intact, repair is advocated; less than 50 per cent tenodesis is recommended. Tendon transfer of flexor digitorum longus to peroneus brevis or an autograft using gracilis can maintain function.

Bony procedures include:

- Deepening of the peroneal groove – using a 4.5 mm drill, a longitudinal hole is made in the posterior third of the tip of fibular, then the posterior cortex is 'stoved in' to deepen the peroneal groove. The retinaculum is then repaired and a calcaneal osteotomy can be performed if required. The tendons can also be rerouted behind the calcaneofibular ligament as an alternative to the deepening procedure.
- A partial thickness distal fibular osteotomy – this is rotated posteriorly (Kelly procedure).
- Distal fibular sliding graft (Duvries modification) can also be carried out (Fig. 13.5).

POSTOPERATIVE CARE AND INSTRUCTIONS

Tubularization of tears/bony procedures (4 weeks plaster of Paris, 4 weeks brace).

RECOMMENDED REFERENCES

Dombek MF, Catanzariti AR. Peroneal tendon tears: a retrospective review. *J Foot Ankle Surg* 2003;**42**:250–8.

Manoli A, Graham B. The subtle Cavus foot. *Foot Ankle Int* 2005;**26**:256–63.

Oyedele O, Maseko C, Mkasi N, *et al.* High incidence of os peroneum in cadavers. *Clin Anat* 2005;**19**:605–10.

Porter D, Torma J. Peroneal subluxation in athletes. *Foot Ankle Int* 2005;**26**:436–41.

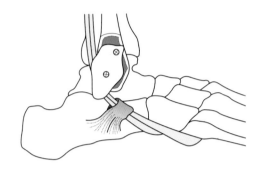

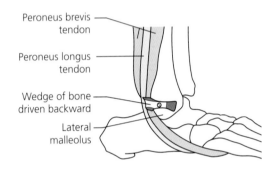

Figure 13.5 *Bone block procedures*

Viva questions

1. What are the indications, benefits and drawbacks of ankle arthrodesis?

2. What are the treatment options for a 40-year-old man with symptomatic osteoarthritis of the ankle?

3. Describe the anatomy of anterior ankle arthrotomy?

4. What complications do you warn the patient about prior to ankle replacement? What are their incidences?

5. What are the contraindications to ankle replacement?

6. Describe the portals used in arthroscopy.

7. How do you perform an ankle arthroscopy?

8. What are the complications of ankle arthroscopy and how can they be minimized?

9. How would you fuse an ankle?

10. Describe the follow up and complications you might expect following ankle arthrodesis?

11. What types of ankle arthroplasty are you aware of?

12. What are the principles of the prosthesis used?

13. Describe the technique of ankle arthroplasty.

14. What are the common pitfalls and how can they be avoided?

15. Describe an approach to the peroneal tendons.

16. How might you address peroneal tendon subluxation operatively?

17. What is the most common approach to the Achilles tendon?

18. Describe the technique for direct repair of the Achilles tendon?

19. How might you augment a tendo-Achilles repair, e.g. in a patient with tendon loss/shortening?

20. What are the common indications for operative management of peroneal and Achilles tendon disorders?

Surgery of the foot

Simon Clint and Nick Cullen

Joint/movement	Range of motion
Subtalar joint inversion	10°
Subtalar joint eversion	5°
Transverse tarsal joint adduction	20°
Transverse tarsal joint abduction	10°
Combined foot supination	30°
Combined foot pronation	15°
First metatarsophalangeal joint flexion	30°
First metatarsophalangeal joint extension	60°

Position of arthrodesis

- The positions of arthrodesis are covered in the relevant sections.

PRINCIPLES OF FOOT AND ANKLE ARTHRODESIS

PREOPERATIVE PLANNING

Arthrodesis is a commonly used technique throughout the foot and ankle. Although the approach, position and fixation used are specific to each joint fused, the principles and techniques are common throughout the region and should be well understood. Individual arthrodeses will be dealt with in the relevant sections.

Indications

- Painful arthropathy of a joint – given the large number of adjacent joints in the foot, it can be useful to localize the source of pain with a radiologically guided injection of the proposed joint preoperatively
- Deformity of a joint affecting the position of the remaining foot – often associated with congenital or acquired tendon or neuromuscular conditions.

Contraindications

- Active infection
- Critical ischaemia
- Multiple adjacent arthrodeses (relative contra-indication).

Consent and risks

- Prolonged postoperative treatment: the joint must be immobilized until union and unprotected weightbearing avoided, which may take about 3 months in the hindfoot or ankle.
- Infection and wound healing problems: dependent on surgical technique and soft tissue handling as well as patient factors.
- Cutaneous nerve damage: given the subcutaneous and variable location of cutaneous

nerves in the foot, inadvertent damage and subsequent painful neuroma formation can occur.

- Non-union: absolute risk is dependent on technical and patient factors. Most patients have a 5–10 per cent risk of non-union and ongoing pain for most procedures. This is increased dramatically in smokers (up to sevenfold), those with poor perfusion, active infection or diabetes
- Malunion: technique dependent. Malunions may be symptomatic, requiring footwear adaptations or revision surgery, or may be asymptomatic and tolerated
- Development of arthropathy in neighbouring joints – common over time but may represent the progression of unrecognized early joint disease
- Alteration of gait – dependent on number and location of arthrodeses

Anaesthesia and positioning

General anaesthesia is usually required. A thigh tourniquet is required to allow exposure of the limb to above the knee. This allows accurate assessment of alignment. A supportive bolster under the calf is useful to allow free access to the foot.

SURGICAL PRINCIPLES

The general principles are to **mobilize the joint to allow correction of any deformity and complete access to the joint surfaces**. The surfaces are prepared, maintaining the joint shape and congruity while exposing bleeding cancellous bone. The joint is then held rigidly in the required position of arthrodesis.

Careful placement of incisions of adequate length is vital to prevent undue soft tissue damage and tension. Most joints are relatively superficial so adequate soft tissue cover is vital.

The capsule and surround soft tissues need to be released to allow full access to the joint and to correct any deformity. Most deformities can be corrected with an adequate mobilization but occasionally bone resection is required.

The joint surfaces need to be carefully prepared. First, any peripheral osteophytes should be removed to expose the true joint. Second, the

cartilage and subchondral plate must be removed, maintaining the contour of the joint. This is best achieved with a variety of sharp chisels working in a methodical manner from superficial to deep. Power tools generate unwanted heat and should be avoided. As the joint is prepared, a laminar spreader is gradually advanced into the joint to open it up. Pituitary rongeurs and Kerrison laminectomy rongeurs are useful to access the deep recesses of the joint safely. Once all joint surfaces are removed, the surface area of bleeding bone should be increased by various methods. Using a chisel to cross-cut the surface and applying a slight twist on removal can produce bone 'petals' to good effect.

The joint should be positioned in the desired position and, if needed, provisionally held with a K-wire. A careful confirmation of the position with respect to the limb alignment and the rest of the foot must be undertaken to ensure a satisfactory outcome. It is unusual, unless bony destruction has occurred, to require supplementary bone graft. If required, sufficient quantities can usually be harvested locally from the calcaneus, medial malleolus or proximal tibia without need to prepare the iliac crest.

Rigid fixation and compression of the joint must be achieved. This is usually done with some form of compression screw or screws. However, in certain situations other forms of fixation, such as staples, intramedullary devices or external fixations may be appropriate. Satisfactory compression can be tested by carefully inserting a fine chisel into the joint and twisting – there should be no give.

Careful, tension-free wound closure is critical. A soft tissue layer should be closed over the joint prior to skin closure. The joint is immobilized in a back-slab to protect the fusion and soft tissues.

POSTOPERATIVE CARE AND INSTRUCTIONS

The leg should be elevated until swelling has subsided. Mobilization should avoid weight-bearing on the joint. In the forefoot, a wedge-type shoe may be sufficient but usually a non-weightbearing cast should be used. Unprotected weightbearing should be avoided until there is clinical and radiological evidence of union.

RECOMMENDED REFERENCE

Hardy MA, Logan DB. Principles of arthrodesis and advances in fixation for the adult acquired flatfoot. *Clin Podiatr Med Surg* 2007; **24**:789–813.

HALLUX VALGUS CORRECTION

PREOPERATIVE PLANNING

There are a multitude of procedures described for the correction of hallux valgus deformity, some considered historical and others in current use. In order to select the correct procedure for a specific patient, an understanding of the spectrum of hallux valgus deformities must exist.

Indications and choice of procedure

The presence of a bunion is not an indication for surgery.

The strongest indication for operative intervention in hallux valgus is pain. This pain is located over the bunion and usually only felt with shod feet. Pain present when barefoot or under the metatarsal head suggests another source of the pain should be sought. Footwear problems due to extreme deformities are a relative indication. Operating solely for cosmetic or fashion reasons is generally not recommended.

On examining the patient, the neurovascular status of the patient must be examined along with the overall hindfoot and foot alignment. Joint mobility is assessed: hypermobility of the first tarsometatarsal joint (TMTJ) is associated with an increased risk of postsurgical recurrence.

Contraindications

Patients with significant pre-existing degenerative change in the metatarsophalangeal joint (MTPJ) will usually not benefit from realignment surgery and should be offered arthrodesis. (See 'First metatarsophalangeal joint arthrodesis', p. 242.)

Patients with hypermobility or instability of the first TMTJ are likely to have a recurrence after a simple osteotomy. These deformities might be best treated with a first TMTJ arthrodesis combined with a lateral release (see Lapidus procedure below).

Consent and risks

There is considerable variation, depending on the specific procedure: details of operation-specific risks are detailed within the operative techniques below. General complications are listed here.

- Foot shape: most procedures will result in a narrower forefoot with a straighter hallux. However, this may still preclude the wearing of many fashionable shoes
- Stiffness: most procedures which violate the MTPJ are associated with varying degrees of postoperative stiffness. This can be particularly troublesome with the Scarf osteotomy due to the degree of soft tissue mobilization
- Recurrence of deformity: usually associated with poor technique, attempting to push the indications of a procedure too far or not recognizing complicating factors (laxity, increased distal metatarsal articular angle [DMAA], congruent joint, etc.)
- Overcorrection and hallux varus: usually occurs due to overenthusiastic soft tissue correction or excessive displacement of the capital fragment. Excessive medial eminence excision or the excision of the fibular sesamoid in a McBride release also predispose to hallux varus.
- Nerve damage and neuroma formation: damage to the dorsomedial or plantar nerves is possible with most procedures and can cause painful neuroma formation
- Transfer metatarsalgia: anything that alters the relationship between the first and lesser metatarsals in the sagittal plane can lead to painful overloading of the lesser metatarsals, usually the second. This can occur in techniques that result in excessive shortening or elevation of the metatarsal head. It can also occur with defunctioning of the hallux, as occurs with a Keller procedure

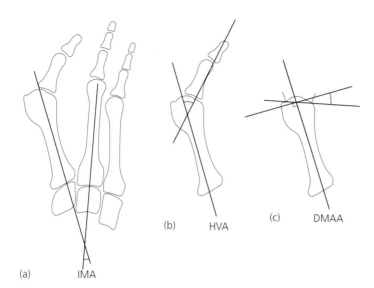

(a) IMA

(b) HVA

(c) DMAA

Figure 14.1 *Radiographic assessment of hallux valgus. (a) Intermetatarsal angle (IMA). (b) Hallux valgus angle (HVA). (c) Distal metatarsal articular angle (DMAA)*

Operative planning

Radiology

All patients presenting with hallux valgus should have *weightbearing* anteroposterior (AP) and lateral radiographs of both feet obtained. Various radiographic angles and measurements are frequently used to define the anatomical location and magnitude of the hallux deformity which can aid surgical planning (Fig. 14.1). These include:

- *Hallux valgus angle (HVA)* – the angle between the anatomical axes of the first metatarsal and the proximal phalanx
- *First–second intermetatarsal angle (IMA)* – the angle between the anatomical axes of the first and second metatarsals
- *DMMA* – the angle between a line drawn from the medial and lateral borders of the articular surface of the distal metatarsal and the anatomical axis of the metatarsal
- *Interphalangeal angle* – angle between the proximal and distal articular surfaces of the proximal phalanx of the hallux
- *Joint congruity* – the medial and lateral borders of the joint surface of the metatarsal and phalanx are identified. The first MTPJ is said to be congruent if the lateral and medial borders of the two joint surfaces align. If they do not, the joint is incongruent (Fig. 14.2)
- *Presence of degenerative changes in the first MTPJ*
- *Signs of first TMTJ instability* – these include

opening up of the first TMTJ on the lateral view and widening of the gap between the first/second metatarsal bases.

- Congruent deformities require an osteotomy that incorporates rotation to correct the relationship of the articular surface to the axis of the metatarsal.
- Mild deformities can be corrected with a single metatarsal osteotomy (e.g. biplanar Chevron or modified Scarf – see below) with or without the addition of a phalangeal osteotomy (Akin osteotomy – see below).
- Severe deformities occasionally require a combined proximal and distal metatarsal osteotomy (see proximal metatarsal osteotomy below).
- Most authors categorize incongruent hallux valgus based on broad categories of severity. Such categories are not absolute but act as general guidelines to help define the limits of certain procedures and to help in the selection of the correct treatment. Table 14.1 shows typical figures.

Anaesthesia and positioning

All hallux valgus surgery can be performed under a regional (ankle) block or general anaesthesia. A bloodless field is provided by a thigh or ankle tourniquet. The patient is positioned supine and the whole foot and ankle prepared.

Table 14.1 Categorization of hallux valgus severity*

Angle measured	Normal	Mild	Moderate	Severe
HVA	<15°	15–20°	20–40°	>40°
IMMA	<9°	9–11°	11–16°	>16°
DMAA	<6°			

*After Coughlin, Mann, Saltzman. Surgery of the Foot and Ankle. Philadelphia: Mosby Elsevier, 2007.

SURGICAL TECHNIQUES

Given the huge range of surgical procedures described for hallux valgus, it is not within the scope of this book to describe them all. We shall therefore concentrate on those procedures commonly performed. Each procedure is described individually but in practice several techniques, such as the metatarsal osteotomy, Akin osteotomy and lateral soft tissue release, may be performed in combination.

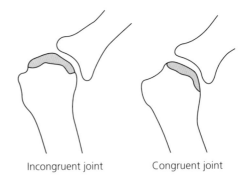

Incongruent joint   Congruent joint

Figure 14.2 *Assessment of first metatarsophalangeal joint congruity*

First metatarsophalangeal joint soft tissue release

A soft tissue release attempts to balance out the soft tissues around the first MTPJ. With a valgus deformity, the medial tissues become attenuated and those on the lateral side contracted. The original McBride procedure was more extensive, including excision of the lateral sesamoid, and was associated with a high rate of hallux varus. The procedure has been altered so many times that the term 'modified McBride' is misleading and should be avoided.

A soft tissue release is rarely performed in isolation. However, it is part of many procedures so a detailed understanding is important.

Specific indications

- Incongruent, mild hallux valgus with normal, or near normal IMA
- In combination with another procedure (see below).

Consent and risks

- Overcorrection and hallux varus: caused by excessive soft tissue release and excessive medial plication
- Excessive medial plication can also lead to joint stiffness
- Nerve damage: the common digital nerve is deep to the inter-metatarsal ligament and can be damaged

Incision

Starting on the medial side, a medial longitudinal incision is made, centred over the metatarsal head and extending from the shaft of the proximal phalanx to the distal shaft of the metatarsal.

Dissection

Structure at risk

- Dorsomedial sensory nerve

Dissection is continued down to capsule and then a dorsal flap is carefully elevated to identify the dorsal nerve adherent to the capsule on the dorsomedial aspect. This is repeated on the plantar side, dissecting around the capsule to create a small pocket. A longitudinal capsulotomy is performed and any adhesions released.

Surgical technique

Unless a distal metatarsal osteotomy is also to be performed, the prominent medial eminence of the head can now be removed. This is done with a fine oscillating saw, aiming to cut in line with the medial shaft starting 2–3 mm from the medial sulcus (Fig. 14.3).

Attention is now turned to the first web space. A 3 cm incision is centred between the metatarsal heads in the first web space then bluntly dissecting down to the level of the heads. Inserting a laminar spreader or self-retainer between the heads allows identification of the lateral sesamoid and the insertion of adductor hallucis into its lateral edge. Using a size 15 blade, the capsule is released from the dorsal aspect of the sesamoid then the blade advanced to the insertion of

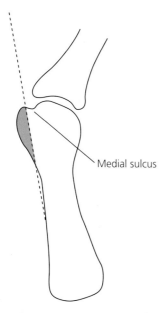

Medial sulcus

Figure 14.3 *Excision of medial eminence of first metatarsophalangeal joint*

adductor hallucis into the phalanx. The insertion of adductor hallucis is released from the phalanx then, working proximally, the remaining tendon is released from the sesamoid. Deep to this is the inter-metatarsal ligament which runs from the second metatarsal to the lateral sesamoid, not the first metatarsal itself. This is carefully divided from the sesamoid, taking care to preserve the neurovascular bundle which lies directly underneath. The lateral capsule (metatarso-sesamoid ligament) is then incised longitudinally, after which the articular surface of the lateral sesamoid can be inspected and should be reducible underneath the metatarsal head. The retractor is removed and confirmation that the toe can be passively overcorrected is sought.

Returning to the medial side, the metatarsal head should be reducible onto the sesamoids. If too much resistance is encountered, a bony procedure is required to correct the deformity. Subsequent capsular plication is designed to take in excess capsule, not pull the sesamoid complex over.

Using an absorbable suture, the excess capsule is 'double-breasted' while holding the MTPJ flexed. This is done by passing a stitch through the dorsal capsule from outside, medial to the extensor tendon and avoiding the identified nerve. The needle is then passed from outside the plantar capsule, just medial to the sesamoid then reversed to come from inside out. It is finished by exiting through the dorsal capsule, near the earlier entry point. As the suture is tightened, the dorsal capsule should double-breast over the plantar capsule. Plication is checked to ensure that it is not too tight by flexing and extending the joint.

Closure

The rest of the capsule is then closed with absorbable sutures prior to skin closure.

Scarf osteotomy

The scarf osteotomy is a powerful and versatile osteotomy allowing correction of all of the axes of the hallux valgus deformity; it is a technically challenging procedure with a steep learning curve. It is named after a joiners' technique, used to connect two beams.

Specific indications

- Moderate or severe hallux valgus
- Hallux valgus with an increased DMAA
- Revision surgery.

Specific contraindications

- Poor bone stock or osteoporosis increasing the risk of fracture.

Consent and risks

- Fracture: given the length of the osteotomy, fracture, either intraoperatively or postoperatively can occur (3–5 per cent)
- MTPJ stiffness: especially if the metatarsal is inadvertently lengthened
- Malunion: care must be taken to ensure all cuts are in the correct direction in all three planes
- Troughing: this occurs when the shaft cortex of one fragment collapses into the cancellous bone of the other fragment (Fig. 14.4). This results in elevation of the metatarsal head and rotation of the osteotomy. It is more common where there is poor bone stock. By ensuring the ends of the osteotomy are in dense metaphyseal bone, rather than the diaphysis, the risk can be reduced

Incision

A medial approach, as described above, is performed. However, the incision continues proximally until approaching the TMTJ.

Dissection

Structures at risk

- Dorsomedial sensory nerve
- Blood supply to first metatarsal head

Dorsally, the capsule and dorsal periosteum is released from the distal half of the bone, exposing the dorsal surface. Plantarwards, great care is taken to not damage the vascular leash entering the head on the plantar surface of the neck (Fig. 14.5).

Surgical technique

The periosteum is only elevated from the proximal third, dissecting away from the neck. A minimal excision of the medial eminence is performed in line with the shaft, aiming to just expose cancellous bone. At this point it is advisable to draw out the planned osteotomy, on the medial aspect of the bone (see Fig. 14.5). The longitudinal arm begins at a point 3 mm from the dorsal cortex, 5 mm proximal to the dorsal articular edge. This then extends proximally and plantarwards to a point 3 mm from the plantar surface and 10 mm from the TMTJ. Two horizontal 60° limbs are then added to the ends to exit the nearby cortices. The distal horizontal limb should be perpendicular to the second metatarsal shaft; we advise drawing a line connecting the

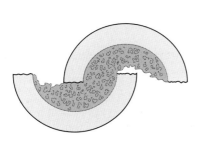

Figure 14.4 *Troughing of Scarf osteotomy*

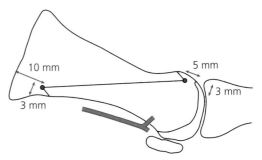

Figure 14.5 *Scarf osteotomy and plantar vascular supply of the metatarsal head*

medial point of origin of the distal first metatarsal cut running perpendicular to the second metatarsal shaft and on through the lateral rays the metatarsal head that it passes through (usually the fourth) can be used as a reference for the cut. Palpating the fourth metatarsal head, another line is drawn on the dorsal surface, from the distal arm across the dorsal surface towards the fourth.

Once satisfied with the planned osteotomy, an oscillating saw is used to score the cortex for the longitudinal arm. After a starting point is made, the blade is angled plantarwards, in the plane of the shafts of the metatarsals. Maintaining this angle, the whole length of the longitudinal arm is cut, penetrating only the medial cortex; the lateral cortex is then softly cut in the same plane. Next the distal arm is cut, maintaining the slight plantar angle and aiming for the fourth metatarsal head as planned. The proximal cut should now be cut parallel or slightly divergent to this – if the cuts converge, the osteotomy will not displace. The osteotomy should now be mobile. If not, all cuts are checked for completion and the two fragments gently freed with a MacDonald dissector, starting proximally.

The osteotomy is now displaced as required. This is facilitated by a 'push–pull' action, grasping the proximal fragment with a towel-clip while pushing the distal fragment laterally. **The osteotomy should displace laterally and plantarwards**. The reduction is then held with a clamp. The reduction is checked by observing the position of the medial sesamoid: it should lie under the medial metatarsal head. Once the reduction is satisfactory, a K-wire is inserted along the lateral edge of the proximal fragment into the head and a stepped bone clamp will prevent displacement.

The osteotomy is secured with two screws – headless, variable pitch compression screws are ideal. The first screw should start from the dorsolateral aspect of the distal end of the proximal fragment and aim towards the medial sesamoid. **This must be intraosseous to avoid sesamoid damage**. A second screw can then be used in a dorsoplantar direction to secure the proximal extent of the osteotomy. The proximal screw should be bicortical.

After fixation, the prominent medial cortex of the proximal fragment can be bevelled flush with the shaft.

Closure

Closure of the capsule should be performed as described previously.

Akin osteotomy

Specific indications

- Hallux inter-phalangeus deformity, where the deformity occurs distal to the MTPJ
- In combination with a metatarsal osteotomy to correct residual phalangeal deformity.

Specific contraindications

Akin osteotomy in isolation will not correct joint incongruity or an increased IMA so should not be used alone in these cases.

Incision

A medial longitudinal incision is performed, starting just proximal to the interphalangeal joint (IPJ) and extended past the medial eminence of the metatarsal. This can be incorporated into the incision for a metatarsal osteotomy if required.

Dissection

A longitudinal capsular incision is made and extended proximally to incise the periosteum of the phalanx. This is then carefully elevated, allowing the placement of retractors superiorly and inferiorly.

Surgical technique

Structure at risk

- Flexor hallucis longus tendon

If required, the medial eminence of the metatarsal can be excised, as above. The osteotomy is a closing wedge osteotomy, performed with an oscillating saw from the medial side; the lateral cortex is left intact. Particular care should be taken to avoid damage to the long flexor inferiorly. It is easy to overcorrect the deformity, so it is wise to underestimate the size of the wedge and check the

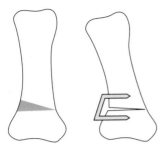 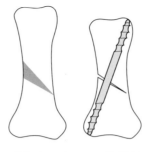

Osteotomy for staple fixation   Osteotomy for screw fixation   Figure 14.6 *Akin osteotomy*

result. The alignment of the osteotomy depends on the planned means of fixation (Fig. 14.6).

If a staple is used, the first cut should be parallel to the proximal joint surface. The second cut is parallel to the base of the nail, aiming to converge before the lateral cortex, leaving it intact. The wedge is removed and the osteotomy closed. If there is resistance, the lateral cortex can be cautiously weakened with the saw, but should not be breached. Using the planned staple as a guide, entry holes are drilled using a fine K-wire and the staple inserted. After insertion the joint is inspected to ensure that it is not penetrated by the staple. Postoperative radiographs can be misleading in this regard because of the convex nature of the joint surface.

If a cannulated compression screw is to be used, the osteotomy will be angled to allow compression. A screw will be inserted over a guidewire passing from the medial edge of the proximal flair of the phalanx, exiting distally in the lateral cortex.

Closure

The capsule is closed with absorbable sutures prior to skin closure. A forefoot dressing is applied.

Chevron osteotomy

The chevron osteotomy is a relatively simple osteotomy for the correction of mild hallux valgus.

Specific indications

- Mild (and moderate – see below) hallux valgus deformity

- Congruent hallux valgus deformity as the osteotomy does not disturb the balance of the joint – using a biplanar chevron (see below).

Specific contraindications

Due to technical limits of the procedure, it should be reserved for deformities with an IMA <12° HVA <30° and DMMA <15°. Attempting to push the indications further increases the risk of avascular necrosis of the capital fragment.

Consent and risks

- Avascular necrosis of the capital fragment: up to 20 per cent in some series. Probably technique dependent with increased avascular necrosis seen with extensive soft tissue stripping and release and with excessive displacements attempted
- Malunion: if the osteotomy is angled too proximally, shortening of the first metatarsal will occur with translation. Similarly, if the osteotomy is angled dorsally the metatarsal head will be elevated. Both of these technical errors will alter the relationship of the first metatarsal head to that of the lesser metatarsals and may lead to transfer metatarsalgia

Incision and dissection

A standard medial approach is made to the metatarsal head (see above).

Surgical technique

The medial eminence is resected in a plane parallel to the medial border of the foot,

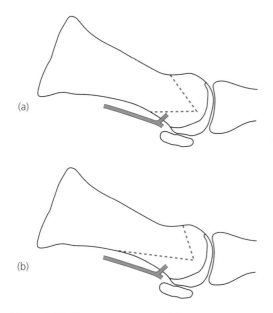

(a)

(b)

Figure 14.7 Chevron osteotomy. (a) Classic chevron osteotomy, risking damage to plantar blood supply to metatarsal head. (b) Modified chevron osteotomy to preserve plantar blood supply to metatarsal head

beginning at the sulcus. A lateral release is not routinely performed due to the increased risk of avascular necrosis. The chevron osteotomy is a V-shaped cut of **approximately 60° with the apex at the centre of the metatarsal head** (Fig. 14.7). Because the plane of the cuts is crucial, it can be useful to place a K-wire in this central point, running parallel to the sole of the foot and the distal articular surface of the metatarsal. This wire can be then be used as a cutting guide to position the limbs of the chevron. The most crucial cut is the plantar limb, which must exit the plantar surface of the metatarsal in an extra-articular position to avoid damage to the sesamoid articulation. Several authors advocate a more horizontal plantar limb (see Fig. 14.7) to attempt to preserve the plantar blood supply (see 'Scarf osteotomy' above). The dorsal limb is then cut at approximately 60° to the first cut. After completion of the cuts, the capital fragment can be translated laterally by up to 30 per cent of its width to correct the hallux valgus.

If there is an increased DMMA, the joint can be reorientated by means of a biplanar chevron. By taking a small (1–2 mm) wedge from the superomedial and inferomedial aspect of the limbs, the fragment can be displaced laterally but rotated medially, correcting the DMMA as may be required in a congruent hallux valgus.

Although inherently a stable osteotomy, most surgeons hold the osteotomy with a K-wire or screw inserted from a dorso-proximal to plantar-distal direction. Care must be taken not to leave any fixation proud of the joint to avoid damage to the sesamoid articulation.

Closure

Capsular closure is as above.

Lapidus procedure

Specific indications

- Hallux valgus deformity in the presence of instability of the first TMTJ
- Moderate to severe incongruent hallux valgus deformity
- Salvage procedure for previous failed hallux valgus surgery
- Arthritis of the first TMTJ.

Specific contraindications

Given the shortening of the first ray that occurs with Lapidus, the procedure should not be performed on patients with short first metatarsals.

Surgical technique

Structure at risk

- Tibialis anterior tendon

The Lapidus procedure involves first TMTJ arthrodesis; this should be performed with the previously described lateral soft tissue release, excision of the medial eminence and plication of the medial capsule. The medial incision for the MTPJ can be continued proximally to the TMTJ. Alternatively, a separate medial incision can be made centred over the joint. The joint is usually deep to a vein, crossing from dorsal to plantar and some authors advocate preserving it to reduce postoperative swelling. The joint can be identified with the aid of a needle and opened to mobilize the joint. Care must be taken to avoid damage to the tendon of tibialis anterior, which lies on the inferomedial aspect of the joint. Using traction on the toe, the joint can be opened and preparation of the joint performed as detailed in 'Principles of foot and ankle arthrodesis' (p. 230). Once the preparation has begun, there is enough room to insert a laminar spreader.

Several authors describe a Lapidus procedure as a closing wedge arthrodesis. However, this is usually not required. By careful preservation of the joint shape the base of the metatarsal can usually be displaced medially and slightly inferiorly with digital pressure, thereby reducing the IMA and overcoming the elevation of the metatarsal head caused by shortening of the joint. A good correction coincides with the appearance of a 'step' on the medial side. Once reduced, the joint is provisionally held with a K-wire before checking the position. If further correction is required, minimal resection of the inferolateral aspect of the metatarsal base is performed.

The arthrodesis can be secured by means of screws or a custom plate. To use screws, a 3.5 mm glide hole is drilled from the dorsum of the metatarsal, starting 15–20 mm from the joint and slightly laterally, aiming for the cuneiform. It is important to avoid aiming too plantarwards, which results in a poor hold on the cuneiform. The cuneiform is then drilled, using a 2.5 mm drill in standard AO fashion. Prior to inserting the screw, an oval groove in the transverse plane should be created (using a small burr or countersink) to accommodate the head of the screw and avoid breaking the dorsal cortical bridge. Once tightened, a second screw can be inserted from the cuneiform to the metatarsal, in a parallel sagittal plane to the first screw.

Closure

The soft tissues are closed over the fusion prior to skin closure.

Specific postoperative instructions

If satisfactory fixation is achieved and the patient is compliant, they may mobilize postoperatively in a forefoot-offloading wedge shoe for 12 weeks.

Otherwise a non-weightbearing cast can be used to protect the arthrodesis.

Proximal (basal) metatarsal osteotomy

The proximal metatarsal osteotomy is usually performed in combination with a lateral soft tissue release, excision of medial eminence and medial capsule closure, as described above.

Specific indications

Correction of moderate to severe hallux valgus, especially when associated with a large IMA. By making an osteotomy at the base of the metatarsal, larger corrections of IMA can be made than by operating more distally.

Specific contraindications

Congruent deformities (if used in isolation) – as the osteotomy does not alter the relationship between the anatomic axis of the metatarsal and the distal articular surface, it will not alter the DMMA. However, it may be of use when combined with a distal osteotomy to correct a congruent deformity with increased IMA (a double osteotomy).

Consent and risks

- Malunion: any misorientation of the plane of the osteotomy can result in significant accidental misplacement of the metatarsal head
- Overcorrection: given the power of this osteotomy to realign the shaft, overcorrection and hallux varus can be troublesome, especially when combined with an aggressive lateral release

Incision

A dorsal incision is made over the base of the metatarsal, avoiding any superficial cutaneous nerves.

Surgical technique

The osteotomy is ideally placed about 1 cm from the TMTJ in metaphyseal bone to provide a broad area for union. A dome osteotomy or closing or opening wedge osteotomies can be performed.

The lateral closing wedge will tend to shorten the metatarsal. There are various plates designed to fix the opening wedge osteotomies.

The coronal plane of the osteotomy is vital – it should be perpendicular to the plane of the metatarsal. If the blade is directed too medially, the head will be elevated and if directed too laterally it will be depressed. In the sagittal plane, the blade should be positioned perpendicular to the sole then angled slightly proximally. Once cut, the osteotomy can provisionally be reduced and the position checked. If satisfactory the osteotomy is fixed with two screws or a screw and wire.

Keller procedure

This involves excision of the medial prominence of the metatarsal and the proximal third of the phalanx to relax the lateral structures and allow correction of the toe, which is then held with a temporary K-wire. Although once commonly performed, its generally unsatisfactory results have caused it to fall out of favour. The patient is left with a floppy great toe and, by defunctioning the hallux, is prone to overload their lesser rays with resultant pain. However, it can be considered in the older, minimally ambulatory patient who has footwear problems or in those patients whose soft tissues or general fitness precludes a more aggressive procedure.

GENERAL POSTOPERATIVE CARE AND INSTRUCTIONS

- The foot is dressed with a standard forefoot dressing, extending above the ankle.
- The foot is elevated for 72 hours to reduce swelling.
- The patient may mobilize, fully weightbearing, in a forefoot-offloading wedge shoe for 6 weeks.
- After skin wounds have healed, the patient is taught passive mobilization of the MTPJ to reduce stiffness.

RECOMMENDED REFERENCES

Barouk LS. Scarf osteotomy for hallux valgus correction. Local anatomy, surgical technique, and combination with other forefoot procedures. *Foot Ankle Clin* 2000;**5**:525–58.

Barouk LS. *Forefoot reconstruction*. Paris: Springer-Verlag, 2005.

Weil LS. Scarf osteotomy for correction of hallux valgus. Historical perspective, surgical technique, and results. *Foot Ankle Clin* 2000;**5**:559–80.

FIRST METATARSOPHALANGEAL JOINT CHEILECTOMY

PREOPERATIVE PLANNING

Hallux rigidus, or degenerative arthritis of the first MTPJ, is a common condition. Although in its early stages it can be managed with conservative measures, such as footwear and activity modifications, patients often require operative intervention. Cheilectomy, from the Greek for lip, *cheilos*, addresses both the pain and stiffness found in this condition.

Indications

- Mild to moderate degenerative changes in the first MTPJ with pain and stiffness, failing to respond to conservative management
- More advanced degenerative changes in a patient unwilling to lose joint movement (patient must be counselled that there may be improvement in movement but only limited improvement in pain)
- Prominent dorsal osteophytes causing footwear problems.

Contraindications

Advanced degenerative changes with loss of joint space.

Consent and risks

- Failure or recurrence of symptoms: especially if the degenerative changes are more extensive than appreciated preoperatively or if insufficient resection is performed
- Instability of first MTPJ: especially if resection exceeds 35 per cent of joint surface
- Damage to dorsal cutaneous nerve and neuroma formation

Anaesthesia and positioning

- Regional or general anaesthesia
- Ankle or thigh tourniquet
- Supine on operating table.

SURGICAL TECHNIQUE

Landmarks

- The MTPJ of the great toe is easily palpable
- Extensor hallucis longus (EHL) tendon.

Incision

A 5 cm dorsal incision is made along the medial border of EHL centred over the first MTPJ.

Dissection

The underlying extensor hood is incised in line with the incision but leaving a cuff of tissue on the medial side of the tendon to avoid violating the tendon sheath and reducing the risk of adhesions. The joint capsule is incised and the joint exposed by dissection medially and laterally. Alternatively, a medial approach, as described in first MTPJ arthrodesis, may be used.

PROCEDURE

A full synovectomy is performed and any loose bodies removed. Flexing the joint fully allows inspection of the joint surface. In mild and moderate disease, the damage is usually limited to the dorsal aspect. Ideally, the resection should extend from just dorsal of the edge of the viable cartilage to just proximal of the dorsal prominence of the head. However, care should be taken to ensure that this resects 20–30 per cent of the joint (Fig. 14.8).

Note on resection level (Fig. 14.8): a common cause for failure of cheilectomy is insufficient resection. **A minimum of 20 per cent of the articular surface** must be removed, even if this includes normal joint surface, to ensure adequate movement. Exceeding 35 per cent is likely to destabilize the joint.

The dorsal prominence is resected with a saw or osteotome and satisfactory dorsiflexion (ideally

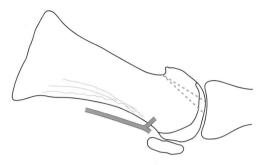

Figure 14.8 First metatarsophalangeal joint cheilectomy – minimum and maximum resection levels

60°) is confirmed. Any prominent osteophytes are removed from the dorsal phalanx and the medial and lateral aspect of the head, and the joint is irrigated to thoroughly wash out. Bone wax can be used sparingly to reduce bleeding and adhesions.

Closure

Careful closure of the capsule with interrupted Vicryl precedes skin closure. A forefoot dressing is applied to above the ankle.

POSTOPERATIVE INSTRUCTIONS

The foot is elevated for 48 hours. The patient fully weightbears on a postoperative shoe and aggressive active and passive mobilization begins once skin healing has occurred

RECOMMENDED REFERENCE

Coughlin MJ, Shurnas PS. Hallux rigidus. Grading and long-term results of operative treatment. *J Bone Joint Surg Am* 2003;**85**:2072–88.

FIRST METATARSOPHALANGEAL JOINT ARTHRODESIS

PREOPERATIVE PLANNING

Once a patient has developed severe hallux rigidus, a cheilectomy is unlikely to address the problem. Although various arthroplasties are available, most either have limited long-term results or are associated with high failure rates. Arthrodesis of the joint provides a reliable solution to the pain of advanced arthritis of the joint.

Indications

- Painful arthropathy of first MTPJ not responding to conservative treatment and not suitable for less invasive treatment (e.g. cheilectomy)
- Severe first MTPJ deformity in the presence of degenerative changes
- Salvage of failed first ray surgery.

Absolute contraindications

- Active infection
- Limb ischaemia or poor perfusion.

Relative contraindication

Previous IPJ arthrodesis or pre-existing IPJ degenerative changes.

Consent and risks

(see also 'Principles of foot and ankle arthrodesis', p. 230)
- Malunion: excessive extension can cause defunctioning of hallux and transfer metatarsalgia. Excessive flexion can cause increased wear and pain in the IPJ. Excessive valgus can cause pressure on the second toe
- Damage to dorsal cutaneous nerve and neuroma formation
- Unable to wear high heels after surgery: this must be stressed to women considering operation
- Minimum of 6 weeks protected weightbearing

Anaesthesia and positioning

- Regional or general anaesthesia
- Ankle or thigh tourniquet
- Supine on operating table.

SURGICAL TECHNIQUE

Landmarks

The MTPJ of the great toe is easily palpable.

Incision

A straight medial midline incision is made, centred over the MTPJ.

Dissection

This is continued straight down to the joint capsule, without developing flaps. The capsule is incised in line with the skin incision and freed dorsally over the metatarsal head and sufficiently around the phalangeal base to allow its surface to be delivered. Alternatively, the approach described for cheilectomy may be used.

Procedure

The surfaces are prepared in a manner outlined in 'Principles of foot and ankle arthrodesis' (p. 231). Given the joint's small size it is not possible, or really necessary, to use a laminar spreader. Furthermore, the concave surface of the phalanx makes the use of chisels difficult; a curette or bone nibbler may be more useful, Various dome-shaped reamers may also be used, but care should be taken to avoid removal of excessive bone, which will lead to shortening.

Note about sagittal position of arthrodesis (Fig. 14.9): several textbooks state a fixed value for the position of first MTPJ arthrodesis, e.g. 25–30° extension. This can be confusing as it may be unclear if this refers to the angle relating to the floor or the metatarsal shaft. Furthermore, the angle to the metatarsal depends on the pitch of the metatarsal, i.e. whether the foot is planus or cavus. It is therefore preferred to arthrodese the joint in a relative position to a simulated floor. Using a flat surface to push up against the sole of the foot, assess the position of the pulp of the hallux with regard to the surface. If a finger can be pushed under the pulp the toe is too extended. If there is no space for any flexion of the IPJ the position is too flexed. An ideal position allows a small amount of movement with downward pressure on the distal phalanx.

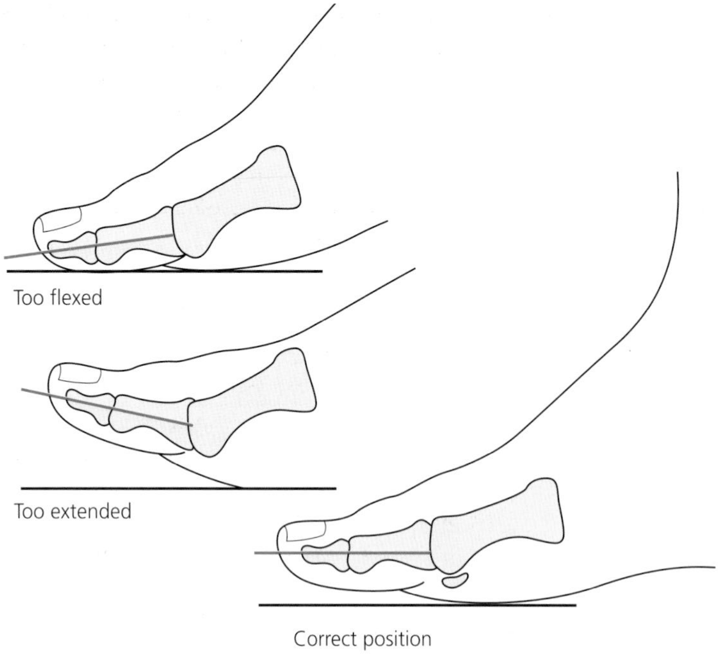

Too flexed

Too extended

Correct position

Figure 14.9 *Coronal position of arthrodesis of the first metatarsophalangeal joint. Note that the phalanges are parallel to floor, allowing clearance of toe pulp*

The joint is positioned as required and provisionally held with a K-wire. The sagittal position of the toe is then assessed with regard to a flat surface as outlined above. The coronal position should be of sufficient valgus to avoid the medial border of the toe rubbing upon the toe-box of a shoe but not so much that there is impingement of the hallux against the second toe; 10–15° HVA is usually appropriate. There should be no rotational deformity.

In primary surgery with good bone stock, the arthrodesis can be secured with two crossed screws. The first is inserted with a lag technique to compress the joint; the second provides a derotational function. Alternatively, a custom-made plate may be used.

Closure

- Careful closure of the capsule with interrupted Vicryl precedes skin closure.
- A forefoot dressing is applied to above the ankle.

POSTOPERATIVE INSTRUCTIONS

The foot is elevated for 72 hours. A reliable patient can mobilize in a wedge shoe to offload the forefoot until evidence of clinical and radiological union. If there is concern about the compliance of the patient, a cast may be used.

RECOMMENDED REFERENCE

Coughlin MJ, Shurnas PS. Hallux rigidus. *J Bone Joint Surg Am* 2004;**86**(Suppl 1):119–30.

INGROWING TOENAIL SURGERY

PREOPERATIVE PLANNING

A multitude of operations exist to deal with ingrowing toenails, or onychocryptosis. Chemical ablation with phenol of either part or all of the nail matrix is associated with lower recurrence rates than surgical ablation in most series.

Indications

Painful onychocryptosis or recurrent infections.

Contraindications

- Severe digital vascular compromise is an absolute contraindication
- Active infection is a relative contraindication.

Recurrence may be better treated with total matrix ablation.

Anaesthesia and positioning

Toenail surgery can be effectively performed under digital block with or without additional sedation. A bloodless field is established with the use of a digital tourniquet secured with an artery forcep.

SURGICAL TECHNIQUE

The affected nail border is elevated from the nail bed and surrounding skin by blunt dissection with forceps. The nail border is then cut using a blade or scissors underneath the ungual fold (Fig. 14.10). Grasping the fragment with an artery forcep and using a rotating movement, the nail border is carefully avulsed in its entirety, complete with the widened germinal base. The nail groove is then carefully curetted.

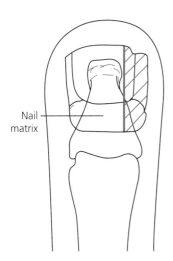

Figure 14.10 *Partial matrix ablation – line of excision for nail border*

All blood is carefully cleared from the field and all exposed skin protected with petroleum jelly. A cotton bud is soaked in phenol and inserted along the exposed nail bed, under the ungual fold, and left for 60 seconds. This process is repeated once more then the whole area irrigated with copious amounts of saline. The tourniquet is released and a toe dressing applied.

POSTOPERATIVE CARE AND INSTRUCTIONS

The foot is elevated for 48 hours then the dressings are reduced. The wound is then washed in tepid boiled salted water twice a day using a baby toothbrush, sweeping in a proximal to distal direction. When showering the patient is instructed to aim the spray directly over the wound.

RECOMMENDED REFERENCE

Herold N, Houshian S, Riegels-Nielsen P. A prospective comparison of wedge matrix resection with nail matrix phenolization for the treatment of ingrown toenail. *J Foot Ankle Surg* 2001;**40**: 390–5.

INTERDIGITAL NEUROMA

PREOPERATIVE PLANNING

Indications

Proven, symptomatic interdigital (Morton's) neuroma in the third (80–90 per cent) or second (10–20 per cent) web space failing to respond to conservative treatment.

Contraindications (relative)

- Vague symptoms or unusual location
- Other causes of metatarsalgia
- Lack of response to accurate injection of lesion.

- Scar pain (especially with plantar incision)
- Interdigital numbness: common but rarely troublesome
- Vascular damage and digital ischaemia: risk if multiple web space explorations are undertaken

Anaesthesia and positioning

May be performed under general or regional anaesthesia. The patient is positioned supine with an ankle or thigh tourniquet to provide a bloodless field.

SURGICAL TECHNIQUE

Landmarks

The dorsal aspect of the affected web space.

Incision

A longitudinal incision is placed over the dorsum of the foot, starting in the web space and extending 3–4 cm proximally. (An insufficient incision is commonly found in recurrent cases and is to be avoided.)

Dissection

Structure at risk

- Dorsal digital nerves

Taking care to avoid the dorsal digital nerves, dissection is carried down to the metatarsal heads and a laminar spreader is used between the metatarsal heads to place the transverse metatarsal ligament under tension. A Macdonald dissector is placed under the ligament which is then divided under direct vision. The laminar spreader is then advanced into the wound to open up the intermetatarsal space.

Procedure

Structure at risk

- Common digital artery

Plantar pressure will usually deliver the neuroma into the wound. Sometimes it will be obscured by a bursa which requires excision. Taking care to protect the common digital artery, the neuroma is retracted proximally and the two true digital nerves are divided. The nerve is then traced as proximally as possible and then divided under traction such that the cut end is proximal to the weightbearing area of the foot. The specimen should be sent for histology for confirmation of the diagnosis.

Closure

After release of the tourniquet, haemostasis is obtained. Skin is closed in a single layer and a forefoot bandage is applied.

POSTOPERATIVE CARE AND INSTRUCTIONS

The patient should elevate the foot for 48 hours. They may mobilize, weightbearing as tolerated, in a postoperative flat shoe.

RECOMMENDED REFERENCE

Mann RA, Reynolds JD. Interdigital neuroma: a critical clinical analysis. *Foot Ankle* 1983;**3**: 238–43.

LESSER TOE DEFORMITIES

PREOPERATIVE PLANNING

The decision-making process for correction of lesser toe deformities must take into account the type of deformity and whether it is fixed or flexible. A detailed examination of the deformity must be made in the awake patient prior to surgery. The position of the toe in the standing and lying position must be noted and any deformity assessed for a fixed component. Any subluxation or dislocation of the MTPJ must be identified. There is some confusion in the literature regarding toe deformity nomenclature. For the purposes of this book we have used the following terms:

- *Mallet toe* – a flexion deformity of the distal IPJ (DIPJ), often resulting in a callosity on the tip of the toe.
- *Hammer toe* – a flexion deformity of the proximal IPJ (PIPJ), often associated with hyperextension of the DIPJ and an accommodative hyperextension of the MTPJ.
- *Claw toe* – a term usually reserved for multiple toes and often associated with an underlying neurological condition. The primary deformity is one of hyperextension of the MTPJ with secondary flexion of the PIPJ.

Indications

- Painful lesser toe deformity not responding to conservative treatment
- Severe lesser toe deformity causing footwear problems and not responding to footwear modification.

Contraindications

- Vascular insufficiency
- Local infection
- Undiagnosed underlying neurological condition (relative).

Consent and risks

- Infection: <1 per cent
- Neurovascular damage: <1 per cent
- Vascular insufficiency of the digit following correction of a severe or long-standing deformity: may require further shortening or accepting a slightly flexed position
- Recurrence of deformity
- Swelling
- Non-union of arthrodesis: 20–50 per cent of PIPJ arthrodeses in some series formed a fibrous union, but this does not correlate with postoperative dissatisfaction
- Malunion of arthrodesis: hyperextension of the joint or varus/valgus deformity often poorly tolerated
- Loss of movement or function of the toe, depending on procedure performed

Anaesthesia and positioning

Anaesthesia can be regional or general. If surgery is limited to the interphalangeal joints a digital block can be used. A supine position is used, with the foot at the end of the table.

SURGICAL TECHNIQUES

Percutaneous flexor digitorum longus tenotomy

Indication
Flexible mallet deformity

Incision
Holding the toe to put the flexor tendon under tension, a size 15 blade (or tenotomy blade if available) is used to make a 2–3 mm incision over the DIPJ flexor crease.

Procedure

Structure at risk

- Neurovascular bundles

With the blade facing away from the neurovascular bundle, the tightened tendon is palpated with the blade and divided. The toe is then released to check the degree of correction.

Closure
Formal closure of the wound is not required.

DIPJ arthrodesis

Indication
Fixed mallet deformity

Incision
An elliptical incision is made over the DIPJ and carried down to bone, excising the extensor tendon. Care is taken to avoid damage to the nail matrix distally.

Procedure

Structure at risk

- Neurovascular bundles

Facing the blade away from the neurovascular bundles the collateral ligaments are divided, allowing deliverance of the condyles of the middle phalanx into the wound. Using a bone cutter, the condyles are excised at the metaphyseal flair. The articular surface of the distal phalanx is then decorticated. Under direct vision, the flexor digitorum longus tendon in the base of the wound is divided and the degree of correction is assessed. A double-ended K-wire is advanced in an antegrade direction through the distal phalanx, aiming to come out just below the nail bed. The joint is then reduced and the wire advanced into the middle phalanx to secure the joint.

Closure

The wound is best closed with non-absorbable mattress sutures to secure the skin and extensor tendon *en masse*.

Flexor tendon transfer (Girdlestone procedure)

The principle of this procedure is to re-create the action of the intrinsic muscles in flexing the MTPJ and extending the IPJs.

Indications

- Flexible hammer deformity
- Flexible claw toe deformity.

Incision

A 5 mm transverse incision is made over the proximal flexor crease.

Procedure

Structure at risk

- Neurovascular bundles

Following blunt dissection down to the flexor sheath, the sheath is incised in a longitudinal manner. Of the three tendons seen, the flexor digitorum longus (FDL) is the central one. A percutaneous FDL tenotomy is performed at the level of the DIPJ (see above) and the FDL is delivered out of the proximal wound. The tendon is split into two halves along its length. On the dorsum of the toe, a longitudinal incision is made over the proximal phalanx. A small artery forcep is used to bluntly dissect down one side of the phalanx, remaining close to the extensor expansion, and exiting the toe through the plantar wound. The forcep is used to grasp one half of the divided FDL tendon and deliver it to the dorsum, repeating the manoeuvre on the other side. Holding the MTPJ in about 20° flexion, both ends of the tendon are sutured to the extensor tendon, using an absorbable suture. The toe is released to ensure that the correction is being held. If there is judged to be some residual tightness in the MTPJ, a dorsal release may be performed (see below). A K-wire may be used to protect the repair.

Closure

Skin wounds are closed with appropriate sutures, usually non-absorbable suture material.

PIPJ arthrodesis

Indication

Fixed hammer deformity or claw toe deformity

Incision

An elliptical incision is made over the PIPJ and carried down to bone excising the extensor tendon.

Procedure

Structure at risk

- Neurovascular bundles

Facing the blade away from the neurovascular bundles, the collateral ligaments are divided, allowing deliverance of the condyles of the proximal phalanx into the wound. Using a bone cutter, the condyles are excised at the metaphyseal flair. Sufficient bone must be removed to allow the toe to be straightened without undue tension on the tissues, especially the neurovascular bundles. The plantar plate is released from the middle phalanx allowing its base to be delivered. The articular surface is then decorticated using a nibbler. A double ended K-wire is advanced in an antegrade direction through the middle and distal phalanges, aiming to come out just below the nail bed. The joint is then reduced and the wire advanced into the proximal phalanx to secure the joint.

Closure

The wound is closed with a non-absorbable mattress sutures to secure skin and extensor tendon *en masse*. If the MTPJ remains extended, a dorsal release (see below) should be included to avoid a 'cock-up' deformity.

MTPJ release

Indication

Hyperextension of the MTPJ with or without subluxation.

Incision

Structures at risk

- Dorsal veins
- Dorsal sensory nerve branches

A 3 cm incision is made in line with the metatarsal, centred over the MTPJ. If two adjacent joints are being addressed, the incision should be made in the web space. Attempt should be made to protect the dorsal veins and sensory nerves.

Procedure

Release of the joint should occur in a stepwise manner and stop when satisfactory release achieved. The extensor digitorum longus (EDL) and extensor digitorum brevis (EDB) to the toe (EDL lies medial to EDB) are identified and their tightness assessed. If tight, the EDB may be divided but the EDL should be z-lengthened. A dorsal capsulotomy is performed then, with the blade facing away from the neurovascular bundles,

progressive capsular and collateral releases are performed both medially and laterally. In long-standing deformities, adhesions may exist between the plantar capsule and the metatarsal head which should be released. Once satisfactory release is achieved, the EDL should be repaired with absorbable suture and the wound closed. If, despite maximal release of the MTPJ, the joint cannot be reduced, **a metatarsal osteotomy should be considered**. (see 'Lesser metatarsal [Weil's] osteotomy', below).

POSTOPERATIVE CARE AND INSTRUCTIONS

After all lesser toe surgery the tourniquet should be released prior to waking the patient and the toe observed. If reperfusion is slow, releasing excessively tight dressings and hanging the foot over the side of the table usually allows the toe to reperfuse. If the toe remains white and a K-wire has been inserted, gently bending the arthrodesed joint will relieve excess tension on the blood vessels.

All patients can fully weightbear on a flat postoperative shoe. K-wires, if used, should be removed at 4–6 weeks.

RECOMMENDED REFERENCE

Coughlin MJ. Lesser-toe abnormalities. *J Bone Joint Surg Am* 2002;**84**:1446–69.

LESSER METATARSAL (WEIL'S) OSTEOTOMY

PREOPERATIVE PLANNING

Historically, the Helal osteotomy was a popular treatment for lesser metatarsal overload and subluxed lesser MTPJs. This has largely been replaced by the Weil osteotomy, as popularized by Barouk.

Indications

- Overload of a metatarsal head secondary to a relatively long metatarsal
- Reduction of a chronically subluxed or dislocated MTPJ.

Contraindications

- Gross deformity of the joint
- Vascular insufficiency or infection.

Consent and risks

- Ongoing forefoot pain: often related to the use of an excessively long screw
- MTPJ stiffness: some degree is very common
- 'Floating toe': stiff hyperextension of the MTPJ preventing the toe from touching the floor
- Infection: <1 per cent
- Avascular necrosis and non-union: rare
- Neurovascular damage: rare

Anaesthesia and positioning

See 'Lesser toe deformities' (p. 247).

SURGICAL TECHNIQUE

Incision

A 4 cm incision is made over the metatarsal, or in the interspace if two adjacent osteotomies are to be performed.

Dissection

Structure at risk

- Neurovascular bundles

The extensor tendons are retracted out of the way and the dorsal capsule of the MTPJ released. Protecting the neurovascular bundles, the collaterals are released to allow the proximal phalanx to be displaced plantarwards.

Procedure

A Macdonald dissector or custom made head elevator is inserted under the metatarsal head. Using a fine saw blade, an osteotomy is made, starting 2 mm below the dorsal surface of the head and continuing proximally, parallel to the sole of the foot (Fig. 14.11). Using a fine osteotome or McDonald, the head fragment is freed up to allow

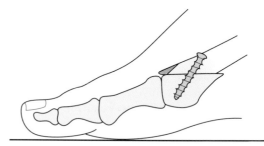

Figure 14.11 *Orientation of Weil osteotomy of the lesser metatarsal and screw placement*

it to retract proximally the desired amount. The fragment can then be fixed with a small screw, the length of which usually decreases from 14 mm in the second metatarsal to 11 mm in the fifth. The excess dorsal bone overhanging the head can then be trimmed to ensure that the proximal phalanx can freely dorsiflex.

POSTOPERATIVE CARE AND INSTRUCTIONS

The patient is asked to mobilize in a heel weightbearing shoe. Once wounds have healed, passive and active range of motion exercises can begin and the toe can be strapped down to prevent hyperextension.

RECOMMENDED REFERENCES

Barouk LS. *Forefoot Reconstruction.* Berlin: Springer-Verlag, 2005.
Helal B. Metatarsal osteotomy for metatarsalgia. *J Bone Joint Surg Br* 1975;**57**:187–92.
Trnka HJ, Mühlbauer M, Zettl R, *et al.* Comparison of the results of the Weil and Helal osteotomies for the treatment of metatarsalgia secondary to dislocation of the lesser metatarsophalangeal joints. *Foot Ankle Int* 1999;**20**:72–9.

FIFTH TOE SOFT TISSUE CORRECTION (BUTLER PROCEDURE)

PREOPERATIVE PLANNING

Indications

- Moderate or severe overriding fifth toe with pain and callosity or footwear problems

- Failure of footwear adaptations and other conservative measures

Contraindications

Digital ischaemia or poor perfusion.

Consent and risks

- Neurovascular damage and risk of toe ischaemia: reduced be careful dissection and avoidance of traction or manipulation of the toe
- Recurrence of deformity: rare

Anaesthesia and positioning

Regional or general anaesthesia is required as digital anaesthesia is insufficient. The patient is positioned supine with an ankle or thigh tourniquet to ensure a bloodless field.

SURGICAL TECHNIQUE

Incision and dissection

Structure at risk

- Neurovascular bundles of the fifth toe

A double-racquet incision is drawn to ensure correct placement. The dorsal limb of the incision should follow the line of tension along the extensor tendon. The plantar limb should be longer and heading laterally (Fig. 14.12). The skin is incised with care and the **neurovascular bundles identified and protected**.

Procedure

The tight extensor tendons are divided then the joint capsule exposed. The tight dorsal capsule and usually the collateral ligaments require release. Sometimes the plantar capsule is adherent and needs to be dissected off. The toe should now assume the required position.

Closure

The skin is closed without tension. The dorsal incision assumes a V to Y position and the plantar incision a Y to V position. The tourniquet must be released to ensure adequate perfusion of the toe prior to the end of anaesthesia. No taping or splintage is required.

POSTOPERATIVE CARE AND INSTRUCTIONS

The patient can mobilize fully weightbearing on a postoperative shoe.

RECOMMENDED REFERENCE

Cockin J. Butler's operation for an over-riding fifth toe. *J Bone Joint Surg Br* 1968;**50**:78–81.

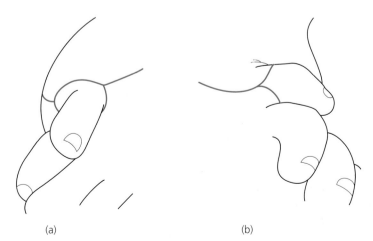

(a)   (b)

Figure 14.12 *Butler procedure – position of skin incision. (a) Dorsal and (b) plantar views*

HINDFOOT ARTHRODESIS

PREOPERATIVE PLANNING

The three joints of the hindfoot, the subtalar (ST), calcaneocuboid (CC) and talonavicular (TN) joints, can be arthrodesed individually or in combination, depending upon the indication. However, as all three joints work in unison, fusion of one will affect the others. As the normal hindfoot swings into varus during gait, Chopart's joints (TN and CC) are locked in position to provide a firm platform. Therefore, a subtalar fusion must avoid varus to leave Chopart's joints relatively mobile and avoid fixed supination of the foot. Similarly, fusion of the TN joint in isolation fixes the CC joint and greatly reduces the movement of the ST joint. Therefore, in arthrodesing one or more of these joints, attention to the position of all three must be taken.

The ultimate aim of any hindfoot fusion is to provide a pain-free, stable hindfoot and a foot that can be placed flat on the floor for weight-bearing.

Indications

(See also 'Principles of foot and ankle arthrodesis', p. 230.)

- Painful arthropathy of one or more hindfoot joints secondary to degenerative, inflammatory or traumatic causes not responding to conservative management. In such cases isolated fusion of the affected joint can be considered.
- Fixed deformity of the hindfoot not amenable to soft tissue correction and/or osteotomy. Historically, this was primarily for paralytic conditions, especially poliomyelitis. Hindfoot fusions are now more commonly performed for tibialis posterior dysfunction, rheumatoid arthritis and congenital neuromuscular disorders. In such cases a double fusion of the TN and CC joints, or a triple fusion of all three joints is indicated.
- Gross instability of the hindfoot with bony destruction, as seen in rheumatoid arthritis or Charcot's joints in people with diabetes.

Contraindications

- Active infection or ischaemia of the limb is an absolute contraindication.
- A more proximal uncorrected deformity is a relative contraindication. It is difficult to judge hindfoot alignment if there is a more proximal deformity. Furthermore, if a proximal deformity is subsequently corrected, the hindfoot alignment may be rendered incorrect. It is therefore prudent to address proximal deformities first.
- Ipsilateral ankle fusion is a relative contraindication – the patient must be counselled that a combined ankle and hindfoot fusion will result in a loss of normal gait and possibly the need for footwear adaptations to walk.

Consent and risks

(See also 'Principles of foot and ankle arthrodesis', p. 230.)
- Non-union: the TN joint is especially prone to non-union. This is likely to be due to its curved surface and extensively cortical composition making adequate visualization and preparation technically difficult. Obtaining adequate rigid fixation can also be difficult compared with the ST joint
- Malunion: due to incorrect positioning or fixation failure. A malunion preventing the patient from placing the foot flat on the floor, often with overload of the lateral border, is very poorly tolerated by the patient and often requires revision

Anaesthesia and positioning

(See also 'Principles of foot and ankle arthrodesis', p. 231.)

For isolated subtalar fusion a lateral decubitus position, with the operative side up, allows excellent access and visualization. For TN or double/triple arthrodeses, a supine position is optimal. The use of a bolster under the calf allows free access around the foot.

SURGICAL TECHNIQUE

Landmarks

- Utility lateral approach – tip of fibula and base of fourth metatarsal
- Anterior approach – EHL and tibialis anterior tendons
- Anteromedial approach – tibialis anterior and posterior tendons.

Incision

Structures at risk

- Sural nerve (utility lateral approach)
- Superficial peroneal nerve (utility lateral approach)
- Saphenous nerve and vein (anteromedial approach)

The incision(s) used will depend upon the joints to be addressed. For isolated TN arthrodesis an anterior approach allows excellent visualization. For isolated ST and/or CC joint fusion, a utility lateral approach is used. For a triple fusion, the utility lateral in combination with an antero-medial approach to the TN joint allows wide skin bridges (Fig. 14.13).

The utility lateral approach allows excellent visualization of the ST and CC joints. It is preferable to the traditional Ollier incision as there is less risk to the branches of the superficial

peroneal nerve. A straight incision is made from the tip of the fibula towards the base of the fourth metatarsal. This should lie between the sural and peroneal nerves but care must be taken, especially distally. The incision can be stopped at the CC joint if access to only the subtalar joint is required.

The anterior approach is an extension of the approach used to access the ankle. A straight incision between the tendons of extensor hallucis longus and tibialis anterior is made over the TN joint and the extensor retinaculum carefully incised. This gives excellent access to the medial and lateral extents of the surprisingly broad TN joint.

Alternatively, if performing a triple fusion, an anteromedial incision between the tendons of tibialis anterior and posterior allows a wider skin bridge. Care must be taken of the saphenous vein and nerve, which lie in this plane. It is harder to access the far lateral extent of the TN joint through this incision and access through the lateral incision may be required.

Dissection

The utility lateral incision is deepened to pass above the peroneal tendons to the subtalar joint. By releasing the insertion of extensor digitorum brevis and elevating this with a distally based flap, the sinus tarsi and CC joint can be visualized. In triple arthrodeses, after preparation of the CC and ST joints, the lateral aspect of the TN joint can be accessed from the lateral side.

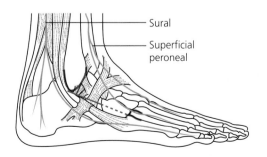 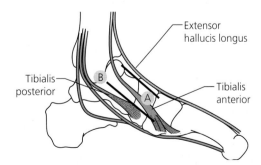

Figure 14.13 *(a) Approaches for hindfoot arthrodesis – utility lateral approach. (b) Approaches for hindfoot arthrodesis – anterior (A) and anteromedial (B) approach to talonavicular joint*

Procedure

Structure at risk

- Tibial neurovascular bundle

Once exposed and mobilized the selected joints should be meticulously prepared as detailed in 'Principles of foot and ankle arthrodesis' (p. 231). With regard to the TN joint, the full extent of the joint must be realized for successful fusion. It is easy not to prepare deep enough (one should see the spring ligament in the depth of the wound) or laterally enough. During subtalar preparation, the posterior facet is prepared first. When the tendon of FHL (identified by moving the toe) is visualized, preparation is deep enough. Great care should be taken, however, as deep to the FHL is the tibial neurovascular bundle. After preparation of the posterior facet, the medial facet can be prepared. Damage to the structures posterior to this, and the head of the talus superiorly, must be avoided. Once all of the required joints have been prepared, they need to be held in the required position of arthrodesis. For the ST joint, the optimum position is 5° of valgus. However, if there is rigidity of the midfoot from a longstanding deformity, 5° of valgus may not allow the foot to be placed flat on the floor. Therefore, the position of the weightbearing foot should be confirmed by using a flat surface prior to fixation of the ST joint. A varus position must be avoided.

The ideal position of arthrodesis of the TN joint is one of 'talar neutral' – that is, with the domed talar head central in the navicular. In this position the long axis of the talus should pass through the long axis of the first metatarsal. Care must be taken not to extend or flex the TN joint and the foot should be perpendicular to the tibia with the ankle in neutral. Again, the position of the foot flat on the floor must be checked and a suboptimal position may have to be accepted to achieve this. The CC joint position will be dictated by the other joints and therefore fixed last.

Various methods of ST joint fixation have been described. Our preferred method is to place a large diameter (8 mm) cannulated compression screw from the posterolateral aspect of the calcaneum into the talus to cross the posterior facet at 90°. This avoids possible impingement problems from a screw inserted from the talar neck. The entry point is in a line down from the lateral margin of the Achilles tendon, just above the plantar skin of the heel. Too plantarwards or central an entry point may cause painful prominence of the screw head. Usually, a single screw is sufficient. The TN joint can be fixed using a retrograde screw from the medial edge of the navicular into the talar neck. Care must be taken to ensure a good bite is obtained medially without intruding upon the NC joint. Further fixation can be obtained with a screw from the anterior surface of the navicular. Screw fixation of the CC joint, antegrade from the anterior process of the calcaneum or retrograde from the cuboid, can sometimes be difficult. In which case, compression staples or a low profile plate can be used.

Closure

All wounds should be carefully closed, ensuring a good soft tissue layer is closed over the joints prior to skin closure. If an anterior approach has been used, the retinaculum must be carefully repaired. The leg is then placed in a back-slab.

POSTOPERATIVE CARE AND INSTRUCTIONS

(See also 'Principles of foot and ankle arthrodesis', p. 231.)

The patient is kept in a non-weightbearing cast for 6 weeks or until early radiological signs of union are seen. They can then begin to gradually increase their weightbearing. A cast should be retained for 3 months or until there is solid radiographical and clinical evidence of union.

RECOMMENDED REFERENCE

Davies MB, Rosenfeld PF, Stavrou P, *et al.* A comprehensive review of subtalar arthrodesis. *Foot Ankle Int* 2007;**28**:295–7.

CALCANEAL OSTEOTOMY

PREOPERATIVE PLANNING

Indications

A calcaneal osteotomy is rarely indicated in isolation. It is usually performed as part of a soft tissue correction of a hindfoot deformity to protect the reconstruction and reconstitute the mechanical axis of the hindfoot. Commonly used examples are a medial displacement osteotomy as part of a tibialis posterior reconstruction and a closing wedge or lateralizing osteotomy as part of a pes cavus correction. Occasionally an osteotomy may be used to correct a post-traumatic deformity of the calcaneum, but this is often done in combination with a subtalar arthrodesis as there is usually associated joint disruption.

Contraindications

- Active infection or critical ischaemia of the limb is an absolute contraindication.
- A more proximal uncorrected deformity is a relative contraindication. It is difficult to judge hindfoot alignment if there is a more proximal deformity. Furthermore, if a proximal deformity is subsequently corrected, the hindfoot alignment may become incorrect. It is therefore advisable to address proximal deformities first.

Consent and risks

- Neurovascular damage: the sural nerve is in the zone of the incision and must be avoided. On the medial extent of any osteotomy, the neurovascular bundle is close by and can be injured with aggressive use of power tools
- Malunion: usually due to technical errors in judging the degree of correction but also due to hardware failure
- Non-union: rare due to large surface area of cancellous bone
- Recurrence of deformity, especially if the deforming soft tissues are not correctly balanced or there is a progressive neuromuscular condition

Anaesthesia and positioning

- General or spinal anaesthesia with a thigh tourniquet allowing exposure to above the knee to judge alignment satisfactorily.
- Most soft tissue procedures require access to both the medial and lateral sides of the hindfoot. Therefore, position the patient supine, with a removable sandbag under the ipsilateral buttock.

SURGICAL TECHNIQUE

The calcaneal osteotomy is usually performed first as part of any soft tissue correction of the hindfoot to avoid accidental damage to the correction.

Landmarks

- Anterior border of tendo-Achilles
- Junction of dorsal and plantar skin of heel.

Incision

Structure at risk

- Sural nerve

Some authors advocate an oblique lateral incision over the line of the proposed osteotomy. Unfortunately, this coincides with the course of the sural nerve and puts it at risk. We therefore advise an extensile lateral incision, commonly used for calcaneal fixation, as the sural nerve is protected in the elevated flap. This also allows better visualization of the calcaneum. The inferior limb of the incision runs along the junction of the plantar and dorsal skin. The superior limb extends superiorly in line with the anterior border of the tendo-Achilles (Fig. 14.14). The extent of the exposure required is less than for calcaneal fixation but the insertion of tendo-Achilles superiorly and plantar fascia inferiorly should be visualized.

Dissection

The incision is carried straight down to bone and the flap elevated in the subperiosteal layer with minimal trauma to the soft tissues.

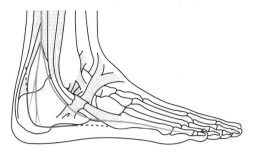

Figure 14.14 *Extensile lateral approach to os calcis*

Procedure

Structures at risk

- Tendo-Achilles
- Plantar fascia

For both medial and lateral displacement and lateral closing wedge osteotomies, the angle of the osteotomy is the same, at about 45° to the plantar surface of the foot (Fig. 14.15). It runs anterior to the insertion of tendo-Achilles to superior to the insertion of the plantar fascia. Trethowan bone levers are placed to protect these two structures and guide the osteotomy line. Using an oscillating saw, the lateral wall is cut and the saw advanced until it reaches the medial wall.

The medial wall is cautiously weakened by bouncing the saw off the wall and the osteotomy completed using of a broad osteotome **with care to avoid any pressure on the medial soft tissues**. Once completed, the osteotome is carefully twisted to mobilize the fragment and a dissector

used to free the medial periosteum. The tuberosity fragment can then be displaced, either medially or laterally; this is performed with the ankle in a plantar flexed position. Displacement will depend upon the degree of correction required, 1 cm is usually sufficient. The position can usually be provisionally 'locked' by holding the foot in a plantigrade position. Once the surgeon is confident with the correction, a guidewire from a cannulated screw system can be inserted, under fluoroscopic guidance, from the lateral aspect of the tuberosity into the anterior fragment. Care must be taken to ensure that the wire enters the anterior calcaneum and does not penetrate medially. Once satisfied with the position, a single cannulated screw is sufficient to hold the osteotomy. Alternatively, a stepped plate may be used.

A lateral closing wedge can be added to the lateral displacement osteotomy, if required, to allow increased correction; the thickness of the wedge will depend upon the correction desired. Using minimal force, an attempt is made to close the wedge prior to fixation.

Closure

Closure of the flap must be meticulous and without tension. Deep Vicryl sutures and interrupted nylon sutures are satisfactory. The leg should be immobilized once the soft tissue component is completed.

POSTOPERATIVE CARE AND INSTRUCTIONS

The leg should be elevated for 72 hours until swelling has subsided. The leg is then placed in a non-weightbearing cast for a duration usually dictated by the soft tissue correction. The osteotomy usually heals within about 6 weeks.

RECOMMENDED REFERENCES

Dwyer FC. Osteotomy of the calcaneum for pes cavus. *J Bone Joint Surg Br* 1959;**41**:80–6.

Evans D. Calcaneo-valgus deformity. *J Bone Joint Surg Br* 1975;**57**:270–8.

Trnka HJ, Easley ME, Myerson MS. The role of calcaneal osteotomies for correction of adult flatfoot. *Clin Orthop Relat Res* 1999;**365**:50–64.

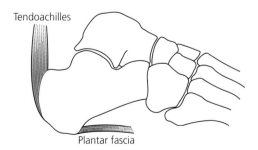

Tendoachilles

Plantar fascia

Figure 14.15 *Alignment of calcaneal osteotomy*

Viva questions

1. Describe how you can maximize the union rate for a midfoot arthrodesis.

2. In the context of hallux valgus deformity, what is congruency and how does it affect your decision-making process?

3. What radiographs do you use to assess hallux valgus deformity, what angles do you measure and how does this influence your choice of operation?

4. What surgical approach do you use for a first metatarsal osteotomy and what are the important structures at risk?

5. Describe the blood supply to the first metatarsal head. How can your choice of hallux valgus procedure affect the blood supply?

6. What structures do you need to identify in performing a lateral release in a hallux valgus deformity?

7. In a scarf osteotomy, what is 'troughing' and how does the design of your osteotomy influence occurrence?

8. Why is a Keller's procedure generally poorly tolerated by patients and when would you consider performing one?

9. What are the key differences between a Weil's and a Helal's osteotomy of the lesser metatarsals?

10. What is the difference between a claw toe, mallet toe and a hammer toe?

11. Describe the mechanics of a Girdlestone tendon transfer for the lesser toes and when you would perform this.

12. How do you assess the severity of hallux rigidus and how does this influence your treatment options?

13. What is the optimum position of arthrodesis of the first metatarsophalangeal joint (MTPJ) and how would you assess this intraoperatively?

14. Describe the anatomy of a toenail. How does this knowledge help in the treatment of ingrowing nails?

15. What is a Morton's Neuroma and where is it most commonly found?

16. How does movement of the subtalar joint in gait affect movement of the Chopart joints (talonavicular and calcaneocuboid)?

17. Describe your understanding of the concept of 'Talar neutral' and why is this useful in assessing foot position?

18. What surgical approach do you use to reach the subtalar joint, what are the landmarks and what structures are at risk?

19. What structures are at risk during a calcaneal osteotomy?

20. When would you consider performing a lateralizing calcaneal osteotomy?

15

Limb reconstruction

Robert Jennings and Peter Calder

PRINCIPLES OF LIMB RECONSTRUCTION

When subjected to slow, steady traction, under the appropriate conditions, living tissue becomes metabolically activated and is able to regenerate. This 'tension-stress' effect was described by Professor Gavril Abramovich Ilizarov from Kurgan in western Siberia, who pioneered the field of limb reconstruction from the early 1950s and developed the highly successful techniques that are still in use today.

Callus, formed at a corticotomy site, can be distracted at speeds of up to 1 mm per day and, reliably, form new bone in the process of 'distraction osteogenesis'. Once the goal length is achieved, a period of consolidation is required before fixator removal. This takes approximately 30–40 days per centimetre of lengthening to prevent bowing or fracture. Anecdotally, the maximum, safe distraction possible per procedure is 20 per cent of the original length of the bone being lengthened.

Distraction osteogenesis requires:
- Stability
- Maintenance of blood supply
- A latency period (5–7 days)
- Appropriate rate of distraction (0.75–1 mm per day)
- Appropriate rhythm (frequency) of distraction (0.25 mm, 6–8 hourly).

BIOMECHANICS

- Monolateral rail:
  - Cantilever loading
  - Concentrated high stress on near cortex
- Circular frame:
  - Beam loading
  - More even distribution of stress across cortices.

Use of all-wire fixation across a diaphysis is less attractive, due to risks to soft tissues. Hence, hybrid fixation with half-pins and wires is preferred.

METHODS TO IMPROVE STABILITY

- Wire:
  - Increase diameter (1.8 mm for adult, 1.5 mm for child)
  - Increase tension (130 Nm for adult, 110 Nm for child)
  - Increase crossing angles (Fig. 15.1)

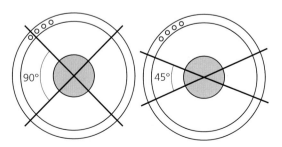

Figure 15.1 'Crossing angles': stability (a) > (b)

- Opposing 'olive' wires
- Increase number of wires
- Half-pin:
  - Increase diameter
  - Hydroxyapatite coating
  - Increase crossing angles (multiplanar)
  - Decrease distance of external construct to bone
  - Near and far positions (Fig. 15.2)
  - Increase number

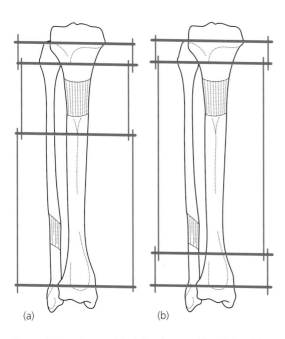

Figure 15.2 'Near and far' fixation: stability (a) > (b)

- Ring:
  - Decrease diameter (note: allow at least 2 cm clearance for swelling)
  - Fix bone in middle (compromise with eccentrically positioned tibia)
  - Near and far positions
  - Increase number (including 'dummy' rings)
- Attachments:
  - Use 'slotted' bolts – high surface area of contact with wire
  - Build ring to wire, if necessary – decrease bend on wire.

SURGICAL TECHNIQUES

PREOPERATIVE PLANNING

Indications

- Tibial/ femoral lengthening
- Long bone deformity correction.

Contraindications

- Non-compliant patient
- Adjacent joint instability
- Skin infection
- Significant soft tissue contractures
- Poor vascularity
- Pregnancy
- Smoker – relative.

Consent and risks

- Duration of treatment must be emphasized (c.40 days/cm)
- Pain: post-surgical, chronic dull ache during distraction is common
- Pin site problems: inflammation; soft tissue infection; osteomyelitis
- Joint stiffness or subluxation
- Soft tissue contractures
- Vascular injury
- Neurological injury: perioperative; postoperative stretching
- Premature/delayed/non-union
- Hardware failure
- Late bowing
- Fracture
- Deep vein thrombosis/pulmonary embolism

Operative planning

Recent radiographs must be available. These should include full leg length views, in the anteroposterior plane, of both lower limbs with the patellae facing forwards and appropriate lateral views. The mechanical and anatomical axes need to be assessed on both legs. If both legs are 'abnormal', standard angles are used for calculations.

Leg length discrepancy

Assessment from history, examination and radiological findings. Care must be taken to differentiate true from apparent causes of leg length discrepancy.

Common causes of apparent leg length discrepancy

- Scoliosis
- Hip instability or dislocation
- Fixed hip adduction
- Fixed knee flexion
- Equinus deformity of the ankle

Angular deformity

Clinical and radiographical examination allows calculation of the centre of rotation of angulation (CORA; Fig. 15.3). This is present at the intersection point of proximal and distal anatomical axes.

A decision is made as to whether the deformity requires surgical correction. This is based on the severity of deformity and the presence or absence of associated factors.

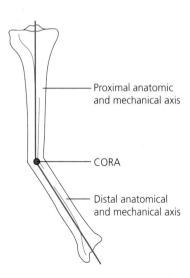

Figure 15.3 'CORA' (centre of rotation of angulation) – mechanical and anatomical axis

Indications for surgical correction of angular deformity

- Mechanical axis deviation (MAD) (Fig. 15.4)
- Rotational malalignment
- Translation
- Leg length discrepancy

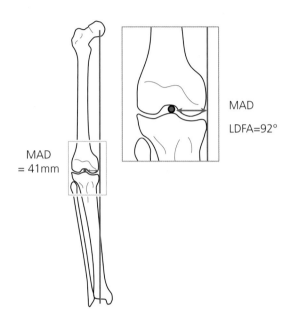

Figure 15.4 Mechanical axis deviation (MAD)

The next decision is the appropriate site for osteotomy. Osteotomy performed at the CORA will not result in translation (Fig. 15.5); osteotomy away from the CORA will produce translation. Note: if the hinge is not on the bisector line (Fig. 15.6) or the CORA is not on the anatomical axis, osteotomy at any level will result in translation.

SURGICAL TECHNIQUE

Wire insertion

- Aseptic 'no hands'/'Russian' technique
- Alcohol-soaked gauze used to coat and hold wire
- Low heat generation is ensured via short, intermittent bursts with the wire driver
- Wire tapped with mallet, when through contralateral skin.

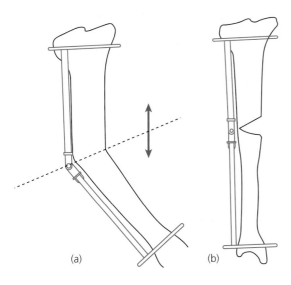

(a)   (b)

Figure 15.5 *With the hinge placed along the 'bisector line of the CORA', there will be no translation*

Half-pin insertion

- Stab skin incision
- Blunt dissection to bone
- Soft tissue protecting drill guide
- Both cortices pre-drilled
- Low heat generation – intermittent drilling
- Saline to cool and wash out swarf (decreases infection risk).

Wire/Half-pin placement

- 'Safe corridors' – avoid neurovascular structures
- Avoid crossing compartments, if possible
- Soft tissues on stretch, e.g. quadriceps in flexion, hamstrings in extension (helps postoperative mobility).

Corticotomy

- Low energy
- Minimal incision, to admit osteotome
- Periosteum incised and preserved, when possible
- A row of holes are pre-drilled with a 4.8 mm drill, with saline used for cooling. This technique allows low heat generation, reducing corticotomy site bone necrosis
- An osteotome is used to join holes, with a twist to break the posterior cortex.

Note: latent period: 5–7 days; quarter turns: 3–4 times per day (0.75–1 mm/day).

FEMORAL LENGTHENING

PREOPERATIVE PLANNING

See 'Principles of limb reconstruction' (p. 259).

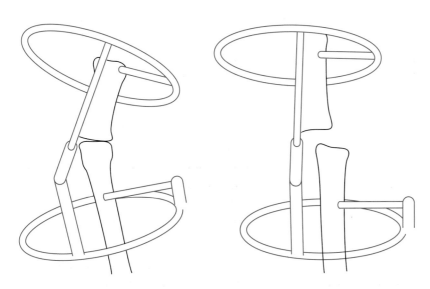

Figure 15.6 *With the hinge placed off the 'bisector line of the CORA', translation will result*

SURGICAL TECHNIQUE

Corticotomy

Landmarks

Junction of the proximal metaphysis and diaphysis – 1.5 cm distal to lesser trochanter.

Incision and dissection

- Image intensifier control
- Adequate longitudinal incision (to admit 8 mm osteotome).

Either:
- Anterior approach – between sartorius and tensor fascia lata (TFL), then through vastus intermedius and rectus femoris

Or:
- Lateral approach – through TFL and split vastus lateralis

Corticotomy technique as above.

Procedure

- Monolateral rail (Fig. 15.7):
  - If no risk of joint subluxation
  - Three half-pins proximal and, at least, three distal to corticotomy.
- Circular frame:
  - If risk of joint subluxation
  - Span knee/pelvis
  - Arches/two-thirds rings to allow mobility
  - Same principles as above.

Lengthening intramedullary nail

Internal lengthening nails have increased in popularity since becoming fully implantable, without the need for an external component for their extension. These newer nails have some advantages over the cumbersome external systems, most notably the lack of pin site associated problems, improved cosmesis and better patient tolerance. However, full weight-bearing is not advisable until the regenerated bone is mature and, inadvertent, rapid extension is a significant risk. Currently, the most popular design of lengthening nail in the UK is the 'ISKD' (Intramedullary Skeletal Kinetic Distractor, Orthofix; Fig. 15.8), with types

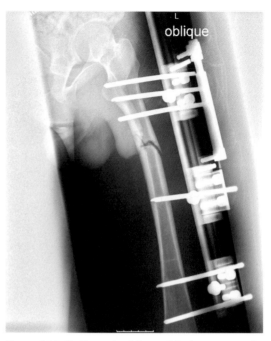

Figure 15.7 *Radiograph of femoral limb reconstruction system (LRS) rail*

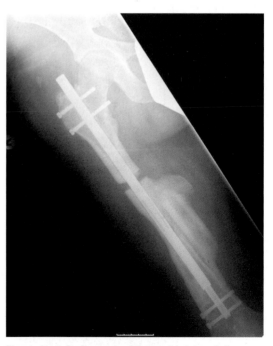

Figure 15.8 *Radiograph of femoral Intramedullary Skeletal Kinetic Distractor (ISKD)*

available for both femur and tibia. Elongation of the internal mechanism is achieved by alternating rotation of the limb and measured with a hand-held monitor.

TIBIAL LENGTHENING (FIG 15.9)

PREOPERATIVE PLANNING

See 'Principles of limb reconstruction' (p. 258).

SURGICAL TECHNIQUE

Corticotomy

Landmarks

Junction of the proximal metaphysis and diaphysis, *c*.1.5 cm distal to tibial tuberosity.

Incision and dissection

- Image intensifier control
- Adequate longitudinal incision over anterior tibial crest (to admit 8 mm osteotome)

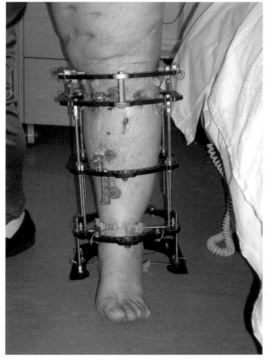

Figure 15.9 *Tibial Ilizarov frame for lengthening*

- Periosteum incised, then lifted off medially and laterally with blunt dissection
- Corticotomy technique as above.

Procedure

- Two rings per bone segment (near and far)
- Two wires/half-pins per ring
- Four connecting, threaded rods between rings (Fig. 15.10)
- Fibular osteotomy
  - Mid-diaphyseal avoids neurovascular structures
- Fix fibula (proximal and distal), to avoid joint subluxation.

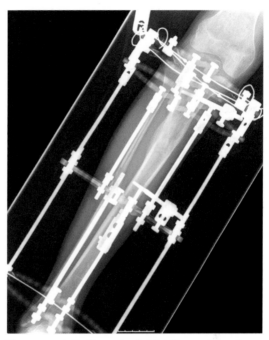

Figure 15.10 *Radiograph of tibial Ilizarov frame for lengthening*

PRINCIPLES OF DEFORMITY CORRECTION

PREOPERATIVE PLANNING

Operative planning

The initial decision is between acute and gradual correction of the deformity:

- Acute
  - Mild deformity
  - Opening or closing wedge
  - Plate and screws
  - Intra-medullary (IM) nail
  - External fixation
- Gradual
  - More severe deformity
  - Less risk of neurological damage
  - Potential for revision of correction protocol
  - Distraction osteogenesis
  - Circular frame e.g. Ilizarov or hexapod type (e.g. Taylor Spatial Frame)
  - Monolateral fixator: on convex side – distraction at osteotomy site (See Fig. 15.5 page 261); on concave side – compression at osteotomy site therefore requires wedge excision.

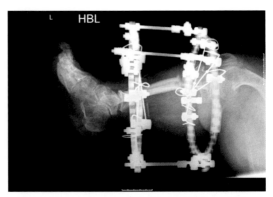

Figure 15.12 *Radiograph of a simple Ilizarov frame construct used to correct deformity in a congenitally short tibia*

SURGICAL TECHNIQUE

Example: Simple, tibial diaphyseal deformity correction with a circular frame.
- Application of proximal and distal rings (see above; Fig. 15.11)
- Osteotomy at CORA (see above)
- Ilizarov method
  - Inter-ring connections with hinges along bisector line of CORA (Fig. 15.12).
- Taylor Spatial Frame (TSF) method (Figs 15.13 and 15.14)
  - Inter-ring connections with six oblique, adjustable struts ('virtual hinge')

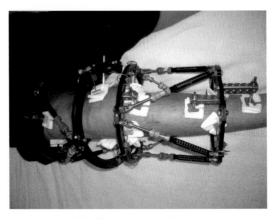

Figure 15.13 *Tibial Taylor Spatial Frame*

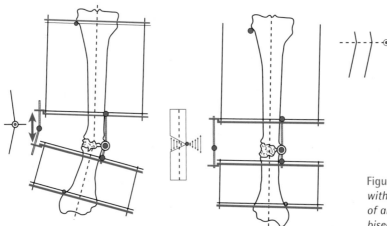

Figure 15.11 *'Near and far' rings with osteotomy at centre of rotation of angulation (CORA), hinge along bisector line*

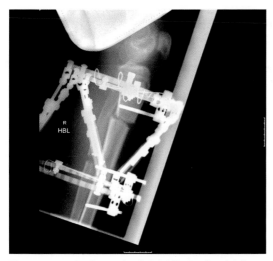

Figure 15.14 *Radiograph of tibial Taylor Spatial Frame for deformity correction*

Online computer programme

- Requires: postoperative radiograph measurements
  - Frame measurements (ring sizes/initial strut lengths)
- Delivers: pre- and post-correction images
  - Corrective protocol.

POSTOPERATIVE CARE AND INSTRUCTIONS

- Latency period (5–7 days)
- Gradual correction period
- Consolidation period
- Removal of frame when clinically and radiologically appropriate.

RECOMMENDED REFERENCES

De Bastiani G, Aldegheri R, Renzi-Brivio L, *et al.* Limb lengthening by callus distraction (Callotasis). *J Pediatr Orthop* 1987;**7**:129–34.

Cole JD, Justin D, Kasparis T, *et al.* The intramedullary skeletal kinetic distractor (ISKD): first clinical results of a new intramedullary nail for lengthening of the femur and tibia. *Injury* 2001;**32**(suppl 4):SD129–39.

Paley D, Herzenberg JE. *Principles of Deformity Correction*. Berlin: Springer, 2001.

Paley D, Herzenberg JE, Tetsworth K, *et al.* Deformity planning for frontal and sagittal plane corrective osteotomies. *Orthop Clin North Am* 1994;**25**:425–65.

Rozbruch SR, Ilizarov S. *Limb Lengthening and Reconstruction Surgery*. New York: Informa, 2007.

Viva questions

1. What are the causes of leg length discrepancy?
2. What problems are associated with leg length discrepancy?
3. How do you assess length discrepancy of the lower limbs?
4. What are the differences between true, apparent and functional leg length discrepancy?
5. What are the treatment options for leg length discrepancy in both adults and children?
6. What are the relative percentage contributions to normal growth of all of the lower limb physes?
7. How can you predict the magnitude of leg length discrepancy at skeletal maturity?
8. What are the problems associated with shoe raises?
9. What problems may occur as a consequence of acute shortening procedures?
10. Who was Professor Gavril Abramovich Ilizarov?
11. What problems may occur due to leg lengthening procedure?
12. What are the prerequisite factors necessary for successful leg lengthening?
13. What are the reasons for leaving a 'latency period' prior to commencing distraction?
14. What are the advantages and disadvantages of lengthening intra-medullary nails?
15. Give the causes of lower limb deformity.

16. How do you assess the degree of lower limb deformity?

17. Draw a 'Selenius graph'.

18. What options are available for correcting lower limb deformity in both adults and children?

19. What are the consequences of hinge misplacement when applying an Ilizarov frame for deformity correction?

20. What are the advantages of using a 'Taylor Spatial Frame' rather than an Ilizarov frame for deformity correction?

16

Paediatric orthopaedic surgery

Russell Hawkins and Aresh Hashemi-Nejad

EPIPHYSIODESIS

PREOPERATIVE PLANNING

Epiphysiodesis involves destruction of the physis to allow equalization of leg length discrepancy (LLD) in children. As **most growth occurs around the knee**, the distal femoral and/or the proximal tibial and fibular physes are targeted depending on the predicted remaining growth.

Indications

- Predicted true LLD 2–5 cm at maturity
- May be used to treat LLD >7 cm through lengthening of the short limb and epiphysiodesis of the long limb.

Contraindications

- Apparent LLD
- LLD <1.5 cm
- Localized infection
- Tumour
- Closed physis.

Consent and risks

- Neurovascular injury: <1 per cent
- Infection: <1 per cent
- Fracture: <1 per cent
- Angular deformity: <1 per cent
- Residual LLD: 80 per cent patients within 1 cm

Operative planning

Various methods exist to determine the LLD at maturity and to guide the timing and type of epiphysiodesis (distal femoral and/or proximal tibial):

- Green–Anderson growth remaining method: estimates growth potential in the distal femoral and proximal tibial physes at various skeletal ages separately for girls and boys.
- Moseley straight line graph: a logarithmic representation of the Green–Anderson method.
- Menelaus arithmetic method: assumes growth of 10 mm/year from distal femur and 6 mm/year from the proximal tibia and that girls reach maturity at 14 and boys at 16 years.
- Eastwood–Cole method: a graphic representation of the arithmetic method but takes into account non-linear changes in LLD. Bone age is more reliable than chronological

age in determining growth remaining and can be calculated using the Greulich and Pyle method. This involves comparison of a left hand and wrist radiograph with a known standard.

Anaesthesia and positioning

General anaesthesia is used, together with intravenous antibiotic prophylaxis. The patient is positioned supine with the knee slightly flexed over a small sandbag. A pneumatic thigh tourniquet is used. An image intensifier is required and a gonadal shield should be appropriately placed.

SURGICAL TECHNIQUE

Landmarks

The image intensifier is used to mark the orientation of the physis in the frontal plane and the midpoint of the physis in the lateral plane.

Approach

A 1–2 cm longitudinal incision is centred over the midpoint of physis medially and laterally. A larger incision is made laterally to identify and protect the common peroneal nerve if performing proximal fibular epiphysiodesis.

Dissection

Sharp dissection is continued down to bone.

PROCEDURE

Physeal cartilage is removed using a 4.5 mm diameter drill under image guidance: a single entry point is made in the lateral cortex in line with the physis on the frontal view and at its midpoint on the lateral view. This minimizes weakening of the cortex and the risk of subsequent fracture. The drill is advanced transversely along the line of the physis in the frontal view until the tip reaches its midpoint (Fig. 16.1).

Using the same entry point each time, the drill is tilted 30° first anteriorly then posteriorly and advanced to the halfway mark to remove a fan-

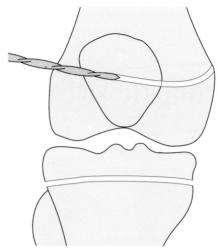

Figure 16.1 *The trajectory of the drill should be checked periodically using the image intensifier to ensure obliteration of the physis*

shaped area of physeal cartilage (Fig. 16.2). This technique is then repeated on the medial side. The swarf should be inspected to ensure removal of physeal cartilage. Further curettage of the epiphyseal surface is performed to remove any remaining physeal cartilage.

Closure

Layered closure using absorbable subcuticular material to skin.

POSTOPERATIVE INSTRUCTIONS

- Mobilize full weightbearing with crutches for comfort for up to 2 weeks.
- Radiographs at 3 months then periodically until maturity to assess physeal closure and leg lengths.

RECOMMENDED REFERENCES

Atar D, Lehman WB, Grant AD, *et al.* (1991) Percutaneous epiphysiodesis. *J Bone Joint Surg Br* 1991;**73**:173.

Eastwood DM, Cole WG. A graphic method for timing the correction of leg-length discrepancy. *J Bone Joint Surg Br* 1995;**77**:743–7.

Menelaus MB. Correction of leg length

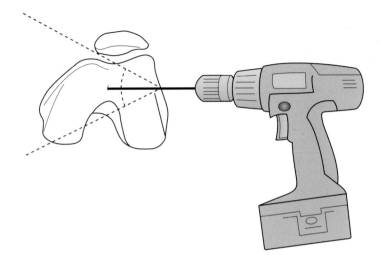

Figure 16.2 *The drill is inserted in the mid-sagittal line of the femur then angled anteriorly and posteriorly by 30° using the same entry point*

discrepancy by epiphyseal arrest. *J Bone Joint Surg Br* 1966;**48**:336–9.

Snyder M, Harcke HT, Bowen JR, *et al.* Evaluation of physeal behaviour in response to epiphysiodesis with the use of serial magnetic resonance imaging. *J Bone Joint Surg Am* 1994;**76**:224–9.

DEVELOPMENTAL DYSPLASIA OF THE HIP – CLOSED REDUCTION

PREOPERATIVE PLANNING

Although often combined with an arthrogram and soft tissue releases, technically this remains a closed procedure as the capsule is not opened. Adductor and psoas releases are performed via an open medial approach, the technical details of which are provided in the 'Developmental dysplasia of the hip – open reduction' section (p. 271).

The optimum timing of reduction is subject to debate: waiting for the capital femoral epiphysis to appear reduces the risk of avascular necrosis although, conversely, early reduction suggests a better long-term outcome.

Indications

- 6–18 months old child with developmental dysplasia of the hip (DDH)
- Failed treatment with Pavlik harness.

Contraindications

Child <6 or >18 months.

Consent and risks

- Application of spica plaster in the human position (Fig. 16.5); subsequent care must be explained to parents
- Avascular necrosis: 5–10 per cent
- Re-dislocation: <5 per cent
- Further surgery: 20 per cent
- Neurovascular injury and infection: <1 per cent (if arthrogram and soft tissue releases performed)
- Risk of conversion to open reduction: 10–20 per cent. Greater risk for high-riding dislocation

Operative planning

Imaging studies are requested depending on the expected presence of the ossific nucleus:
- Dynamic ultrasound if <6 months to determine alpha and beta angles, reducibility and capsular laxity.
- Plain anteroposterior (AP) pelvis and frog lateral radiographs if >6 months. Note any delayed appearance of ossific nucleus, Shenton, Hilgenreiner and Perkins lines, acetabular index and Tonnis grade.

Anaesthesia and positioning

General anaesthesia is used. The patient is positioned supine at the end of a radiolucent table, to allow image intensifier access. The surgeon stands between flexed, abducted and externally rotated hips.

SURGICAL TECHNIQUE

Examination under anaesthesia (EUA) and arthrogram are first performed to assess reduction and the need for adductor longus, gracilis and psoas release.

Landmarks

Adductor longus muscle – palpable in the child's groin (Fig. 16.3).

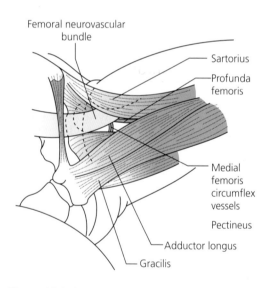

Figure 16.3 *Adductor longus and its relationships*

Procedure

A 22G spinal needle is introduced beneath the palpable adductor longus tendon in the groin and advanced cranially towards the ipsilateral scapular until the tip is felt to traverse the hip capsule. The position is confirmed with image intensifier before instilling 0.5 mL of diluted contrast.

The hip is reduced with a combination of flexion, abduction and anterior displacement without excessive force. Soft tissue releases should be considered if this does not occur easily. If the head appears to stand out from the acetabulum on the arthrogram, this suggests a block to reduction such as an infolded labrum. A conversion to open reduction may therefore be required.

The stability is assessed within the safe zones of flexion and abduction. Typically, a stable position is 90° of flexion and 30–50° of abduction. Extreme positions increase the risk of avascular necrosis and must be avoided.

A well-padded spica plaster is carefully applied in the human position before final radiographic confirmation of reduction (Fig. 16.4).

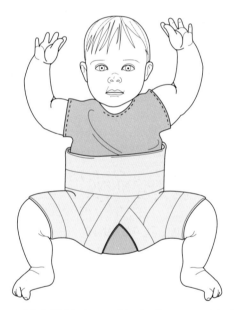

Figure 16.4 *Child plastered in the 'human position'*

POSTOPERATIVE INSTRUCTIONS

- Plaster check prior to discharge.
- Limited slice CT at 2/52 to confirm maintenance of reduction.
- Convert to abduction brace at 10/52.
- Wean out of brace after further 6/52. Depending on acetabular development, night time bracing may continue for up to 1 year.

RECOMMENDED REFERENCES

Harcke HT, Kumar SJ. Current concepts review – the role of ultrasound in the diagnosis and management of congenital dislocation and developmental dysplasia of the hip. *J Bone Joint Surg Am* 1991;**73**:622–8.

Kalamchi A, MacEwen GD. Avascular necrosis following treatment of congenital dislocation of the hip. *J Bone Joint Surg Am* 1980;**62**:876–88.

Malvitz TA, Weinstein SL. Closed reduction for congenital dislocation of the hip. Functional and radiographic results after an average of thirty years. *J Bone Joint Surg Am* 1994;**12**:1777–92.

Ramsey PL, Lasser S, MacEwen GD. Congenital dislocation of the hip: use of the Pavlik harness in the child in the first six months of life. *J Bone Joint Surg Am* 1978;**58**:1000–4.

Severin E. Contribution to knowledge of congenital dislocation of the hip joint: late results of closed reduction and arthrographic studies of recent cases. *Acta Chir Scand Suppl* 1941;**63**:1–42.

DEVELOPMENTAL DYSPLASIA OF THE HIP – OPEN REDUCTION

PREOPERATIVE PLANNING

Open reduction deals directly with soft tissue obstruction facilitating relocation of the hip without excessive force.

Indications

- Children 6–18 months with: obstruction to closed reduction (psoas tendon, contracted capsule, ligamentum teres, transverse acetabular ligament, and inverted limbus), an unstable safe zone, previous failed closed or open reduction
- Children presenting over 18 months.

Contraindications

Children less than 6 months old.

Consent and risks

- Application of spica plaster; subsequent care must be explained to parents
- Neurovascular injury: <1 per cent
- Infection: <1 per cent
- Avascular necrosis: 5 per cent
- Re-dislocation: 1 per cent
- Further surgery for dysplasia or LLD: 10–15 per cent

Operative planning

Radiographs as per closed reduction.

Anaesthesia and positioning

General anaesthesia with intravenous antibiotics. The patient is positioned supine at the end of a radiolucent table. The surgeon stands between the patient's legs for a medial approach or on the operative side for an anterior approach. An image intensifier is required.

SURGICAL TECHNIQUE

A medial approach is used if the patient is less than 12 months old; an anterior approach, via a bikini incision, is preferred if the child is older.

MEDIAL APPROACH

Landmarks

Adductor longus tendon – palpable in the groin, approximately 2 cm lateral to the labia/scrotum.

Incision

A 2.5 cm, vertical skin crease incision is centred on the palpable tendon of adductor longus.

Superficial dissection

Structures at risk

- Anterior and posterior divisions of obturator nerve

The fascia overlying the tendons of adductor longus and gracilis is opened along their length and fractional lengthening tenotomies are performed. Adductor magnus and brevis are exposed with blunt dissection. Branches of the obturator nerve are identified on the superficial surface of the adductor brevis and are protected.

Deep dissection

Structure at risk

- Medial circumflex femoral artery

The plane between the adductor magnus and brevis is dissected to access the lesser trochanter. A psoas tenotomy is performed under direct vision avoiding the medial femoral circumflex vessels which pass over the medial surface of the psoas tendon distally.

A medial arthrotomy is made above the vessels and the acetabular attachment of the ligamentum teres is divided and used as a traction aid to relocate the femoral head. It is then sutured to the anterior inferior capsule.

ANTERIOR APPROACH

Landmarks

- Anterior superior iliac spine (ASIS)
- Pubic tubercle.

Incision

The line of the inguinal ligament is marked between the ASIS and the pubic tubercle. A second line is then dropped vertically downwards from the ASIS. Next, a 5 cm bikini line incision is marked 2 cm inferior and parallel to the inguinal ligament, one-third of it medial and two-thirds lateral to the vertical line.

Superficial dissection

Structure at risk

- Lateral cutaneous nerve of the thigh

The interval between sartorius and tensor fascia lata is developed to reach the rectus femoris and gluteus medius.

Deep dissection

The interval between the rectus femoris and gluteus medius is dissected and the straight head of the rectus femoris is detached from the anterior capsule. It may then be retracted medially to allow psoas tenotomy and L-shaped anterior arthrotomy (see Figure 16.5).

PROCEDURE

Obstructions to reduction are removed as necessary; pulvinar is extracted, the transverse ligament is released and the ligamentum teres excised if obstructive. Adductor releases are performed, via a separate groin incision, to facilitate reduction as required.

The redundant capsule is tightened with capsulorrhaphy following reduction. Using the image intensifier, the position of maximum stability is identified; the hip is placed in 30° of

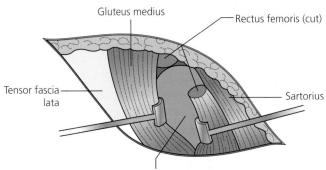

Figure 16.5 *Anterior approach to the right hip*

internal rotation, flexion and abduction then each of these positions is removed in sequence to determine positioning in plaster and the need for future surgery.

Femoral osteotomy or an acetabular procedure may be undertaken concomitantly if severe dysplasia is present in an older child.

Closure

- Layered closure ensuring reconstruction of rectus femoris.
- Skin is closed with absorbable subcuticular material followed by a waterproof dressing.

A well-padded spica plaster is carefully applied in the stable safe zone of flexion and abduction before final radiographic confirmation of reduction. This should be in greater than 90° of flexion without forced flexion and abducted between 30° and 60°.

POSTOPERATIVE INSTRUCTIONS

- Plaster check prior to discharge.
- Limited slice CT at two weeks to confirm maintenance of reduction.
- Spica removal at ten weeks and mobilization allowed.
- Follow up at three months with radiographs.

RECOMMENDED REFERENCES

Ferguson AB Jr. Primary open reduction of congenital dislocation of the hip using a median adductor approach. *J Bone Joint Surg Am* 1973;**55**:671–81.

Morcuende JA, Meyer MD, Dolan LA, *et al.* Long term outcome after open reduction through an anteromedial approach for congenital dislocation of the hip. *J Bone Joint Surg Am* 1997;**79**:810–17.

Tonnis D. An evaluation of conservative and operative methods in the treatment of congenital dislocation of the hip. *Clin Orthop* 1976;**119**:76–88.

Zadeh HG, Catterall A, Hashemi-Nejad A, *et al.* Test of stability as an aid to decide the need for osteotomy in association with open reduction in developmental dysplasia of the hip. A long term review. *J Bone Joint Surg Br* 2000;**82**:17–27.

DEVELOPMENTAL DYSPLASIA OF THE HIP – PELVIC OSTEOTOMY

Various techniques exist for pelvic osteotomy in DDH and an account of them all is beyond the scope of this chapter. Therefore, only the Salter and Pemberton types will be described further.

SALTER OSTEOTOMY

Preoperative planning

Indications

- Acetabular dysplasia; acetabulum faces anterolaterally causing deficient anterior coverage in extension and deficient superior coverage in adduction
- Congruent hip
- 18 months to 6 years (as it requires flexibility of symphysis pubis).

Contraindications

- Bilateral DDH (uncovers contralateral hip)
- Congruent reduction not achievable on EUA arthrogram.

Consent and risks

- Overall risks: <5 per cent
- Neurovascular injury: 1 per cent
- Limited weightbearing/crutches
- Infection: <1 per cent
- LLD: gains 1 cm with Salter osteotomy
- Triradiate cartilage growth arrest (Pemberton osteotomy)
- Failure of graft
- Hardware breakage
- Residual dysplasia (retroversion)
- Secondary degeneration: lateralization of joint increases joint reaction force (Salter)
- Further surgery (removal of hardware, salvage procedures)

Operative planning

Congruency confirmed with EUA arthrogram.

Anaesthesia and positioning

General anaesthesia is used, together with intravenous antibiotics. The patient is positioned supine with an ipsilateral sandbag in a position suitable for image intensifier access.

Surgical technique

Anterosuperior coverage is achieved at the expense of posterior coverage by flexing the acetabular fragment. Typically, the lateral centre edge angle will increase by 10°. It is performed via an anterior approach (see 'Developmental dysplasia of the hip – open reduction', p. 272) extending the bikini incision proximally over the iliac crest to allow splitting of the iliac apophysis and subperiosteal exposure of the ilium to reach the sciatic notch.

Procedure

Structures at risk

- Sciatic nerve – Rang retractors are placed in the sciatic notch keeping them closely applied to bone to protect the nerve
- Devascularization/denervation of abductors

An osteotomy is performed between the sciatic notch and midway between the ASIS and anterior inferior iliac spine (AIIS) using a Gigli saw. This should appear to be parallel to the acetabular surface on AP images. Hinging on the symphysis pubis, the acetabulum is rotated anteriorly and laterally to gain coverage while avoiding retroversion.

A wedge of bone from the iliac wing is inserted perpendicular to the weightbearing axis. The 'winking sign' should be noted on an image intensifier (foreshortening of ipsilateral obturator foramen) and the position held with two threaded Schantz pins across the osteotomy. Image guidance is used to advance the pins proximodistally beginning just proximal to the ASIS and aiming for the triradiate cartilage (Figs 16.6 and 16.7).

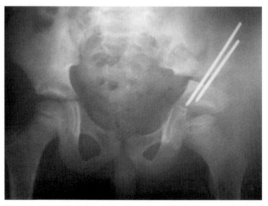

Figure 16.7 *Radiograph showing left Salter osteotomy and 'winking sign'*

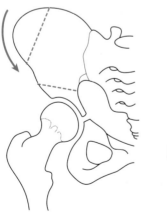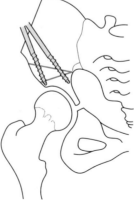

Figure 16.6 *Salter osteotomy*

Closure

- Layered closure ensuring repair of the iliac apophysis
- Absorbable subcuticular material to skin.

Postoperative instructions

Plaster spica for those under 6 years. Limited weightbearing with crutches for 6–8 weeks if over 6.

PEMBERTON OSTEOTOMY

Preoperative planning

Indications

- Double diameter dysplastic acetabulum
- Congruent hip
- Open triradiate cartilage
- Close to normal range of motion
- No degeneration
- Normal proximal femoral morphology
- Paralytic hip disorders/Ehlers–Danlos syndrome (posterior coverage is maintained, conferring stability).

Contraindications

- Poor range of motion (flexion, abduction and internal rotation will be further diminished)
- Closed triradiate cartilage
- Congruent reduction not achievable
- Centre of rotation of head and acetabulum coincide.

For consent and risks/preoperative preparation/anaesthesia and positioning, see Salter osteotomy (p. 273).

Surgical technique

The Pemberton osteotomy reduces the volume of a large-diameter acetabulum making the centre of rotation of both femoral head and socket coincident. The acetabulum is displaced forwards and laterally hinging on the triradiate cartilage (Fig. 16.8). The autograft is stable and fixation is therefore not required. The approach and exposure are performed as per the Salter osteotomy.

Procedure

The osteotomy is made 10–15 mm superior to the AIIS passing a curved osteotome posteriorly to reach the ilioischial and iliopubic limb of the triradiate cartilage (midway between sciatic notch and posterior acetabular rim). The acetabulum is hinged on the triradiate to improve coverage. Corticocancellous graft is harvested from the iliac wing and inserted into the osteotomy site. Posterior stability negates the need for internal fixation.

Closure

As per Salter osteotomy.

Postoperative instructions

As per Salter osteotomy.

RECOMMENDED REFERENCES

Colemann SS. The incomplete pericapsular (Pemberton) and innominate (Salter) osteotomies. *Clin Orthop* 1974;**98**:116–23.
Pemberton PA. Pericapsular osteotomy of the ilium for treatment of congenital subluxation and

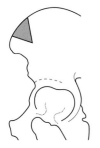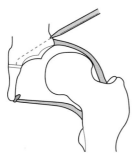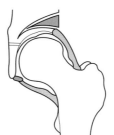

Figure 16.8 *Pemberton osteotomy*

dislocation of the hip. *J Bone Joint Surg Am* 1965;**47**:65–86.

Salter RB. Innominate osteotomy in the treatment of congenital dislocation and subluxation of the hip. *J Bone Joint Surg Br* 1961;**43**:518–39.

Thomas SR, Wedge JH, Salter RB. Outcome at forty five years after open reduction and innominate osteotomy for late presenting developmental dysplasia of the hip. *J Bone Joint Surg Am* 2007;**89**:2341–50.

DEVELOPMENTAL DYSPLASIA OF THE HIP – PROXIMAL FEMORAL OSTEOTOMY

The varus derotation osteotomy (VDRO) is the commonest type performed for DDH.

PREOPERATIVE PLANNING

Indications

- Persistent dysplasia following DDH (coxa valga, anteversion)
- Congruent reduction in abduction and internal rotation
- Reasonable sphericity (lateral portion of head intact).

Contraindications

- Limited range of motion (abduction and internal rotation)
- Active infection
- Pelvic procedure more appropriate (centre-edge angle [CEA] <15°)
- Previous avascular necrosis is a relative contraindication with less predictable results
- Be aware that VDRO will compound an existing negative LLD.

Consent and risks

- Plaster spica if under 6 years
- Limited weightbearing with crutches if over 6 years
- Bleeding

- Neurovascular damage: 1 per cent
- Infection: <1 per cent
- Delayed/non-union: 1–5 per cent (greater risk with increasing age)
- Failure of hardware: <1 per cent
- Incomplete correction
- LLD: inevitable with closing wedge varus osteotomy
- Joint degeneration
- Further surgery (removal of hardware, complex arthroplasty)

Operative planning

An EUA and arthrogram is performed to confirm adequate range of motion and concentric reduction; >15° abduction is required for a varus femoral osteotomy. The type of fixation device and degree of fixed angle is decided (e.g. blade plate/Coventry pin and plate; 90° or 130° angle).

Anaesthesia and positioning

- General anaesthesia
- Supine with ipsilateral buttock sandbag
- Intravenous antibiotic prophylaxis
- Image intensifier.

SURGICAL TECHNIQUE

A lateral approach to the subtrochanteric region of the proximal femur is used to avoid compromise to the vascular supply to the femoral head.

Landmarks

The predicted trajectory of the chosen device along the femoral neck is planned and marked using the image intensifier.

Incision

A 10 cm longitudinal wound is used, running along the lateral aspect of the proximal femur from the metaphyseal flare of the greater trochanter to the proximal femoral diaphysis.

Superficial dissection

The longitudinal incision is continued through superficial fat and the fascia lata, in line with the skin incision.

Deep dissection

Structures at risk

- Perforating branches of profunda femoris artery – these should be identified and cauterized where necessary

The posterior insertion of vastus lateralis is detached from the posterior intermuscular septum and reflected anteriorly to expose the lateral surface of proximal femur. The periosteum is incised longitudinally and elevated at site of the predicted osteotomy.

PROCEDURE

Beginning from the lateral cortex just inferior to the flare of the greater trochanter, a guidewire is passed up the femoral neck, under image control, without breaching the physis. The trajectory should aim to restore a normal neck-shaft angle of 130°.

The wire is measured and over-drilled before insertion of the cannulated lag screw. Under image guidance, the proximal osteotomy is made perpendicular to the shaft in the subtrochanteric region using an oscillating saw.

The second osteotomy is made beginning at same entry point on the lateral cortex with the saw tilted inferiorly creating a medially based wedge with a lateral apex. The medial cortex is

then completed using an osteotome. A guidewire is inserted transversely into the anterolateral cortex distal to the future position of the plate.

The leg is adducted to close the varus osteotomy and the guidewire is used as a joystick to externally rotate the distal shaft into a satisfactory position on fluoroscopy (Fig. 16.9). Congruent alignment of the lateral cortices should be checked to ensure seating of the plate. The plate is applied over the lag screw and the distal shaft is reduced onto the plate and held with a Hey–Groves clamp while maintaining correct orientation. Four bicortical screws are inserted to fix the plate before removal of the guidewire. The degree of correction and position of hardware is confirmed with imaging.

Closure

- Layered absorbable closure of vastus lateralis then fascia lata.
- Subcuticular absorbable material to skin.

POSTOPERATIVE INSTRUCTIONS

- Mobilize partial weightbearing
- Increase weightbearing status at 6–8 weeks after union confirmed clinically and radiographically.

RECOMMENDED REFERENCES

Blockey NJ. Derotation osteotomy in the management of congenital dislocation of the hip. *J Bone Joint Surg Br* 1984;**66**:485–90.

Kasser JR, Bowen JR, MacEwen GD. (1985) Varus derotation osteotomy in the treatment of persistent dysplasia in congenital dysplasia of the hip. *J Bone Joint Surg Br* 1985;**67**:195–202.

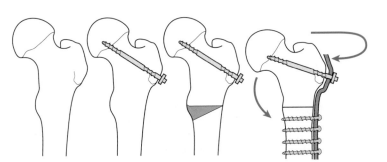

Figure 16.9 *Stages in varus derotation osteotomy. (a) Valgus, anteverted proximal femur. (b) Screw placed under image guidance. (c) Medially based closing wedge osteotomy performed from lateral side. (d) Varus producing osteotomy closed and held with plate following derotation*

Williamson DM, Benson MKD. Late femoral osteotomy in congenital dislocation of the hip. *J Bone Joint Surg Br* 1988;**70**:614–8.

SLIPPED UPPER FEMORAL EPIPHYSIS – PINNING

Manoeuvres to reduce the epiphysis are associated with a high incidence of avascular necrosis (40 per cent); pinning *in situ* therefore aims to prevent further displacement, promote physeal closure and minimize future secondary degeneration.

Slips are described as stable if weightbearing is possible or unstable if weightbearing is not possible even with crutches.

PREOPERATIVE PLANNING

Indications

- Grade I–II slip (Southwick angle <60°). Bilateral pinning is performed if there is:
  - Evidence of bilateral slip
  - Endocrinopathy
  - Younger end of age spectrum (10 years – girls, 12 years – boys).

Contraindications

- Advanced avascular necrosis
- Active infection.

Consent and risks

- Limited weightbearing/crutches
- Avascular necrosis: 0–5 per cent but higher if unstable slip
- Chondrolysis: 10 per cent (greater risk for African Caribbeans, females and poor technique)
- Fracture: <1 per cent
- Infection: <1 per cent
- Failure of hardware
- Further slip (associated with inadequate screw advancement)
- LLD: 1.5 cm difference on average
- Joint degeneration
- Further surgery (removal of hardware/osteotomy/arthrodesis/complex arthroplasty)

Operative planning

- An AP and Billings lateral of both hips – it is bilateral in 25 per cent of cases (Figs 16.10 and 16.11)
- Endocrine work up if at younger end of age spectrum

Anaesthesia and positioning

- General anaesthesia is used.
- Patient is positioned supine on a radiolucent table; care is taken when transferring, preparing and draping the unstable hip to prevent further displacement.
- Intravenous antibiotic prophylaxis is given.
- Image intensifier.

SURGICAL TECHNIQUE

An aspiration of the hip is first performed under image guidance for pain relief and to decompress the retinacular vessels.

Landmarks

The image intensifier is used to delineate the joint and proximal femur.

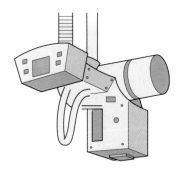

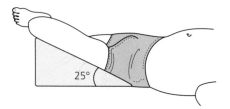

Figure 16.10 *Patient positioning for Billings lateral radiograph. The hip is abducted, externally rotated and elevated 25° on a foam wedge*

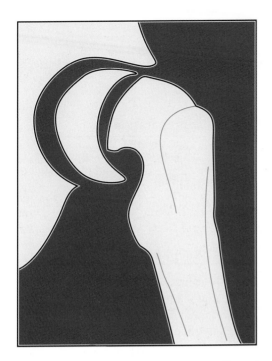

Figure 16.11 *Illustration of Billings lateral radiograph showing slip*

Incision

As pinning is performed percutaneously, the planned trajectory of the screw is marked in two planes using the image intensifier bearing in mind the course of important neurovascular structures. The entry point of the screw should not be distal to the lesser trochanter as this creates stress risers and increases the incidence of fracture. Preoperative marking also limits the number of guidewire passes necessary to achieve a satisfactory screw position, further decreasing the chance of guidewire misplacement and minimizing the risk of fracture. Because the epiphysis is relatively posterior and inferior to the neck, a more anterior entry point is required. Optimum screw position, should avoid the posterior neck and posterior superior epiphysis to preserve the blood supply to the femoral head and minimize the risk of avascular necrosis.

Dissection

Tissues are dissected bluntly down to bone.

PROCEDURE

A guidewire is passed under image intensifier control to avoid malposition and joint penetration. After measuring and over-drilling the wire, a partially threaded 6.5–7.5 mm diameter cannulated screw is inserted. A reverse cutting thread is used for easier subsequent removal. Despite an increase in shear strength across the physis using multiple screws, the use of a single screw diminishes the risk of chondrolysis and avoids the disproportionate complication rate of multiple screws.

The passage of guidewire, drill and screw should be performed under image guidance to avoid joint penetration. The screw tip should reach the centre of the epiphysis, 5 mm from the articular surface with a minimum of three to four threads crossing the physis to provide adequate fixation. At completion, live screening of the hip is performed to ensure solid fixation of the epiphysis and confirm screw position.

Closure

Subcuticular absorbable material is used to close the stab incision.

POSTOPERATIVE INSTRUCTIONS

Range of motion exercises are begun on the first postoperative day. Mobilization is then:
- Fully weightbearing with crutches for 2–3 weeks if slip is stable
- Partial weightbearing until healed if unstable.

Assessment is carried out at 6–8 weeks for clinical and radiological evidence of union and to ensure that there has not been any further slip. Sporting activities are prohibited until physeal closure occurs. Following physeal closure, screw removal is recommended.

RECOMMENDED REFERENCES

Givon U, Bowen JR. Chronic slipped femoral epiphysis: treatment by pinning *in situ*. *J Pediatr Orthop B* 1999;8:216–22.

Loder RT, Aronson DD, Dobbs MB, *et al.* Slipped capital femoral epiphysis. *Instr Course Lect* 2001;**50**:555–70.

Loder RT, Richards BS, Shapiro PS, *et al.* Acute slipped capital femoral epiphysis. The importance of physeal stability. *J Bone Joint Surg Am* 1993;**75**:1134–40.

Phillips SA, Griffiths WEG, Clarke NMP. The timing and reduction of the acute unstable slipped upper femoral epiphysis. *J Bone Joint Surg Br* 2001;**83**:1046–9.

SLIPPED UPPER FEMORAL EPIPHYSIS – OSTEOTOMY

An open reduction with osteotomy serves to restore the head-neck angle with subsequent improvement in hip biomechanics. This aims to provide good future function, minimize or delay the onset of painful secondary degeneration and normalize proximal femoral anatomy for future hip replacement. Osteotomy can be performed at various levels (intracapsular and extra capsular neck, intertrochanteric and subtrochanteric) with greater correction achievable at the site of deformity (more proximally). Although these proximal osteotomies have been associated with a greater risk of avascular necrosis, a Dunn or Fish cuneiform osteotomy performed with meticulous technique, as described below, can achieve excellent results.

PREOPERATIVE PLANNING

Indications

- Slip >60°
- Chronic/acute on chronic or unstable slip
- Open physis.

Contraindications

Closed physis (Southwick intertrochanteric osteotomy may be more appropriate).

Consent and risks

- Avascular necrosis: 10–48 per cent
- Chondrolysis: 10–12 per cent
- Infection: <1 per cent

- Slip progression
- LLD: 1–2 cm shortening
- Further surgery (removal of hardware/complex arthroplasty)

Preoperative preparation

Preoperative AP and lateral radiographs are used to confirm the degree of slip and plan orientation of the osteotomy. Slings and springs are used preoperatively for three weeks if acute or acute on chronic.

Anaesthesia and positioning

- General anaesthesia
- Intravenous antibiotic prophylaxis
- Supine on radiolucent table
- Image intensifier.

SURGICAL TECHNIQUE

Landmarks and approach

The osteotomy is performed via an anterior approach (see 'Developmental dysplasia of the hip – open reduction', p. 272). Particular care must be taken not to disturb the posterior capsule or forcefully manipulate the slip to preserve vascularity to the femoral head.

PROCEDURE

Following longitudinal capsulotomy, the epiphysis must be correctly identified as the anteriorly displaced neck may be mistaken for it. Two osteotomies are required:

- First, an osteotomy is performed perpendicular to the neck at the level of the physis taking more anteriorly to create a wedge. The aim is to leave a convex surface for later reduction and shorten the neck by 3–4 mm. Over-shortening will lead to instability. Care must also be taken to avoid driving instruments into the posterior capsule, compromising the blood supply.
- Second, an osteotomy is made in the long axis of the neck to remove the bony beak on the side of the slip, again taking care not to breach the posterior capsule. Any remaining callus is

carefully removed with a spoon from the posterior capsule.

Shortening the neck, removing the beak and elevating the posterior capsule allows tension-free reduction of the epiphysis. The epiphysis is reduced onto the neck by placing the leg in flexion, abduction and internal rotation. If insufficient bone has been removed, the epiphysis will not reduce easily and posterior structures will be placed under tension increasing the risk of avascular necrosis. Shortening and wedging of the neck should cause the epiphysis to overlap the neck anteriorly giving a mushroom appearance. Restoration of the Shenton line and a valgus head–neck angle of 20° should be ensured using the image intensifier.

While an assistant maintains position, a lateral stab incision is made according to the predicted trajectory of cannulated screw followed by blunt dissection down to the lateral cortex of the proximal femur. A guidewire is then advanced across the osteotomy to hold the epiphysis. Images are checked in two planes to confirm a satisfactory position before definitive screw insertion. Similar to pinning *in situ*, the entry point should not be below the lesser trochanter and screw tips should be 5 mm short of the articular surface.

Dynamic screening allows confirmation of both a solid fixation and satisfactory positioning of hardware.

Closure

- Layered closure including capsular repair with absorbable material
- Subcuticular absorbable material to skin.

POSTOPERATIVE INSTRUCTIONS

- Bed rest with slings and springs for 5 days.
- Mobilize 15 kg weightbearing 8 weeks. Increase weightbearing status at 8 weeks, after confirming union clinically and radiographically.

RECOMMENDED REFERENCES

Biring GS, Hashemi-Nejad A, Catterall A. Outcomes of subcapital cuneiform osteotomy for the treatment of severe slipped capital femoral epiphysis after skeletal maturity. *J Bone Joint Surg Br* 2006;**88**:1379–84.

Dunn DM, Angel JC. Replacement of the femoral head by open operation in severe adolescent slipping of the upper femoral epiphysis. *J Bone Joint Surg Br* 1978;**60**:394–403.

Fish JB. Cuneiform osteotomy of the femoral neck in the treatment of slipped capital femoral epiphysis. *J Bone Joint Surg Am* 1984;**66**:1153–68.

Loder RT. Unstable slipped capital femoral epiphysis. *J Pediatr Orthop* 2001;**21**:694–9.

TENDO-ACHILLES LENGTHENING

PREOPERATIVE PLANNING

Various methods for tendo-Achilles lengthening (TAL) exist and may be used in conjunction with other procedures. Percutaneous methods such as the Hoke and DAMP (distal anterior, medial proximal, also called a White slide) technique and open methods such as the Baker and Vulpius techniques are described (Figs 16.12–16.14). The choice depends on the cause, the individual patient and the surgeon's preference.

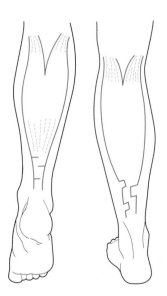

Figure 16.12 *Hoke percutaneous tenotomy*

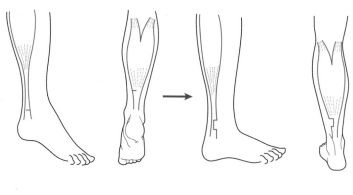

Figure 16.13 *Distal anterior, medial proximal (DAMP) procedure*

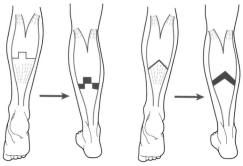

Figure 16.14 *Diagram demonstrating two techniques of gastrocnemius recession. (a) Baker slide (b) Vulpius technique*

Indications

- Fixed equinus deformity, defined as an inability to dorsiflex the ankle sufficiently to allow heel contact without compensation in the remainder of the limb or spine. Often, this correlates with dorsiflexion less than 5° and is seen in various conditions such as cerebral palsy, congenital talipes equinovarus (CTEV), congenital vertical talus, Charcot–Marie–Tooth (CMT), pes planus and intractable toe-walkers
- Failure of conservative treatment
- To achieve stump coverage during Chopart's amputation for congenital malformation of the foot.

Contraindications

- Rigid bony deformity
- Pseudoequinus: a false clinical appearance of equinus caused by plantar flexion of the mid and forefoot (plantaris deformity).

Medical co-morbidity is not a contraindication as percutaneous techniques can be performed under local anaesthesia.

Consent and risks

- The most predictable outcome following TAL is in patients with spastic hemiplegia. The least predictable scenario is seen with percutaneous procedures in patients with diplegia. The two most frequently encountered problems are over-lengthening and recurrence. The former tends to occur following percutaneous procedures on the conjoined tendon whereas recurrence is associated with recession of the gastrocnemius or soleus aponeurosis.
- Neurovascular damage: the sural nerve in particular is at risk
- 1 per cent for percutaneous techniques
- 5 per cent for open techniques
- Plaster immobilization/limited mobility
- Complete tendon rupture (percutaneous)
- Wound problems/infection (open): 1 per cent
- Recurrence (Baker and Vulpius): <5 per cent
- Over-lengthening leading to crouched gait: more likely following percutaneous procedures and associated with uncontrolled lengthening in an older child
- Repeat lengthening: more likely in a younger child and patients with hemiplegia
- Further surgery (hamstring, psoas or selective gastrocnemius lengthening most often required in patients with diplegia)

Preoperative assessment

Silverskiold test under anaesthetic differentiates between pure gastrocnemius tightness (increased ankle dorsiflexion with knee flexion) and combined tightness of gastrocnemius and soleus (limited dorsiflexion in knee flexion and extension).

Anaesthesia and positioning

- General anaesthesia or local anaesthesia for percutaneous techniques
- Prone for open or supine for percutaneous techniques
- High pneumatic thigh tourniquet.

SURGICAL TECHNIQUE

Percutaneous techniques

Both Hoke and DAMP procedures are used to treat combined gastrocnemius–soleus tightness. The advantages are improved healing and the option of local anaesthesia. However, these techniques are associated with an increased incidence of over-lengthening and inadvertent complete tenotomy.

Hoke technique

Structures at risk

- Tibial nerve – at risk proximally
- Sural nerve – laterally
- Flexor hallucis longus muscle – distally

Three points are marked on the tendo-Achilles at 1 cm, 3 cm and 6 cm from its calcaneal insertion. A no. 15 blade scalpel is inserted longitudinally in the midline of the tendon at each marked level then turned through 90° in the desired direction to perform the hemisection while the ankle is dorsiflexed to control the correction. The hemisections are performed on the medial half proximally and distally and the lateral half in the middle incision (see Fig. 16.12, p. 281).

DAMP technique

Two 1.5 cm skin incisions are made postero-medially, one 2 cm from the calcaneal insertion and another 5 cm proximal to it. The anterior two-thirds of the tendon is divided distally and the medial half to two-thirds proximally. (This is because of the 90° rotation of tendon fibres in the distal third of the leg.)

The tendon is divided progressively while tensioning the tendo-Achilles until it yields 5–10° of dorsiflexion. The medial fibres slide over the lateral fibres, giving length in continuity with a thinned portion of tendon distally and a square cut proximally (see Fig. 16.13, p. 282).

OPEN TECHNIQUES

These have the advantage of controlled lengthening but carry a greater risk of recurrence.

Incision

Structures at risk

- Sural nerve
- Short saphenous vein

A 7 cm longitudinal incision is made, 10 cm proximal to the calcaneal insertion positioned 1 cm medial to the midline to avoid the sural nerve.

Dissection

The sural nerve and short saphenous vein are retracted if encountered or may be avoided altogether by raising a full thickness lateral flap. The paratenon is incised longitudinally in the midline to avoid the skin incision, and the medial and lateral edges of the gastrocnemius aponeurosis are exposed.

BAKER SLIDE PROCEDURE

Although considered a selective gastrocnemius lengthening, fibres of the soleus aponeurosis are also incised distally. However, this does not lead to over-lengthening as seen in procedures on the conjoined tendon owing to controlled lengthening and inherent stability.

The medial and lateral thirds of the aponeurosis are incised transversely 12 cm above the calcaneal insertion. A similar incision is then performed across the middle third at least 3 cm proximally to allow side to side contact after lengthening. A tongue and groove pattern is created by joining the proximal and distal cuts with two longitudinal incisions (see Fig. 16.14, p. 282). Dorsiflexion of the ankle allows slide-lengthening of the aponeurosis and reveals any remaining fibres which require incision.

The underlying muscle fibres of soleus are revealed as the aponeurosis is lengthened. Further lengthening should not be performed once 10° of dorsiflexion is achieved on the table, and 3/0 absorbable sutures are placed across the longitudinal portions of the aponeurosis.

VULPIUS PROCEDURE

This is used to treat combined gastrocnemius-soleus tightness when plaster immobilization is not desirable. Instead of a tongue and groove lengthening, an inverted 'V' incision is made in the aponeurosis of both the gastrocnemius and the soleus (see Fig. 16.14, p. 282).

Closure

- Tension-free layered closure with buried knots to avoid skin irritation.
- Subcuticular absorbable material to skin.

With the exception of the Vulpius technique, a below knee plaster is applied in a plantigrade position. A dorsiflexed position must be avoided to prevent a calcaneus deformity.

POSTOPERATIVE INSTRUCTIONS

Mobilize weightbearing as tolerated in cast for four weeks if used. Convert to night-time splint at four weeks and continue for six months. Use guided physiotherapy to maintain position and prevent recurrence.

RECOMMENDED REFERENCES

Baker LD. Surgical needs of the cerebral palsy patient. *J Bone Joint Surg Am* 1956;**38**:313–23.

Borton DC, Walker K, Pirpiris M, *et al.* Isolated calf lengthening in cerebral palsy. *J Bone Joint Surg Br* 2001;**83**:364–70.

Graham HK, Fixsen JA. Lengthening of the calcaneal tendon in spastic hemiplegia by the white slide technique. *J Bone Joint Surg Br* 1988;**70**:472–5.

CONGENITAL TALIPES EQUINOVARUS CORRECTION

PONSETI TECHNIQUE

Preoperative planning

Indications

Flexible CTEV.

Contraindications

- Rigid clubfoot
- Age over 7 years is a relative contraindication as results are notably worse.

Consent and risks

- Neurovascular injury (any open procedure)
- Complete Achilles tenotomy
- Plaster impingement/skin ulceration
- Infection (open procedures)
- Stiffness
- Recurrent deformity: long-term splintage required
- Deformity due to incorrect or incomplete correction, overcorrection or recurrence, e.g. cavus, rocker-bottom, longitudinal breach, flattening and lateral rotation of talus
- 1 cm limb shortening, 2 cm decreased calf girth and smaller shoe by 1 or 1/2 sizes are common sequelae

Do not expect a completely normal foot; although the Ponseti technique yields good clinical results, foot malformations still exist and can be seen radiographically.

Operative planning

The deformity can be graded using various methods. Dimeglio suggests a 20-point scoring system with four grades of severity which correlates with an increasing resistance to correction. The Pirani score helps to predict the need for Achilles tenotomy and is based upon the severity of deformity in the midfoot and hindfoot with a total maximum score of 6. Eighty-five per cent of patients with scores over 5 will require tenotomy.

Anaesthesia and positioning

No anaesthesia or sedation required unless the patient is extremely uncooperative. An assistant is essential.

Surgical technique

Casting is performed weekly, correcting all three components of the deformity in a predetermined sequence prior to additional operative procedures. At least three toe to groin casts are required over a period of 7–10 weeks depending on the severity of deformity.

Castings

- *Cavus:* caused by a relative pronation of the forefoot due to a plantar flexed first ray. The first ray is elevated with pressure beneath the first metatarsal head to supinate the forefoot and align it with the varus hindfoot. Forced pronation of the foot is avoided as this will worsen the cavus.
- *Varus and adductus:* Correction of the abnormally internally rotated calcaneus is achieved by external rotation using the lateral talar head as the fulcrum. The cuboid and anterior calcaneus are displaced laterally by applying medial pressure to the navicular anterior to the ankle and pushing the posterior calcaneus medially by lateral pressure posterior to the ankle, ensuring the talar head does not externally rotate. In severe cases, the navicular may not fully reduce although abduction of the cuneiforms more distally will allow correction and the navicular–cuneiform joints will remodel. Once the calcaneocuboid alignment is restored with the anterior calcaneus lateralized, correction of varus can be achieved. The cast must be toe to groin with the knee in 90° of flexion to maintain abduction and external rotation. This will also treat any

associated internal tibial torsion if present. Midfoot pronation must again be avoided to prevent cavus deformity and a midfoot breach.
- *Equinus:* With the hindfoot varus corrected, serial casts are applied in a progressively dorsiflexed position. This usually requires two to three casts to achieve 15° of dorsiflexion and 60° of external rotation. Dorsiflexion is achieved via pressure beneath the midfoot rather than the metatarsals to avoid rocker-bottom feet.

Additional procedures

Tendo-Achilles lengthening: If dorsiflexion of 15° is not achieved, then a percutaneous tenotomy under local anaesthesia is indicated. This is preferable to posterior ankle and subtalar capsulotomy as contraction of scar tissue in this region will lead to progressive loss of dorsiflexion.

Lateral transfer of the tibialis anterior tendon to the lateral cuneiform may be required for persistent supination.

Postoperative care and instructions

The final cast is left *in situ* for three weeks then assessment made for residual equinus; 90 per cent of patients will require Achilles tenotomy.

Denis Browne boots are worn fulltime for 2–3 months then at night only for 2–4 years or until age 7. These maintain 15° of dorsiflexion (to avoid equinus) and 60° external rotation (to prevent varus, adductus and in-toeing). High-top shoes are worn during the day to maintain position.

Periodic evaluation should be performed by an experienced clinician to assess the relationship between the hindfoot and forefoot, the attitude of the heel, and range of ankle motion. Anteroposterior and lateral radiographs should also be obtained.

EXTENSIVE SOFT TISSUE RELEASE VIA THE CINCINNATI INCISION

Preoperative planning

Indications

- Failed Ponseti treatment: 50 per cent may relapse at an average age of 2.5 years.

Remanipulation and casting with or without Achilles tenotomy followed by splintage may be successful although extensive soft tissue releases are required in resistant cases

- Rigid clubfoot
- Walking on lateral border of foot/internally rotated gait
- Posteriorly placed lateral malleolus (a reflection of uncorrected internal calcaneal rotation)
- Parallelism of talus and calcaneus on AP and lateral radiographs.

Contraindications

Previous releases via alternative incisions.

Consent and risks

- Neurovascular damage: see below
- Plaster immobilization/impaired mobility/long-term splintage
- Residual deformity
- Recurrence and further surgery
- Wound irritation over the Achilles tendon, particularly rubbing on shoes
- Avascular necrosis of the talus
- Arthritis of the hindfoot and midfoot
- Ankle and subtalar stiffness

Preoperative assessment

- AP and lateral radiographs required for assessing the talocalcaneal angle.
- Dimeglio and Pirani scores.

Anaesthesia and positioning

General anaesthesia is used with addition of an intravenous prophylactic antibiotic. The patient is positioned prone with a high thigh tourniquet.

Surgical technique

Landmarks

The base of the first metatarsal, medial malleolus and lateral malleolus is palpable.

Incision (the Cincinnati incision)

An 8–9 cm extensile, transverse incision across the posterior ankle (at the level of the tibio-talar joint) is created. This begins at the base of the first metatarsal, curves below the medial malleolus, rises slightly to traverse the Achilles tendon and continues over the lateral malleolus to terminate distal and medial to the sinus tarsi.

Superficial dissection

Structures at risk

- Sural nerve laterally
- Superficial venous structures below the lateral malleolus

The proximal subcutaneous flap is raised off underlying tissues for around 3 cm to allow proximal visualization.

Deep dissection

Structures at risk

- Posterior tibial nerve and vessels
- Deep tibiotalar portion of the deltoid ligament
- Medial and lateral plantar nerves

This begins laterally with incision of the calcaneofibular ligament and superior peroneal ligament to allow dissection of the peronei off the calcaneus without damaging them. The lateral talocalcaneal ligament and lateral capsule of subtalar joint are then released. The posterior tibial neurovascular bundle is retracted anteriorly to allow further release of the posterior ankle and subtalar capsule and the posterior talofibular ligament. Subsequent posterior retraction of the tibial neurovascular bundle allows division of the superficial tibiocalcaneal part of deltoid. The deep portion of the tibiotalar portion of the deltoid ligament is left intact to prevent excessive subtalar translation and flat foot deformity.

The tibialis posterior tendon sheath is opened along its length from above the medial malleolus to the navicular to allow Z-lengthening of the tendon at least 2.5 cm proximal to the medial malleolus. The nearby posterior tibial neurovascular bundle is protected to avoid its transection.

Dissection continues medially, into the arch of the foot, to release the lacinate ligament, the plantar aponeurosis and small plantar muscles, including abductor hallucis. Beneath the navicular, the master knot of Henry (intersection of the flexor hallucis longus [FHL] and flexor digitorum longus [FDL]) is taken down, taking care not to damage the medial and lateral plantar nerves either side of it. The sheaths of the FDL and FHL are opened and tendon Z-lengthening performed to prevent flexion contracture of the toes when the ankle is dorsiflexed. This is done sufficiently proximally to allow the lengthened portions to be covered by tendon sheath. Conjoint lengthening is an alternative if the tendons are too small to perform Z-lengthening. This step may be unnecessary as toe contractures will often stretch out over time.

The talonavicular joint is freed to mobilize the navicular laterally and releasing all of its attachments; keeping hold of it via the distal end of tibialis posterior tendon will avoid handling the articular cartilage. The dorsal talonavicular ligament and the spring ligament can then be released. Release of the bifurcate ligament and the talocalcaneal interosseous ligament will allow external rotation of the anterior calcaneus.

Finally, the quadratus plantae is stripped off the calcaneus to release the long plantar ligament, the plantar calcaneocuboid ligament and inferior medial capsule of the calcaneocuboid joint without damaging the peroneus longus tendon. The extensive soft tissue releases should result in the plane of the foot being at 90° to the bimalleolar axis with the talus beneath the tibia and slight hindfoot valgus. If the mortise is not fully reduced, tibiofibular ligament release then tibiofibular syndesmosis release can be carried out if the talus is too wide anteriorly. Stabilization with K-wires is the final stage, one passing along the medial column to hold the talonavicular joint and one across the lateral column to hold the calcaneocuboid joint.

Closure

Tendon sheaths over all over-lengthened tendons are closed. The medial and lateral extensions of the Cincinnati incision are closed, without tension, using absorbable sutures to the subcutaneous and subcuticular layers. The posterior, central portion of the wound is left open to heal by secondary intention. If blanching of wound edges following tourniquet release is noted, position in less dorsiflexion.

Apply plaster of Paris from the toes to the mid-thigh with a neutral or slightly plantar flexed foot and the knee flexed to 90°.

Postoperative care and instructions

The cast is changed at 10 days after surgery, to inspect wound. It is removed, along with the K-wires, at 6 weeks. Denis Browne boots are prescribed for the next 12–18 months.

Physiotherapy (for mobility, to promote tarsal growth and preserve cartilage) is continued for at least 6 months.

RECOMMENDED REFERENCES

Ponseti I. *Congenital Clubfoot: Fundamentals of Treatment*. USA: Oxford University Press, 1996.

Crawford AH, Marxen JL, Osterfield DL. The Cincinnati incision: a comprehensive approach for surgical procedures of the foot and ankle in childhood. *J Bone Joint Surg Am* 1982;**84**:1355–8.

Dimeglio A, Benshahel H, Souchet P, *et al*. Classification of clubfoot. *J Pediatr Orthop B* 1995;**4**:129–36.

McKay DW. New concept of and approach to clubfoot treatment: section II – correction of the clubfoot. *J Pediatr Orthop* 1983;**3**:10–21.

Pirani J, Outerbridge HK, Sawatzky B, *et al*. A reliable method of clinically evaluating a virgin clubfoot. 21st World Congress of SICOT, Sydney, Australia, 18–23 April, 1999.

SURGICAL TREATMENT OF PERTHES DISEASE

Perthes disease occurs as a result of a temporary cessation in the blood supply to the femoral head leading to avascular necrosis. It is commonly seen between the ages of 4 and 8 years although should be suspected from 2 to 12 years of age. Although more common in boys by a factor of four, it may be more severe in girls.

Presenting symptoms comprise hip or referred knee pain, stiffness, limping and a short leg. The disease progresses through the four phases of ischaemia (causing collapse and sclerosis), fragmentation, reossification and remodelling, which take place over a 4-year period.

However, development of the hip is frequently abnormal leading to incongruency, altered biomechanics and accelerated secondary degeneration. Prognosis is dependent on age and severity of disease at presentation, and treatment falls into the three broad categories of observation, containment and salvage, depending also on the phase of disease.

PREOPERATIVE PLANNING

Indications

The type of treatment largely depends upon the capacity to remodel and therefore age. Below the age of 6 years, there is high potential for remodelling and therapy therefore tends to be conservative. Above 8 years, further remodelling is limited and treatment is more aggressive in order to correct deformity and extend the longevity of the native hip.

Between the ages of 6 and 8 years, the indications for either a conservative approach or containment procedures depend upon bone age and remodelling potential, the presence of 'at-risk' signs for the viability of the femoral head and whether the hip is congruent or containable. The surgical options for containable hips are a varus osteotomy of the proximal femur and/or a Salter type pelvic osteotomy.

Salvage procedures are indicated if hinge abduction occurs (Fig. 16.15), where the overgrown and uncontained anterolateral portion of the femoral head abuts the lateral rim of the acetabulum. In this situation valgus extension osteotomy (VGEO) of the proximal femur is indicated, which will medialize the centre of rotation of the hip and make it congruent in the weightbearing position. The medial column must be of sufficient height after reossification and a better outcome is expected in younger patients where the triradiate cartilage remains open. This will allow deformity correction, a better functional range of movement, improvement of leg length and abductor function.

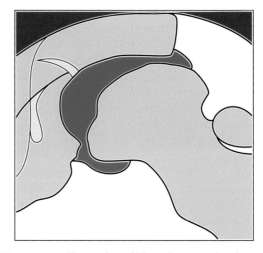

Figure 16.15 *Illustration of hip arthrogram showing hinge abduction, where dye pools medially in abduction*

Contraindications

Containment procedures are contraindicated if hips are not congruent or containable.

Consent and risks

The natural history of the disease must be explained to the child and parents. It should be emphasized that the aim is to improve symptoms and to achieve a spherical and contained femoral head to maximize and prolong native joint function. However, secondary degenerative changes may continue to occur at an unpredictable and accelerated rate ultimately leading to total joint arthroplasty or arthrodesis.

- An older presentation, particularly in girls, is associated with a worse outcome
- Stiffness/contractures
- Other risks pertain to the type of procedure being performed. See the relevant sections on DDH for the risks associated with pelvic and femoral osteotomies

Operative planning

Various classification systems exist to guide treatment and predict the prognosis of Perthes disease.

Catterall grouped patients as I–IV, although large intra- and inter-observer error has been shown with this method. The Herring classification correlates with prognosis according to the degree of collapse of the lateral capital femoral epiphysis during the fragmentation phase using the AP radiograph of the pelvis.

The Stulberg classification (1–5) is made during the reossification phase and predicts the end result of Perthes dependent on the relative shapes of the femoral head and acetabulum. Increasing grade correlates with the likelihood of secondary osteoarthritis with Stulberg 5 hips likely to require total hip replacement before age 50 years.

Head at risk signs include Gage's sign (a lytic 'rat bite' at the periphery of the physis), calcification lateral to the epiphysis, lateral subluxation of the femoral head and horizontal inclination of the physis.

Arthrography will determine the congruency of the hip in various positions and whether an appropriate range of movement is possible to perform the relevant femoral osteotomy (Fig. 16.15). Significant abduction is required for a varus osteotomy and adduction for a valgus osteotomy.

Anaesthesia and positioning

- General anaesthesia
- Supine
- Intravenous prophylactic antibiotics.

SURGICAL TECHNIQUE

- For varus osteotomy, the technique as described in the section 'Developmental dysplasia of the hip – femoral osteotomy' (p. 276) is used, employing the derotation component if required.
- For valgus osteotomy, a similar technique is used as for varus osteotomy, the difference being the orientation of the osteotomy to give a laterally based wedge to achieve the desired realignment.
- Pelvic osteotomy – see 'Salter osteotomy' (p. 273).

POSTOPERATIVE INSTRUCTIONS

As per the type of procedure performed. Regular periodic clinical and radiographic review is required to determine the presence of deterioration and the need for further surgery.

RECOMMENDED REFERENCES

Bankes MJK, Catterall A, Hashemi-Nejad A. Valgus extension osteotomy for 'hinge abduction' in Perthes disease: results at maturity and factors influencing the radiological outcome. *J Bone Joint Surg Br* 2000;**82**:548–54.
Catterall A. The natural history of Perthes disease. *J Bone Joint Surg Br* 1971;**53**:37–53.
Coates CJ, Paterson JMH, Catterall A, *et al.* Femoral osteotomy in Perthes disease. Results at maturity. *J Bone Joint Surg Br* 1990;**72**:581–5.
Herring JA, Kim HT, Browne R. Legg–Calvé–Perthes disease. Part I: classification of radiographs with use of the modified lateral pillar and Stulberg classifications. *J Bone Joint Surg Am* 2004;**86**:2103–20.
Herring JA, Kim HT, Browne R. Legg–Calvé–Perthes disease. Part II: prospective multicentre study of the effect of treatment on outcome. *J Bone Joint Surg Am* 2004;**86**:2121–34.

PRINCIPLES OF SURGERY IN CEREBRAL PALSY

PREOPERATIVE PLANNING

Cerebral palsy results from an insult to the immature brain and its effects are variable. It may be classified anatomically (hemiplegic, diplegic or total body involvement) or physiologically (spastic, athetoid, ataxic or mixed). The spastic form is most common; a combination of muscle weakness and spasticity leads to a progressive sequence of dynamic deformity, fixed contractures, bony deformity and joint subluxation or dislocation. Depending on the severity, intervention may be indicated at any point during this continuum to optimize energy consumption during gait, to perform activities of daily living, to facilitate standing or seated transfer and to maintain hygiene. Maximum function requires a straight spine over a level pelvis, congruent, mobile hips, mobile knees and plantigrade feet.

Cerebral palsy is typically treated in one of three phases:
- Dynamic contractures – casting and/or botulinum toxin (BTX) injection
- Fixed contractures – muscle balancing techniques such as releases, lengthening and transfers
- Bony deformity and joint incongruence – osteotomies.

Decisions around timing of surgery are difficult. Allowing maturation will improve certainty about the gait pattern and reduce the risk of recurrent deformity at the price of an increased chance of fixed deformities and multilevel operations being required. Surgery in the younger child may be less technically demanding but can lead to repeat surgery year on year. In addition, single level operations may reveal further problems: a common example is a crouched gait occurring after Achilles tendon release due to unrecognized, concomitant tight hamstrings. Throughout all stages physiotherapy helps to reduce fixed deformity and occupational therapy can adapt equipment to accommodate existing deformity.

SURGICAL TECHNIQUES IN MUSCLE CONTRACTURES

Botulinum toxin A injections

Botulinum toxin A inhibits the release of acetylcholine from the nerve terminal at the neuromuscular junction, causing decreased muscle activity in a dose-dependent manner. It may be administered under local or general anaesthesia or sedation. It should be placed deep to the muscle fascia in a dose appropriate for the patient and the number of injection sites required. The injection volume must be sufficient to allow diffusion to end-plate zones which may be scattered, particularly in the sartorius and gracilis.

Localize injection sites using palpation and anatomical knowledge; accuracy is improved with electrical stimulation or ultrasound guidance. Combine injection with casting, orthoses and guided physiotherapy to maximize the benefits.

Contraindications

- Myasthenia gravis

- Aminoglycoside antibiosis
- Non-depolarizing muscle relaxants
- Pseudobulbar palsy
- Gastro-oesophageal reflux or frequent chest infections.

Consent and risks

- Local: pain, temporary weakness in adjacent muscles
- General: mild generalized weakness, urinary incontinence, constipation, dysphagia and aspiration pneumonia

Parents and patients should be warned of its temporary effect of 12–16 weeks and the risk of recurrence and further procedures.

SURGICAL TECHNIQUE

Muscle balancing techniques

Adductor psoas and gracilis release is commonly indicated for the classic flexion adduction contracture and scissoring gait seen in cerebral palsy. Muscle imbalance combined with infrequent weightbearing causes structural changes at the hip (increased anteversion, posterolateral acetabular dysplasia) leading to posterolateral migration, pelvic obliquity and scoliosis. This is more commonly seen in quadriplegic patients and releases are performed early (3–4 years) to prevent deterioration. Muscles should be released sequentially during the procedure and performed bilaterally to prevent a windswept deformity. Releases are also commonly combined with proximal varus femoral osteotomy at age 5.

Hamstrings may be released proximally or distally to improve flexion contracture at the knee. Equinus deformity at the ankle is very common and is treated with tendo-Achilles release (see p. 281 for details). Knee and ankle releases are performed in a walking child between 4 and 6 years old.

Another common problem is the thumb in hand deformity treated with adductor pollicis release and is performed in the older child. Tendon transfers such as tibialis anterior or tibialis posterior are often used in balancing the foot in combination with bony surgery.

OSTEOTOMY AND JOINT CONTAINMENT

Hip containment

Quadriplegic patients should be monitored regularly for hip subluxation and dislocation, which tends to occur between 18 months and 6 years. Hips at risk are those with limited abduction with uncovering of <50 per cent on radiography. At-risk hips may be treated with adductor, psoas and hamstring release although a more aggressive approach may be considered. Subluxed hips (>50 per cent uncovered) are treated with soft tissue releases and varus proximal femoral osteotomy.

Early dislocated hips may be treated with open reduction; however, this may not be possible and poor conformity between the head and acetabulum may lead to early failure. A varus derotational osteotomy with soft tissue releases and/or shortening may be more appropriate. This can be combined with pelvic osteotomy.

Late dislocations require either resurfacing or total joint arthroplasty; a large articulation is preferred to confer stability. Alternatively, a Girdlestone excision arthroplasty may be considered.

Triple arthrodesis of the ankle

Various foot and ankle deformities are seen in cerebral palsy such as planovalgus, equinovalgus, equinovarus and calcaneovalgus. Triple arthrodesis is indicated for symptomatic degeneration and uncontrolled deformity. Despite frequent complications such as residual deformity, pseudarthrosis, pain and progressive intertarsal and tarsometatarsal arthritis, the response to surgery is good.

Scoliosis surgery

Scoliosis is more common in quadriplegic and non-ambulatory diplegic patients. The risk of progression is related to age at presentation and hip problems. Curves are likely to reach 50° if present by age 5. Bracing is seldom preventive. Nutrition must be optimized preoperatively and patients must be monitored closely postoperatively for respiratory complications.

Indications for surgery are curves >40° or progression >10° per annum. Ambulatory patients receive posterior fusion whereas non-ambulatory patients require additional anterior fusion and pelvic fixation.

RECOMMENDED REFERENCES

Gage JR. *The Treatment of Gait Problems in Cerebral Palsy*. Cambridge: Cambridge University Press, 2004.

McCarthy JJ, D'andrea LP, Betz RR, *et al*. Scoliosis in the child with cerebral palsy. *J Am Acad Orthop Surg* 2006;**14**:367–75.

Owers KL, Pyman J, Gargan MF, *et al*. Bilateral hip surgery in severe cerebral palsy. *J Bone Joint Surg Br* 2001;**83**:1161–7.

Ramachandran M, Eastwood DM. Botulinum toxin and its orthopaedic applications. *J Bone Joint Surg Br* 2006;**88**:981–87.

Skoff H, Woodbury DF. Management of the upper extremity in cerebral palsy. *J Bone Joint Surg Am* 1985;**67**:500–3.

Viva questions

1. What are the clinical signs of hip instability in the newborn?

2. What are Hilgenreiner and Perkins lines and what is their relevance?

3. What are the relative advantages and disadvantages of the anterior and medial approaches to the paediatric hip in developmental dysplasia of the hip?

4. Describe the Smith–Petersen approach to the paediatric hip?

5. What are the indications for varus proximal femoral osteotomy in developmental dysplasia of the hip?

6. How does a varus proximal femoral osteotomy affect range of hip movement and leg lengths?

7. What structures are at risk during a Salter pelvic osteotomy?

8. What are the indications and contraindications of the Pemberton pelvic osteotomy?

9. What is the ideal screw position when pinning a slipped upper femoral epiphysis? What risks are associated with this procedure?

10. What are the indications for prophylactic pinning of the contralateral hip in slipped upper femoral epiphysis?

11. How does the blood supply to the femoral head change throughout childhood?

12. What are the treatment options for avascular necrosis following slipped upper femoral epiphysis?

13. What is your approach to the treatment of Perthes disease in a 7-year-old child?

14. What classification systems do you know for grading the severity and predicting the prognosis of Perthes disease?

15. What are the component deformities of club foot and which structures are tight?

16. Which structures are at risk during extensive soft tissue release of congenital talipes equinovarus via the Cincinnati approach?

17. How would you distinguish between a tight tendo-Achilles complex and gastrocnemius tightness?

18. What methods can you describe to determine when epiphysiodesis should be performed?

19. How much growth per year can be expected from each of the four main physes in the lower extremity in adolescence?

20. What is your approach to the orthopaedic assessment and treatment of the child with cerebral palsy?

Amputations

William Aston and Rob Pollock

Ideal amputation stump lengths, including the shortest and longest to allow adequate prosthetic fitting and the increased energy expenditure by level

Amputation	Ideal level – shortest (S)/longest (L)	Increased energy expenditure
Transradial	Proximal 2/3 – distal 1/3 junction S – 3 cm distal to biceps insertion L – 5 cm above wrist joint	*Not applicable*
Transhumeral	Middle 1/3 of humerus S – 4 cm below axillary fold L – 10 cm above olecranon	*Not applicable*
Transfemoral	Middle 1/3 of femur S – 8 cm below pubic ramus L – 15 cm above medial joint line	*65 per cent*
Transtibial	8 cm for every 1 m of height S – 7.5 cm below medial joint line L – Allow adequate soft tissue coverage	*25 per cent*

ABOVE KNEE AMPUTATION

PREOPERATIVE PLANNING

Indications

'Dead, dangerous or damn nuisance' (Apley). This essentially means that if a limb is not viable due to disease or trauma, a danger to the patient due to infection, crush injury or tumour, or non-functional as a result of a congenital abnormality or trauma and not amenable to other treatment modalities, then amputation should be considered.

Indications by percentage are:

- Peripheral vascular disease – 55 per cent

- Diabetes – 25 per cent
- Trauma – 10 per cent
- Tumour – 5 per cent
- Infection/congenital – 5 per cent.

Contraindications

Inability to gain consent in a well-orientated patient in time, place and person.

Consent and risks

- Neurological pain
- Phantom limb sensation
- Flap demarcation and necrosis necessitating stump revision or vac pump application

- Dermatological problems related to the scar and the skin–prosthesis interface
- Problems with prosthetic fitting related to the size/shape/length of the stump and the associated soft tissues
- Joint contractures
- Choke syndrome: venous outflow obstruction in the distal part of the stump due to prosthetic constriction

Operative planning

Anteroposterior and lateral radiographs are used for templating to determine the necessary bone resection level and clinical examination is vital to plan satisfactory soft tissue closure with skin that is sensate and that will heal normally. A **priority is adequate blood supply to the soft tissues** to enable this. Ideal and minimal resection levels should be taken into account (see p. 293). Flap lengths and their positioning, may have to be altered to accommodate skin problems or tumour excision. By doing this it may be possible to prevent a more proximal amputation.

Anaesthesia and positioning

General anaesthesia is used, with the patient positioned supine. There is some evidence to suggest (and is the authors' preference) that epidural anaesthesia, local anaesthetic infiltration of the nerves prior to transection and good analgesia in the immediate postoperative period, is effective in reducing the significant problem of postoperative neurological pain.

If a tourniquet can be used in the non-ischaemic limb then it should, but must be deflated prior to wound closure to ensure that adequate haemostasis has been achieved. A tourniquet should not be used in an ischaemic limb.

SURGICAL TECHNIQUE

Landmarks and incision

The bone transection point is marked as per planning/templating. Equal anterior and posterior flaps are marked on the thigh, with their apices at

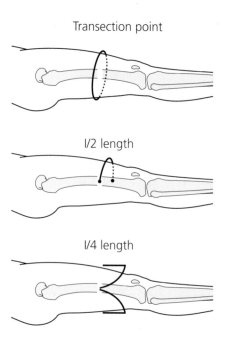

Figure 17.1 *Amputation flap marking for equal anterior and posterior flaps. (a) Measurement of circumference of limb at bony transection point with a suture – length. (b) Marking medial and lateral apices. (c) Marking extent at flaps*

the midpoint medially and laterally, at the level of anticipated bony transection. The **lengths of the flaps combined must be greater than the width of the limb**.

An easy way to do this (Fig. 17.1) is to pass a suture length around the limb at the level of transection. This length is then halved and placed around the anterior portion of the thigh at the transection level, then mark the medial and lateral apices of the flaps at the ends of the suture. The suture is then halved in length again and measured distally from the transection point in the midline anteriorly and posteriorly to mark the maximal extent of the flaps. By marking a quadrant of a circle between each of these four points, two semicircular flaps of correct length are drawn onto the anterior and posterior aspects of the leg.

Superficial dissection

The incision follows the line as marked vertically down through the skin, subcutaneous fat and through the deep fascia to form the skin flaps. At all times careful soft tissue handling techniques should be used.

Deep dissection

The quadriceps muscle is divided, straight down to bone, in the line of the incision. The femoral canal is identified medial to the femur and the artery and vein ligated within it. These should be **double tied proximally and if necessary a transfixion suture used**. The periosteum is incised at the level of resection and the femur transected using a saw, ensuring protection of the soft tissues. A rasp is used to smooth the sharp edges of the cut bone and prevent high pressure areas in the stump. The sciatic nerve is identified and transected, with a sharp blade under gentle traction, so that the end retracts proximally. Any cutaneous nerves encountered should also be transected in a similar fashion. The sciatic nerve has a significant artery running within it and therefore should be ligated, but this is not necessary for other nerves. The hamstring compartment is divided and the leg removed. The wound should be washed thoroughly and the tourniquet released to ensure adequate haemostasis.

Assessment of the flaps is carried out and any necessary trimming of muscle. In a non-ischaemic limb the quadriceps and the hamstrings can be sutured (myodesis) through drill holes, to the bone, under slight tension. The deep muscle fascia is sutured together over the end of the bone (Fig. 17.2). A drain is inserted and the superficial fascial, fat and skin layers closed separately. The skin can be closed with absorbable or non absorbable sutures as tissue healing should be normal.

In the ischaemic limb care should be taken to keep the skin and muscle flap as one myocutaneous flap and any tension on the tissues should be avoided, due to potential compromise of the vascular supply and therefore myodesis should not be used. Instead the muscle can simply be sutured to the periosteum (myoplasty) or the deep fascial layers of the muscle masses be sutured together over the end of the bone. Drain insertion and layered closure is as above, except the skin should be closed under no tension and interrupted non-absorbable sutures used.

A suitable stump dressing should be securely applied, and this should remain in place for the first 5 days.

Technical aspects of procedure

In order to avoid large amounts of redundant soft tissue the muscle flaps and skin flaps should be debrided as appropriate. However, a cylindrical, soft, well-padded soft tissue mass over the stump is desirable. In some cases, such as when atypical flaps are used, the stump may be left large on purpose to allow for possible skin demarcation and the potential for refashioning and closure. To avoid large dog-ears a stepwise approach to closing the flaps is advised, starting by opposing

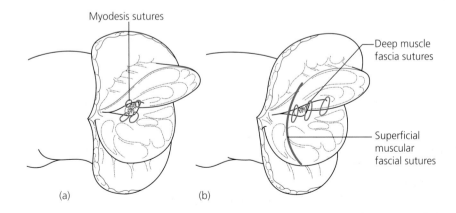

Figure 17.2 *Femoral amputation stump – closure in layers. (a) myodesis sutures to bone. (b) Muscle fascial layer closure*

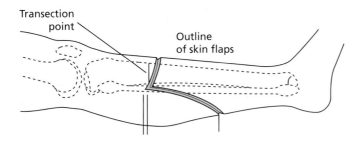

Figure 17.3 *Tibial – long posterior flap*

the middle of the flaps and subsequently halving the distance between sutures for each layer. Scars placed directly over bony prominences with little or no intervening soft tissue must be avoided as it will lead to scar adherence to the bone and skin breakdown.

Closure

As described above.

POSTOPERATIVE CARE AND INSTRUCTIONS

- The drain is taken out when there is minimal drainage, typically 48–72 hours.
- Dressings to be changed, under aseptic precautions at 3–5 days, looking specifically for signs of infection or skin flap demarcation.
- Specialist physiotherapy referral for stump bandaging and rehabilitation should be made preoperatively and start as soon as the wound is satisfactory.
- Prosthetic referral can also be made preoperatively or postoperatively if appropriate.
- Definitive prosthetic fitting is often 4–6 months after surgery, when the stump has matured.
- A temporary prosthesis can be used within a week of surgery.

BELOW KNEE AMPUTATION

PREOPERATIVE PLANNING

Similar principles as for above knee amputation with specific reference to the ideal stump lengths set out above (see p. 293).

SURGICAL TECHNIQUE

Landmarks and incision

In the non-ischaemic limb, equal flaps are marked out in a similar way to above knee amputation; in the ischaemic limb a long posterior flap (Fig. 17.3) is used as the posterior blood supply is significantly better.

Superficial dissection

As for above knee amputation.

Deep dissection

Generally as for above knee amputation. The anterior tibial artery and vein are encountered, with the deep peroneal nerve in the anterior compartment, the superficial peroneal nerve in the lateral compartment and the posterior tibial and peroneal artery and veins with the tibial nerve in the deep posterior compartment. Nerves and vessels should be ligated and/or transacted as for above knee amputation.

Technical aspects of procedure

The same rules regarding soft tissue reconstruction and closure apply in the ischaemic and non-ischaemic limb as for above knee amputation.

The fibula should be transacted obliquely approximately 2 cm proximal to the tibial transection and the ends smoothed.

Closure

As for above knee amputation.

POSTOPERATIVE INSTRUCTIONS

As for above knee amputation.

COMPLICATIONS

As for above knee amputation.

LESSER TOE AMPUTATION

PREOPERATIVE PLANNING

Similar principles as for above knee amputation.

SURGICAL TECHNIQUE

Landmarks and incision

For an amputation at the base of the toe/proximal phalanx a tennis racquet incision can be used (Fig. 17.4). More distally the principle of a short dorsal and longer plantar flap is applied.

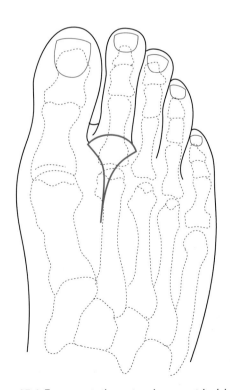

Figure 17.4 *Toe amputation – tennis racquet incision*

Dissection

Full thickness myocutaneous flaps are created, down to periosteum. Division of the flexor and extensor tendons allows them to retract proximally. The neurovascular bundles are sought to allow transection of stretched digital nerves and tying off of the vessels. The bone is transected and smoothed off with a rasp. Care must be taken with closure of the muscle and fascia over the stump.

Technical aspects of procedure

When amputating the second toe it is best to try to leave as much of the proximal phalanx as possible to avoid drift of the hallux into valgus.

Hallux amputation

As for lesser toe except a posteromedially based flap is used to swing into the defect.

Closure

Interrupted non-absorbable sutures.

POSTOPERATIVE INSTRUCTIONS

Dressings are changed, with aseptic precautions, at 3–5 days, looking specifically for signs of infection or skin flap demarcation.

FOOT/RAY AMPUTATIONS

PREOPERATIVE PLANNING

Similar principles as for above knee amputation.

SURGICAL TECHNIQUE – DEPENDENT ON TYPE/LEVEL OF AMPUTATION

Border ray amputation – first or fifth ray

Landmarks and incision

A tennis racquet incision is used, based on the metatarsal (Fig. 17.5). With the proximal extent of the incision coming up to the level of the tarsometatarsal joint.

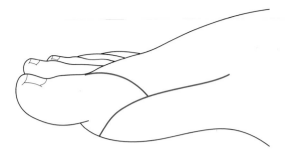

Figure 17.5 *Tennis racquet incision for excision of first ray*

Dissection

Create one full thickness flap, down to bone, to prevent devascularization of the flap. Once the bone has been reached, subperiosteal dissection continues. The bone is transected, at the base of the appropriate metatarsal, sloping the cut to the shape of the foot and to minimize pressure on the skin. Tendons are cut under tension and allowed to retract, ligate arteries and transect nerves.

Technical aspects of procedure

Removal of the ray may be made easier if the metatarsophalangeal joint is disarticulated first and the metatarsal is removed separately. Note, during disarticulation of the first metatarsophalangeal joint, the penetrating branch of the dorsalis pedis should be preserved (approximately 1 cm distal to the joint).

Closure

A single layer of non-absorbable suture is used.

Central ray amputation

Landmarks and incision

Dorsal incision with tennis racquet around the toe.

Superficial dissection

Skin and fat to bone.

Deep dissection

Subperiosteal dissection is done. Transection of the base of the metatarsal leaving a remnant is technically easier than disarticulation at the

cuneiform joints. Dissect out from proximal to distal removing the intrinsics either side.

Technical aspects of procedure

If two rays are to be removed then place the incision between the metatarsals. The second ray is relatively immobile and therefore if the third and forth rays are to be removed then an osteotomy at the base of the fifth may be required to enable closure of the wound. Protected weightbearing for 4 weeks should be performed.

Closure

Interrupted non-absorbable sutures.

Transmetatarsal (midtarsal) amputation

Landmarks and incision

A long plantar and shorter dorsal flap is used (Fig. 17.6). The dorsal flap begins at the level of the intended transection and curves distally as comes medially. The plantar flap starts at the level of the metatarsal heads and curves to meet the dorsal incision medially and laterally.

Dissection

Skin and fat are incised in line with the skin. The metatarsophalangeal joints should be disarticulated and toes removed. The levels of transection of the metatarsals are marked and cut and edges smoothed. The tendons are stretched and cut so that they retract proximally. Similarly, the nerves are divided proximally and the digital arteries ligated then divided.

Technical aspects of procedure

Longer flaps are required medially, due to increased thickness of the foot.

Closure

Interrupted non-absorbable single layer closure is all that is required.

Midfoot amputations

These amputations use exactly the same principles as above. As opposed to a midtarsal amputation, these amputations do not leave any

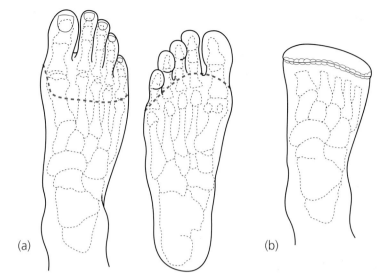

Figure 17.6 *Transmetatarsal amputation: (a) incision; (b) after closure*

of the metatarsals behind. The Lisfranc amputation is at the level of the tarsometatarsal joints and the Chopart amputation at the level of the midtarsal joints. Lisfranc and Chopart amputations have a tendency to go into an equinovarus deformity with time.

Hindfoot amputation – Syme amputation

When considering performing a Symes amputation, a below knee amputation must also be considered. A below knee amputation gives a superior cosmetic result, enables better prosthetic fitting and subsequent function. However, what a Symes does provide is a short leg and a stump which can be used to mobilize short distances, such as going to the bathroom in the middle of the night, without having to hop or apply a prosthesis.

Landmarks and incision

A single posterior heel flap is used. The incision is from the tip of the lateral malleolus across the ankle joint to 2 cm below the medial malleolus. It continues vertically down around the heal, and back to the tip of the lateral malleolus (Fig. 17.7).

Dissection

Skin and fat are incised in line with the skin. All structures are then transected down to bone. The talus is excised by placing the foot in equinus and sequentially dividing the anterior capsule, deltoid ligament and calcaneofibular ligament, taking care to preserve the posterior tibial artery. After division of the posterior capsule and the tendo-Achilles, the foot is removed by shelling out the calcaneus and preserving the posterior flap.

The distal tibia is transected 0.6 cm from the joint line, cut so that it will be parallel to the ground, and the edges rounded off (see Fig. 17.7). The tendons are cut and allowed to retract proximally, as are the medial and lateral plantar nerves. The anterior tibial and posterior tibial arteries are ligated just proximal to the edges of the flap. The heal pad is brought forward, over the

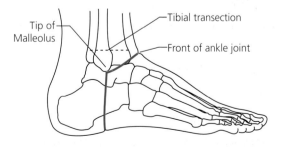

Figure 17.7 *Syme amputation: incision and tibial transection point*

cut surface of the tibia, and sutured through drill holes on the anterior surface of the tibia.

Technical aspects of procedure

The skin flap should not be excessively trimmed as it may devascularize it. The dog-ears will resolve over time, with bandaging or further procedure.

Closure

A drain is inserted and the skin closed over it, using interrupted nylon sutures.

POSTOPERATIVE CARE AND INSTRUCTIONS (FOR ALL FOOT/RAY AMPUTATIONS)

- Partial or non-weightbearing is dependent on the procedure.
- Physiotherapy/prosthetic referral is recommended at an early stage.

RECOMMENDED REFERENCES

Byrne RL, Nicholson ML, Woolford TJ, *et al.* Factors influencing the healing of distal amputations performed for lower limb ischaemia. *Br J Surg* 1992;**79**:73–5.

Falstie-Jensen N, Christensen KS, Brochner-Mortensen J. Long posterior flap versus equal sagittal flaps in below-knee amputation for ischaemia. *J Bone Joint Surg Br* 1989;**71**:102–4.

Hagberg E, Berlin OK, Renstrom P. Function after through-knee compared with below-knee and above-knee amputation. *Prosthet Orthot Int* 1992;**16**:168–73.

Halbert J, Crotty M, Cameron ID. Evidence for the optimal management of acute and chronic phantom pain: a systematic review. *Clin J Pain* 2002;**18**:84–92.

Harris RI. Syme's amputation: the technique essential to secure a satisfactory end-bearing stump. *Can J Surg* 1964;**7**:53–63.

Hudson JR, Yu GV, Marzano R, *et al.* Syme's amputation. Surgical technique, prosthetic considerations, and case reports. *J Am Podiatr Med Assoc* 2002;**92**:232–46.

Malawer MM, Sugarbaker PH. *Musculoskeletal Cancer Surgery Treatment of Sarcomas and Allied Diseases*. London: Kluwer Academic Publishers, 2001.

Pardasaney PK, Sullivan PE, Portney LG, *et al.* Advantage of limb salvage over amputation for proximal extremity tumours. *Clin Orthop Relat Res* 2006;**444**:201–8.

Viva questions

1. What are the indications for amputation?

2. What are the ideal amputation levels in long bones and why?

3. How does the surgical technique differ when performing an amputation on an limb with vascular disease?

4. How would you decide on the appropriate level for an amputation?

5. Describe above or below knee, or toe or foot/ray amputations.

6. How do you transect a nerve?

7. What are the complications associated with amputation? How can these complications be minimized?

8. What measures would you take to minimize postoperative pain?

9. How would you decide between a Syme and a below knee amputation?

Index